SOCIAL ISSUES, JUSTICE AND STATUS SERIES

SOCIAL EPILEPTOLOGY: UNDERSTANDING SOCIAL ASPECTS OF EPILEPSY

Social Issues, Justice and Status Series

Risk and Social Welfare
Jason L. Powell and Azrini Wahidin (Editors)
2009. ISBN: 978-1-60741-691-3

Handbook on Social Change
Brooke H. Stroud and Scott E. Corbin (Editors)
2009. ISBN: 978-1-60741-222-9

Social Development
Lynda R. Elling (Editors)
2009. ISBN: 978-1-60741-612-8

Low Incomes: Social, Health and Educational Impacts
Jacob K. Levine (Editor)
2009. ISBN: 978-1-60741-175-8

Social Epileptology: Understanding Social Aspects of Epilepsy
Jaya Pinikahana and Christine Walker
2009. ISBN: 978-1-60876-228-6

SOCIAL ISSUES, JUSTICE AND STATUS SERIES

SOCIAL EPILEPTOLOGY: UNDERSTANDING SOCIAL ASPECTS OF EPILEPSY

JAYA PINIKAHANA
AND
CHRISTINE WALKER
EDITORS

Nova Science Publishers, Inc.
New York

For permission to use material from this book please contact us:
Telephone 631-231-7269; Fax 631-231-8175
Web Site: http://www.novapublishers.com

Library of Congress Cataloging-in-Publication Data

Social epileptology : understanding social aspects of epilepsy / [edited by] Jaya Pinikahana, Christine Walker.
p. ; cm.
Includes bibliographical references and index.
ISBN 978-1-60876-228-6 (hardcover : alk. paper)
1. Epilepsy--Social aspects. I. Pinikahana, Jaya. II. Walker, Christine, Ph. D.
[DNLM: 1. Epilepsy. 2. Attitude to Health. 3. Culture. 4. Socioeconomic Factors. WL 385 S6747 2009]
RA645.E64S63 2009
362.196'853--dc22

2009028874

Published by Nova Science Publishers, Inc. ✦ New York

CONTENTS

PREFACE

Epilepsy is neither an illness nor a disease, but a brain disorder, frequently associated with neurological and psychosocial difficulties. It is not a purely 'neurological phenomenon' and it requires a juxtaposition of both the neurological and sociological components to elucidate the 'unexplored' dimensions of this disorder. Although clinical, neurological, biological, psychiatrical and even therapeutic aspects of epilepsy have been fairly consistently reviewed, relatively little is known about psychosocial aspects of this condition. Social research into epilepsy has been a 'shadow-dweller' for too long and a publication on these lines is long overdue. This book fills a gap in the literature in social context of epilepsy. The main objective of this book is to advance our understanding of social aspects of epilepsy; to encourage further research that draws on reported studies in epilepsy; to introduce the targeted audiences to applied social research into epilepsy and to illustrate the benefits of such research for health policy change and practice. This book demonstrates the significance of social aspects of epilepsy by presenting a series of articles on topics that have not largely been discussed in 'neurological circles'. Thematically, this volume focuses on 'psychosocial' context of epilepsy with particular emphasis on 'social' context of the disorder.

The history of epilepsy has been described by some writers as '4000 years of ignorance, superstition and stigma, followed by 100 years of knowledge, superstition and stigma'. It has been with us for thousands of years and it will remain so for a few more thousands of years. Throughout history, epilepsy has been subject to many interpretations ranging from supernatural causes to neurological explanations. It is the most common serious brain disorder and perhaps one of the most universal of all medical disorders. About 50 million people worldwide are living with epilepsy averaging 1% of the population. Epilepsy is a condition that affects people of all ages, races and levels of social status, though as shall be seen through the pages of this book, epilepsy does not affect everyone iin the same way or to the same extent.

The weight of ignorance, superstition and stigma means that epilepsy cannot be seen just as a neurological condition that only needs to be treated with anit-epileptic drugs. Although clinical, neurological, biological and psychiatric aspects of epilepsy have been fairly consistently reviewed, relatively little has been investigated on social aspects of this condition. This book presents a collection of some new findings of social research into epilepsy from around the world. Its aim is to show the extent to which social aspects, including beliefs, practices and politics about epilepsy impact on epilepsy as well as to demonstrate that the experience of epilepsy varies according to the social contexts in which it occurs.

This collection has been made possible through the innovative direction undertaken by the Epilepsy Foundation of Victoria, Australia. In 2005 The Epilepsy Foundation of Victoria established a program of applied social research which aims to provide an evidence base to argue for improved policies and services at government and community level. Overall the aim of such an applied social research program is to enhance the quality of life of all people with epilepsy. Each of the chapters therefore concentrates on an important social aspect of epilepsy either for the individual, or the community.

Chapter 1 defines the various epilepsy syndromes and seizure types, with a focus on the common clinical presentations and their associated features. It provides a detailed overview of the medical evaluation of the patient with epilepsy, as well as the patient with their first seizure. A summary of currently accepted drug treatments for epilepsy is provided, with specific indications, requirements for monitoring, and common adverse effects of antiepileptic drugs.

Chapter 2 discusses how epileptic seizures are perceived, evaluated and acted (not acted upon) by people in different cultures throughout a greater part of human history. The author elaborates various ethno-cultural explanations to demonstrate how epilepsy remains a profound social condition compounded by historical and socio-cultural interpretations. It is a fascinating article with a readable length.

Chapter 3 addresses the impact of the diagnostic label itself to a wider consideration of the various disadvantages associated with living with epilepsy. A review of literature on epilepsy and stigma is presented with a six-point research program for a future sociology of epilepsy.

Chapter 4 explores the 'treatment gap' in relation to the economics of the developed Western world and other developing economies. The author argues that the 'treatment gap' cannot be closed by simply making more anti-epileptic drugs available in developing countries. All economies are complex structures which affect the distribution of medicines. In many cases those monst in need may not have access to treatment unless social inequalities are addressed.

Chapter 5 focuses on women with epilepsy addressing their health issues in relation to epilepsy. The authors discuss puberty and menstruation, gender specific side-effects of anti-epileptic drugs, catamenial epilepsy, pregnancy and delivery, fertility, effects of epilepsy on pregnancy, effects of pregnancy on epilepsy, breastfeeding, sexual function, menopause, cosmetic issues, and osteoporosis with special reference to epilepsy.

Chapter 6 is about injuries in epilepsy. The authors of this chapter discuss various aspects of the medical risks relating to epilepsy, including total and cause-specific mortality, accidents and injuries in patients with epilepsy and mortality related with seizures. This chapter reviews the best available epidemiological information about injuries, including incidence and risk factors associated with these injuries, and specific types of injuries such as fractures, burns, concussions, and dislocations.

Chapter 7 is a brief review on law, driving and epilepsy. The author introduces the topic and then discusses the issues of advocacy and social consequences of the law for people with epilepsy. The understanding of these issues allows one to explore the relationship between epilepsy and the law regarding such activities as driving, employment or social interaction.

Chapter 8 addresses the social, cultural and environmental context of epilepsy in Cameroon. The authors explore how the condition affects the daily lives of people with epilepsy and how external, and contextual factors interact with the lived experience. This includes the experience of gender differences in living with epilepsy in Cameroon.

Chapter 9 is a comprehensive article on knowledge, attitudes and epilepsy. An extensive search of international literature, particularly in USA, Europe, Germany, Africa, the Middle East and India, Asia and South Korea presents a detailed review of knowledge of and attitudes toward epilepsy. Teacher attitudes and beliefs towards students with epilepsy in USA and Canada, Europe, South America, Asia, the Middle East and India, are Africa are also reviewed. The perceptions of epilepsy, and obstacles for people with epilepsy in non-Western societies are discussed using some research findings. The authors also discuss the inaccurate depictions in the media, patient education, and education for key social groups.

Chapter 10 reviews the clinical and psychosocial variables affecting employment of people living with epilepsy. The authors discuss the societal stigma and employment, epilepsy and the workplace, legislation, epilepsy and work, driving and work, vocational training and job placement programs and improving employment opportunities for people with epilepsy.

Chapter 11 discusses epilepsy and physical exercise. The authors discuss the risk and benefits of physical activity for people with epilepsy. They describe the risk of sports participation, psychological benefits of exercise, and antiepileptic drugs and exercise. The authors use some animal models and experimental models to discuss the benefits of exercise training for people with epilepsy.

Chapter 12 focuses on economic and psychosocial burden of epilepsy in developing countries. The author discusses the stigma, treatment gap, economic burden , psychological burden, quality of life, social issues using some findings from developing countries.

Chapter 13 is a detailed and graphic account of media and epilepsy. The author argues that epilepsy continues to be portrayed as associated with victimization, fear, secrecy, possession and violence. 'Seizures are depicted, most often on television, in ways that will titillate, captivate and draw the audience to watch a particular show' says the author.

About the Contributors

Jaya Pinikahana MSc, PhD is the Principal Researcher/head, research division at the Epilepsy Foundation of Victoria, Australia. Since completing his PhD in 1990, he has gained research experience in numerous areas including chronic illness, mental illness and ageing. He was the chief investigator for a WHO funded study on malaria transmission in Sri Lanka in early 90s. He swapped life in Sri Lanka as a senior university lecturer to being a senior researcher in Western Australia. Prior to coming to the Epilepsy Foundation of Victoria, he worked as a research fellow at National Ageing Research Institute in Melbourne and as a senior research fellow in nursing at Monash University, Victoria. He has published more than 30 papers in national and international journals. Jaya has been extensively involved in teaching general sociology, health sociology, and research methods for arts, medical and nursing students in Sri Lanka, United Kingdom, New Zealand and Australia. He is a regular reviewer of manuscripts for health and nursing journals and funding bodies.

Christine Walker PhD is a member of the Management Committee of the Epilepsy Foundation of Victoria and the vice chair of Epilepsy Australia. She is an experienced social researcher specializing in the area of health policy and health services that relate to the needs of people with chronic illnesses. She is currently a Chief Investigator in several Australian National Health and Medical Research Council research grants on diabetes and heart disease. Having conducted research into the value of chronic disease self-management as a strategy to prevent chronic diseases, she has published the results in national and international journals. More recently she has written several reports on the status of epilepsy in the Australian community. She has co-edited a book on chronic illness which presents the most recent thinking about approaches to the care of people with chronic illnesses in Australia. In April 2007 Christine received an award from University of New South Wales Research Centre for Primary Health Care and Equity for her contribution to chronic disease care. She is currently the CEO of the Chronic Illness Alliance, Australia.

Graham Scambler is Professor of Medical Sociology and Director of the Centre for Sociological Theory and Research on Health at University College London. He is the author and editor of a number of books on aspects of health and society, including the textbook 'Sociology as Applied to Medicine' (now in its 6th.Ed), and has well over 100 academic publications. He is co-editor of the international journal 'Social Theory and Health'.

Mark Cook is Professor and the Director, Department of Neurology and the University of Melbourne, St. Vincent's Hospital Melbourne, Victoria, Australia. He is also the President of the Epilepsy Foundation of Victoria, Australia

Jordan Kamel MBBS, BMedSc is graduated from the University of Melbourne medical school in 2006, and currently undertaking his medical residency at St Vincent's Hospital, Melbourne. He has an advanced medical science degree in medical humanities with the Centre for Health and Society, School of Population Health, the University of Melbourne.

Jose F. Tellez-Zenteno, MD, PhD is Associate Professor of Neurology and Director of the Epilepsy program, University of Saskatchewan, Royal University Hospital, Saskatoon, SK, Canada. Dr. Tellez graduated from he National University of Mexico in medicine and completed a PhD in clinical epidemiology in the same University. He completed the residencies of internal Medicine and Neurology at the National Institute of medical Sciences and Nutrition in Mexico City. He did post-graduate training in epilepsy in the epilepsy centers of the University of Western Ontario and the University of Calgary in Canada. His research interest includes health-related outcomes in epilepsy care, epidemiology of epilepsy, clinical epilepsy, epilepsy surgery and neuroepidemiology. He has published more than 80 peer-reviewed articles that can be found in several peer-reviewed journals such as neurology, epilepsia, brain, epilepsy research, seizure and epileptic disorders.

Rita Nguyen is a third year medical student at the School of Medicine of the College of Medicine - University of Saskatchewan. She is interested in the field of neurosciences and worked with Dr. Tellez in the chapter of epilepsy and injuries.

Roy G. Beran, MBBS, MD, FRACP, FRACGP is a Conjoint Associate Professor of Medicine at the University of New South Wales and Professor in the School of Medicine at Griffith University, Queensland. He has been the President of the Australian College of Legal Medicine since 2002. He is trained as a consultant neurologist and practices as such though recently was accredited also as a sleep physician. He is the Australian Governor and Secretary General of the Board of Governors of the World Association for Medical Law. He is a Member and past Board Member of the Australian and New Zealand Institute of Health Law and Ethics and a member of the Australian Academy of Forensic Sciences and an Honorary Fellow of the Faculty of Forensic and Legal Medicine of the Royal College of Physicians (London). Within the neurological domain, he is a Member of the Australian and New Zealand Association of Neurologists and a Corresponding Fellow of the American Academy of Neurology.

Line Sveberg Røste MD, PhD is a Consultant Neurologist and chief of emergency and intensive care unit., Department of Neurology, Rikshospitalet University Hospital at the University of Oslo. Thesis on Sex hormones and gonadal function during antiepileptic drug treatment. Scientific focus: Women and men with epilepsy, deep brain stimulation. Editor of consensus document on women and epilepsy, Norwegian Medical Association, (Neurologists and Gynecologists from University Hospitals in Norway). Engaged in the pharmaceutical committe at Rikshospitalet University Hospital; head of drug side-effect comittee, involved in education of staff and the purchase of drugs at Rikshospitalet University Hospital. Full time position as consultant in neurology with focus on general and acute neurology and also part of the clinical interdisciplinary team on women and epilepsy at Rikshospitalet University Hospital.

Erik Taubøll is Professor of Neurology and Deputy departmental head, Department of Neurology, and head of Section for adult epileptology at the National centre for Epilepsy, Division for Clinical Neuroscience, Rikshospitalet University Hospital. Main interest of research has been in gender issues in epilepsy studying the complex interaction of hormones, epilepsy and antiepileptic drugs. In the Laboratory of Experimental Neurology at Rikshospitalet University Hospital, a wide variety of experimental models ranging from *in vitro* techniques including cell cultures and hippocampal slices, *to in vivo* whole animal models have been used. In addition, several human studies have been performed on the effects of antiepileptic drugs on endocrine function. The Epilepsy Research Group at Rikshospitalet University Hospital has also research interests in bone health, status epilepticus, Sudden unexplained death in epilepsy (SUDEP), epilepsy and genetics and deep brain stimulation.

Sanjeev V. Thomas is Professor of Neurology at The Sri Chitra Tirunal Institute for Medical Sciences and Technology, Trivandrum in India. He has a number of research papers on Epilepsy and related issues. He has won several awards in recognition of these works. He has made important contributions to the study of epilepsy in India, particularly, its economic burden psychosocial impact and quality of life. He had been focusing on the gender specific issues of epilepsy. Dr. Thomas is the principal investigator of the registry of epilepsy and pregnancy in Kerala, which is operational for the past eleven years. This is the first of its kind in any developing country. He is the editor of the Annals of Indian Academy of Neurology and a member of the National Executive Committees of the Indian Epilepsy Society and Indian Epilepsy Association.

John O. Elliott MPH is a clinical researcher in the epilepsy division at the Ohio State University's Department of Neurology. His research focuses on epidemiology, health behavior, health education and preventative measures for persons with epilepsy. He earned a master's in public health in community health education from Temple University in Philadelphia.

Sheri Hart MD, PhD is an Assistant Professor of Neurology at the Ohio State University. She completed a combined medical scientist program at The Ohio State University, USA. She has also completed a residency training in Neurology and fellowship training in Clinical Neurophysiology. Currently her research interests include epilepsy, mood disorders and autonomic function.

Christine Charyton, PhD is a Licensed Psychologist. She completed postdoctoral training specializing in pervasive and behavioral childhood disorders. Currently, she is a lecturer in the Department of Psychology and has a courtesy appointment in the Department of Neurology at the Ohio State University. Her research interests include the aesthetic science of creativity and innovation; cognitive risk taking, positive and strength-based psychology for epilepsy and other neurological disorders.

Toba Schwaber Kerson is Mary Hale Chase Professor in Social Sciences and Social Work and Social Research at Bryn Mawr College, Bryn Mawr, Pennsylvania, U.S.A., holds a Master of Social Science degree from the Columbia University School of Social Work, and a Doctor of Social Work and a Ph.D, in Sociology from the University of Pennsylvania. Author of many articles and books including Boundary Spanning: An Ecological Reinterpretation of Social Work in Health and Mental Health Systems (Columbia, 2002), she is currently writing what will be a fourth edition of Social Work in Health Settings: Practice in Context. Professor Kerson sits on several editorial boards and is Book Review Editor of Social Work in Health Care. She has written extensively on the subject of seizures and epilepsy in film and on television including Implacable images: Why epileptiform events continue to be featured in film and television (with L.A. Kerson), Epileptic Disorders (2006).

Ramon Edmundo D. Bautista, M.D., M.B.A. is Associate Professor of Neurology and Director of the Comprehensive Epilepsy Program, University of Florida Health Science Center in Jacksonville, Florida. Dr. Bautista graduated from the University of the Philippines College of Medicine and completed his residency in neurology at Washington University in St. Louis, Missouri. He did post-graduate training in clinical neurophysiology and epilepsy at Emory University in Atlanta, Georgia and Yale University in New Haven, Connecticut. Dr. Bautista is a member of the *American Academy of Neurology* and the *American Epilepsy Society*. His research interests include clinical epilepsy and neurophysiology as well as health-related outcomes of epilepsy care. His publications can be found in various peer-reviewed journals such as *Neurology*, *Epilepsia*, *Epilepsy and Behavior*, and *Seizure*.

Logan A Crews is a second year student at the University of Florida College of Pharmacy in Gainesville, Florida. He received his AA degree from the University of Florida. His research interests include the pharmacoepidemology of epilepsy and health-related outcomes of epilepsy care.

Pascale Allotey is currently Professor of Race and Diversity in Health with an international research focus on the health and human rights of populations marginalised by gender, ethnicity, disease and disability.

Daniel Reidpath is a social epidemiologist and currently Professor of Public Health. His areas of expertise are in the measurement of population health, and the social determinants of health.

Ricardo Mario Arida Ph.D is Professor at the Department of Physiology – Laboratory of Neurophysiology and Exercise Physiology - Universidade Federal de São Paulo in Brazil. He did his postdoctoral research on the role of central fadigue hypothesis at Oxford University, UK. He continued his research on the effect of physical activity in epilepsy in the Laboratory of Experimental Neurology at Universidade Federal de São Paulo – Brazil, from 2001-2006. Specifically, his research is focused on the mechanisms by which physical activity affects epilepsy. His has special concern to the effects of exercise in the developing brain of animals submitted to brain insults such as status epilepticus early in life.

Esper Abrão Cavalheiro PhD is Professor of Experimental Neurology at the Universidade Federal de São Paulo, Brazil. His PhD in Neuroscience was gained in 1978 in Universidade Federal de São Paulo. He had his post-doctoral training at the Centre Nationale de la Recherche Scientifique (CNRS) – France (1980-1982) and at the Universitá di Roma – Italy – (1982-1983). His research interests include experimental models of epilepsy and translational application, epilepsy education and social aspects of epilepsy. His most important national and international services include the Establishment of the Brazilian Association of Epilepsy, the Brazilian branch of the IBE in 1987, Dean, Graduate Students at the Universidade Federal de São Paulo, Brazil (1992-1999), Secretary for the Ministry of Science and Technology from Brazil(1999-2001), President of the Brazilian National Research Council (CNPq) (2001-2003), Chair of the ILAE Neurobiology Commission (2001-2005), IBE Secretary General (2001-2005),

Member of the ILAE Educational Commission (2005-present) and Life/Health Sciences Advisor for the Presidency of the Brazilian Center for Strategic Studies (2006 – present). He has published extensively in this area with more than 200 peer-reviewed publications on different aspects of experimental epilepsy and neurosciences.

Fulvio Alexandre Scorza Ph.D. is Professor at the Department of Neurology and Neurosurgery – Universidade Federal de São Paulo in Brazil. He had his postdoctoral training at Harvard Medical School from 2001 to 2003. He is involved in research into the mechanisms of sudden unexpected death in epilepsy. His peer-reviewed research publications include the impact of exercise in the central nervous system, alternatives therapies for epilepsy treatment and sudden unexpected death in epilepsy.

In: Social Epileptology
Editors: J. Pinikahana and C. Walker

ISBN 978-1-60876-228-6

Chapter 1

EPILEPSY: DEFINITION, SYNDROMES, AND TREATMENT

Jordan Kamel and Mark Cook *
Department of Neuroscience and University of Melbourne,
St. Vincent's Hospital Melbourne, Victoria, Australia

ABSTRACT

This chapter defines the various epilepsy syndromes and seizure types, with a focus on the common clinical presentations and their associated features. It provides a detailed overview of the medical evaluation of the patient with epilepsy, as well as the patient with their first seizure. The appropriate indications for referral to specialist services are also discussed. An up to date summary of currently accepted drug treatments for epilepsy is provided, with specific indications, requirements for monitoring, and common adverse effects to be aware of. The particular management issues of using antiepileptic drugs in pre-menopausal women, as well as non-pharmacological treatments (i.e. surgical interventions) for refractory epilepsy are reviewed. Finally, the major psychosocial implications for patients living with epilepsy are mentioned, including associated psychiatric illnesses such as depression, as well as social and occupational restrictions imposed by this disease.

INTRODUCTION

Epilepsy is common group of disorders that are characterised by the occurrence of at least two unprovoked seizures that are greater than 24 hours apart [1]. Seizures are defined by the manifestation of abnormal hypersynchronous discharges of cortical neurons, which can be recorded by the electroencephalogram (EEG). The clinical features of a seizure depend on the specific location of epileptic discharges in the cortex, and the extent and pattern of propagation of epileptiform activity in the brain [1]. Epilepsy should be considered as a

* Correspondence: Professor Mark Cook, Director, Department of Neurology, St. Vincent's Hospital, Fitzroy, Victoria 3065, Australia. Ph: +613 9288 3068; fax: +613 9288 3091. mark.cook@svhm.org.au

syndrome or disease, where seizures are best regarded as the particular symptoms of the epilepsy. This chapter is intended to familiarise the reader with the evaluation and management of epilepsy, as well as highlight the psychosocial issues that surround this disease.

SEIZURE TYPES

In 1981, the International League Against Epilepsy (ILAE) developed a classification of epileptic seizures that divides seizures into two major classes: partial-onset seizures and generalised-onset seizures (see Table 1). Partial-onset seizures begin in a focal area of the cerebral cortex, whereas generalised onset seizures have an onset that occurs simultaneously in both cerebral hemispheres. Some seizures are difficult to fit into a single class and are considered as unclassified seizures. This system is based on the strict correlation between clinical ictal semiology and EEG findings, and still remains widely accepted [2]. Other classifications have also been proposed, such as the semiological seizure classification advanced by Lüders et al. This patient-oriented classification of epileptic seizures is based purely on ictal semiology [3]. National Institute for Clinical Excellence (NICE) guidelines stress the importance of accurately diagnosing both the seizure type(s) and epilepsy syndrome, as well as aetiology, as failure to do so can lead to inappropriate treatment and persistence or even worsening of seizures [4].

Table 1. Classification of seize types

Partial-onset seizures
Simple partial seizures (SPS)*
Complex partial seizures (CPS)*
Secondarily generalised tonic-clonic seizures*
Generalised-onset seizures
Absence seizures*
Myoclonic seizures*
Primary generalised tonic-clonic seizures*
Clonic seizures
Tonic seizures
Atonic seizures
Based on the International League Against Epilepsy classification

*Common seizure types that will be discussed further.

Partial-Onset Seizures

Partial-onset seizures are further classified as simple partial seizures, complex partial seizures, or secondarily generalised tonic-clonic seizures [1]: Simple partial seizures (SPS), also known as auras, are defined by the preservation of consciousness during the seizure. A reliable history identifies the seizure as partial-onset and not generalised [5]. They occur in approximately 80% of temporal lobe seizures, and usually last less than a couple of minutes.

SPS are subdivided into four categories according to the symptoms present; motor, sensory, autonomic and psychic. Motor symptoms can vary and include focal movements, posturing and vocalisation. Sensory symptoms include all five senses and a vertiginous sensation. They are usually characterised by experiences of abnormal olfactory or gustatory experiences, or even visual and auditory hallucinations. Autonomic symptoms include the common rising epigastric sensation, typically observed in mesial temporal lobe epilepsy, and other symptoms such as mydriasis and vasomotor phenomena. Psychic symptoms are characterised by various experiences involving memory (e.g. déjà vu or jamais vu), affect (e.g. fear or pleasure), or other complex psychic phenomena such as illusions. The aura type depends on the cortical region involved. The diagnosis is based on the repeated, stereotyped occurrence of the same experience in association with focal EEG changes. It may lead on to a complex partial seizure or secondarily generalised event, in which the aura may serve as a warning of impending disturbance of consciousness.

Complex partial seizures (CPS) are distinguished from SPS solely on the basis of the patient's state of consciousness. This is usually assessed by the ability of the patient to respond to external stimuli. This is intact in SPS and impaired in CPS [6]. Again, the exact symptomatology depends on the seizure focus. A complex partial seizure of temporal lobe origin may start with a wide-eyed, motionless stare, dilated pupils, and behavioural arrest. Oral alimentary automatisms such as lip smacking, chewing and swallowing may be noted. Manual automatisms or unilateral dystonic posturing may also be observed. These are involuntary, repetitive but often coordinated motor activities. Patients may have reactive automatisms, in which they continue their ongoing motor activity or react to their surroundings in a semi-purposeful manner, although they are not aware of this (e.g. slicing a loaf of bread). A typical complex partial seizure lasts around 30-120 seconds and is followed by brief postictal confusion. However, generalised weakness and fatigue may persist for longer.

Secondarily generalised seizures often begin with an aura (a simple partial seizure) that may evolve into a complex partial seizure with loss of awareness, and then into a generalised tonic-clinic seizure with epileptiform activity spreading throughout both cerebral hemispheres. This may not be clinically evident, as rapid spread from the point of origin, or seizure focus occurring in a clinically silent area of the brain may result in generalised tonic-clonic events without any premonitory features. In addition, the patient is frequently amnesic for their aura, highlighting the importance of an eye witness account of seizure semiology to elicit any lateralising features.

Generalised-Onset Seizures

Generalised-onset seizures are classified into six major categories: absence seizures, tonic seizures, myoclonic seizures, clonic seizures, primary generalised tonic-clonic seizures and atonic seizures [1]:

Absence seizures, also known as petit mal seizures, are brief episodes of impaired consciousness with no aura or postictal confusion. They typically last less than 30 seconds (usually 5-10 seconds) and may be accompanied by simple automatisms. Facial automatisms are the most common type, especially repetitive blinking, or mouthing movements. Hyperventilation or photic stimulation may precipitate events, at least in children. These seizures typically begin during childhood or adolescence, and may persist into adulthood. However, new onset absence seizures in adulthood are most uncommon. As their clinical features may be relatively subtle, absence seizures may go unrecognised for many years in a child. Patients may subsequently develop generalised tonic-clonic seizures (see below), which is often the first symptoms that brings them to medical attention. If absence seizures in children occur very frequently, they may present with a decreased performance in school.

Myoclonic seizures consist of brief, shock-like jerking movements that last less than a second. They often occur in clusters within a few minutes, frequently on waking. They may evolve into clonic seizures.

Clonic seizures are continuous, rhythmic, jerking movements that occur with or without impaired consciousness. They can be of focal or generalised onset, the latter typically involves both upper and lower extremities.

Tonic seizures consist of sudden stiffening of muscles of the head, trunk and/or extremities in either flexion or extension, lasting several seconds. Typically, these seizures occur during periods of drowsiness, shortly after falling asleep or on waking. They are frequently associated with other neurological abnormalities.

Atonic seizures consist of brief loss of postural tone, often resulting in 'drop attacks'. They also tend to occur in patients with clinically significant neurological abnormalities. Tonic-clonic seizures, commonly referred to as grand mal seizures, consist of several motor behaviours. They typically begin with generalised tonic extension of the extremities lasting for several seconds, followed by clonic rhythmic convulsions. During this phase the patient may bite their cheek or tongue, and become incontinent. The clonic phase usually terminates within minutes, and is followed by a prolonged period of postictal confusion. Generalised-onset tonic-clonic seizures are not preceded by an aura, which is the main clinical feature that differentiates them from secondarily generalised tonic-clonic seizures. However, as the aura that precedes secondarily generalised seizures is often not noted, as mentioned above, differentiation between the two may be problematic based on the semiology alone.

Table 2. Classification of epileptic syndromes

Partial epilepsies
Symptomatic
Temporal lobe epilepsy*
Idiopathic
Benign childhood epilepsy with centrotemporal spikes
Generalised epilepsies
Primary generalised
Childhood absence epilepsy*
Juvenile absence epilepsy*
Juvenile myoclonic epilepsy*
Symptomatic generalised
West syndrome (infantile spasms)
Lennox-Gastaut syndrome
Based on the International League Against Epilepsy classification

*Common epilepsies that will be discussed further.

EPILEPSY SYNDROMES

The patient's prognosis for disability and recurrence of epileptic seizures depends the type of epilepsy syndrome that they have [1]. The common epilepsies will be addressed (see Table 2).

Generalised Epilepsies

The primary, or idiopathic generalised epilepsies (PGE/IGE) represent a group of epileptic syndromes that are characterised by generalised-onset seizures without any underlying or associated neurological condition. They are common, and are important to identify, as they are generally easier to treat than other epilepsy syndromes. This is in contrast to the symptomatic generalised epilepsies, which typically occur in early childhood and tend to be more difficult to control. The most common seizure types that occur in PGE include absence, myoclonic and generalised tonic-clonic seizures, and various combinations of these manifestations are seen. Age at onset is often used to classify these seizure types:

Absence seizures are seen in childhood absence epilepsy (CAE), juvenile absence epilepsy (JAE), and juvenile myoclonic epilepsy (JME). As mentioned previously, patients with absence seizures may also develop generalised tonic-clonic seizures (GTCS). These seizures may occur well after patients appear to have achieved good control. Thus, a long seizure-free period of several years is often recommended before discontinuation of therapy is considered [7]. Sudden death does not result directly from absence seizures. However, accidents from driving or operating dangerous machinery during absence episodes may result in death indirectly. The morbidity from typical absence seizures is related to the frequency and duration of events, as well as the patient's daily activities. Educational and behavioural problems are consequences of frequent, unrecognised seizures [7]. Effective treatment of seizures can improve learning and developmental issues in children.

The remission rate for CAE is about 80%. Good prognostic signs include early onset of absence seizures, quick response to therapy, and a normal EEG. However, generalised tonic-clonic seizures may develop in about 40% of children with CAE, and it is these patients that are also more likely to have persistence of seizures. The remission rate for JAE is less favourable than that for CAE. JAE also carries a greater risk of subsequently developing generalised tonic-clonic seizures, perhaps as high as 80%.

Juvenile myoclonic epilepsy is a very common seizure type to begin in adolescence. Typically upper limb myoclonus on waking has been present for some months prior to the first generalised tonic-clinic seizure that draws attention to the situation. It is particularly sensitive to sleep deprivation. Patients with JME usually can achieve excellent control with relatively small doses of medications. However, they generally need to be treated for life, as relapse rates after medication withdrawal are high, up to 80-90% [1]. Careful attention to lifestyle issues and avoidance of seizure precipitants (e.g. avoiding sleep deprivation, abstinence from alcohol, compliance with medications) is particularly important. JME also carries a high risk of developing generalised tonic-clonic seizures.

For patients who have generalised tonic-clonic seizures (GTCS), the morbidity and mortality is higher if there is no aura, as in primary GTCS, but also some cases of secondarily

GTCS (as previously discussed). Patients can sustain posterior shoulder dislocations, and fractured bones. The incidence of sudden death is more than 20 times higher in persons with epilepsy, compared to the general population. Some of the risk factors for sudden unexpected death in epilepsy (SUDEP) include generalised tonic-clonic seizures, frequent seizures, younger age of disease onset, and treatment with multiple anticonvulsants [5]. The overall incidence of SUDEP is 1.21 per 1,000 patient-years and is higher among women, causing up to 18% of all deaths in patients with epilepsy (8).

Partial Epilepsies

Temporal lobe epilepsy (TLE) is the most common partial epilepsy syndrome that is characterised by focal-onset seizures arising from the medial or lateral temporal lobe, which is the most epileptogenic region of the brain. Morbidity and mortality are increased compared with those in the general population due to increased accidents from episodes of impaired consciousness. About 47-60% of patients become seizure free with medical treatment. However, after two first line anti-epileptic drugs (AEDs) have failed, the chance for seizure freedom is only 5-10%. Surgery in well-selected patients with refractory TLE yields a seizure-free outcome rate of 70-80% (9). A seizure free period in the first year after anterior temporal lobectomy is predictive of long-term seizure-free outcome [10]. Mortality also occurs in TLE from SUDEP. Patients with refractory TLE have an increased risk of sudden death that is 50 times greater than the general population. Patients with refractory TLE involving the dominant hemisphere often have impaired language function as demonstrated by reduced naming ability on the Boston Naming Test [9].

Indications for Referral to Specialist Services

Although most patients can have their medications re-prescribed by a general practitioner, if seizures are not controlled or there is diagnostic uncertainty, the patient should be referred to tertiary services (see Table 3 for indications for referral) [4]. In children, the diagnosis and management of epilepsy within the first few years of life may be particularly challenging. Clinicians should have a lower threshold for referring children with suspected epilepsy to tertiary services, as severe developmental, behavioural and psychological disturbances may develop in consequence to uncontrolled seizures. An individual who has a prolonged convulsive seizure (lasting more than five minutes), or serial seizures (three or more seizures in an hour) in the community should receive urgent medical care and treatment [4].

Table 3. Indications for referral to specialist services

The epilepsy is not controlled with medication within 2 years
Seizure control after two drugs is unsuccessful
The patient is aged under two years
The patient experiences, or is at risk of, unacceptable side effects from medication
There is a unilateral structural lesion
There is psychological and/or psychiatric co-morbidity
There is diagnostic doubt as to the nature of the seizures and/or epilepsy syndrome
Based on the NICE Clinical Guidelines

Evaluating The Patient

Clinical History

Obtaining an account of the seizure semiology is arguably the most useful part of the diagnostic evaluation of a patient that presents with seizures. The events before, during and after the seizure should be enquired about. An eyewitness history can be most useful, and specific, focussed questioning may yield a better description of the circumstances. The clinical features of the different common seizure types have previously been discussed.

It is always useful to enquire about seizure triggers. Common precipitants include sleep deprivation, menstruation, acute illness and stress. Some patients have seizures triggered by flashing lights or exercise. Identification of avoidable factors may form an integral part of a patient's management plan.

The patient's past medical history may be relevant. A history of head injury, stroke, intracranial malignancy or infection may provide vital clues as to the aetiology of seizures. Potential reversible causes of provoked seizures such as drug withdrawal, diabetes, and thyroid disease are also important to ascertain, and may refute a diagnosis of epilepsy. A family history of seizures is also relevant, particularly if there is a family history of absence or myoclonic seizures.

Neurological Examination

A full neurological examination should be performed, although it is usually unremarkable. It should evaluate the patient for lateralising signs that imply a focal abnormality. A baseline cognitive assessment should also be performed.

Laboratory Investigation

Plasma prolactin levels within 10-20 minutes of a GTCS are elevated 5-30 times the baseline value [5], and can help with the differentiation from non-epileptic seizures. However, this technically challenging to measure, and generally not recommended.

Metabolic (e.g. electrolytes, liver-function testing, blood glucose level), toxic and infectious screens may be indicated in certain situations to exclude any readily reversible causes of seizures. Seizures provoked by these causes, by definition, do not confer a diagnosis of epilepsy.

Electroencephalography

Electroencephalography (EEG) may be performed in patients with relevant histories. It should be performed only to support a diagnosis of epilepsy in adults whose clinical history suggests that the seizure is likely to be epileptic in origin [4], rather than be used in isolation. The pattern and location of epileptiform activity can identify specific epilepsy syndromes, such as the classic generalised 3 Hz spike-wave complexes seen with absence epilepsy. In individuals presenting with a first unprovoked seizure, unequivocal epileptiform activity shown on EEG can be used to assess the risk of seizure recurrence. Although the formal diagnosis of epilepsy requires two unprovoked seizures to occur, some clinicians may diagnose epilepsy when one unprovoked seizure occurs in the setting an interictal EEG with epileptiform discharges [1]. Repeated EEGs may be helpful when the diagnosis of the epilepsy syndrome or seizure type remains unclear. Provocation of seizures using photic stimulation and hyperventilation remain part of the standard EEG assessment. When a standard EEG has not contributed to classification, a sleep deprived EEG can be performed, as this may give a higher yield of capturing epileptiform activity. Long-term video or ambulatory EEG monitoring may be useful in those patients who present diagnostic difficulties.

Neuroimaging

Neuroimaging should be used to identify structural abnormalities that cause certain epilepsies, and are essential in partial epilepsies, or if the epilepsy cannot be classified on clinical and EEG grounds. As computerised tomography (CT) will not detect most types of relevant structural brain abnormalities, magnetic resonance imaging (MRI) is the imaging modality of choice [4]. MRI is particularly important in patients who develop epilepsy before the age of two years or in adulthood, who have any suggestion of focal-onset seizure on history, examination or EEG, and in patients whose seizures continue despite first-line medication. Although MRI is more sensitive, CT is still being used where MRI is not available or contraindicated, and is appropriate for emergency situations [11].

Neuropsychological Assessment

Neuropsychological assessment should be considered in individuals in whom it is important to evaluate learning disability and cognitive dysfunction, particularly in regards to language and memory. Referral for neuropsychological assessment is indicated when an individual with epilepsy is having educational or occupational difficulties, or complains of memory or other cognitive issues, and when an MRI has identified abnormalities in cognitively important brain regions [4]. It is also essential as part of any pre-surgical evaluation for the treatment of epilepsy, as shall be discussed later.

Seizure Recurrence after the First Seizure

Estimates of the risk of seizure recurrence in the two years after a first unprovoked seizure range from 15-80%. The main high risk factors include an abnormal brain MRI, an abnormal EEG, and partial-onset seizures. A patient with none of these factors has a recurrence risk of approximately 15%, and thus is not treated. A patient with all three risk factors has a recurrence risk of around 70%, and thus warrants treatment. The major unresolved question is whether to treat patients with only one of these factors, when the recurrence risk is 30-50% [1].

The First Seizure Trial Group randomly selected 397 patients with unprovoked, generalised tonic-clonic first seizure to take a conventional anticonvulsant (i.e. sodium valproate, carbamazepine, phenytoin or phenobarbital) or no treatment. At one year, 18% of treated patients had seizure recurrence, compared with 39% of untreated patients [12]. However, the likelihood of being seizure free at 3-5 years is similar whether drugs are started after the first seizure, or deferred until after a seizure recurs [13]. The risks and benefits of commencing therapy should be carefully weighed against each other and discussed with the patient and their family or carers. A number of other factors often significantly influence the decision, particularly driving status and affect on employment or other potentially hazardous activities, and for women of childbearing years the potential teratogenicity of the various therapies.

Currently Accepted Treatments

Antiepileptic Drugs

Antiepileptic drugs (AEDs) should be individualised according to the seizure type, epilepsy syndrome, other concurrent medication, patient co-morbidities, as well as the individual's lifestyle and preference. The ultimate goal of treatment is to achieve a seizure-free status without adverse effects. This is achieved in more than 60% of patients with epilepsy who require treatment with AEDs [1]. However, many people still suffer from adverse effects of anticonvulsants, or have seizures that are refractory to medical therapy.

AEDs are the mainstay of therapy for people with unprovoked seizures, and are generally recommended if the patient has had more than one seizure. As discussed, patients that present with their first unprovoked seizure should have a tailored decision based on their risk factors for recurrence such as an abnormal brain MRI, abnormal sleep-deprived EEG, and evidence of the seizure to be focal-onset in nature. It is recommended that patients should be treated with a single antiepileptic drug (monotherapy) wherever possible, to minimise adverse effects. If the initial treatment is unsuccessful, then monotherapy with a different drug should be tried. Combination therapy with more than one AED should only be considered when several attempts of monotherapy have not resulted in adequate seizure control. The best regimen that balances seizure reduction with tolerability of side effects should be chosen.

The newer AEDs include gabapentin, pregabalin, lamotrigine, levetiracetam, oxcarbazepine, tiagabine, topiramate and vigabatrin. Within their licensed indications, they are recommended for the management of epilepsy in people who have received no benefit from treatment with the older AEDs such as carbamazepine, sodium valproate and phenytoin. These older drugs may also be unsuitable because of intolerable side effects, or specific contraindications.

Some anticonvulsants have multiple mechanisms of action (e.g. lamotrigine, topiramate, sodium valproate, zonisamide), while others have only one known mechanism (e.g. phenytoin, carbamazepine, ethosuximide). They can be divided into eight groups based on their mechanisms (see Table 4).

Table 4. Classes of anticonvulsants (1)

Blockers of repetitive activation of sodium channels	Phenytoin, carbamazepine, oxcarbazepine
GABA enhancers	Phenobarbital, benzodiazepines
Glutamate modulators	Topiramate, lamotrigine, felbamate
T-calcium channel blockers	Ethosuximide, valproate
N- and L-calcium channel blockers	Topiramate, lamotrigine, zonisamide, valproate
H-current modulators	Gabapentin, lamotrigine
Carbonic anhydrase inhibitors	Topiramate, zonisamide
Blockers of unique binding sites	Levetiracetam, gabapentin, pregabalin

AEDs in Women

Women of childbearing age present specific management issues. Hepatic enzyme inducing AEDs such as phenytoin, phenobarbital, carbamazepine and oxcarbazepine increase clearance of the OCP, thus reducing its effectiveness. Non-hormonal methods of contraception should be advised if women on the pill are using these agents.

AEDs are potentially teratogenic. Women with epilepsy taking anticonvulsants have 2-3 times the risk than other women of having a baby with a fetal abnormality, including neural tube defects [14]. Certain agents such as sodium valproate have been particularly implicated. In addition, treatment with multiple agents should be avoided, with monotherapy at the lowest possible dose aimed for. The risks of potential teratogenic effects must be balanced against the risk of uncontrolled seizures during pregnancy. Folic acid supplementation should be recommended for all women to take three months before and after conception, where possible. Sodium valproate has also been associated with reproductive endocrine disorders including polycystic ovarian syndrome, anovulatory cycles and hyperandrogenism.

Medical Treatments for Specific Types of Seizures and Epilepsy Syndromes (1): (See Tables 5 and 6)

Absence seizures: If absence seizures alone are present, most neurologists use sodium valproate, although ethosuximide is still used in children and less often adults. Absence seizures may be present with other types of seizures (e.g. GTCS, myoclonic seizures), for which lamotrigine and topiramate are other options.

Table 5. Drug options by seizing type

Seizure type	First-line drugs	Second-line drugs	Other drugs that may be considered	Drugs to be avoided (may worsen seizures)
Generalised tonic–clonic	Sodium valproate Lamotrigine Topiramate	Clobazam Levetiracetam Oxcarbazepine	Acetazolamide Clonazepam Phenobarbital Phenytoin Primidone	Tiagabine Vigabatrin Gabapentin/Pregabalin
Absence	Ethosuximide Lamotrigine Sodium valproate	Clobazam Clonazepam Topiramate		Carbamazepine Gabapentin/Pregabalin Oxcarbazepine Tiagabine Vigabatrin
Myoclonic	Sodium valproate (Topiramate)	Clobazam Clonazepam Levetiracetam Piracetam Topiramate Lamotrigine		Carbamazepine Gabapentin/Pregabalin Oxcarbazepine Tiagabine Vigabatrin
Tonic	Lamotrigine Sodium valproate	Clobazam Clonazepam Topiramate Levetiracetam	Acetazolamide Phenobarbital Phenytoin Primidone	Carbamazepine Oxcarbazepine
Atonic	Lamotrigine Sodium valproate	Clobazam Clonazepam Levetiracetam Topiramate	Acetazolamide Phenobarbital Primidone	Carbamazepine Oxcarbazepine Phenytoin
Focal with/without Secondary Generalisation	Carbamazepine Lamotrigine Oxcarbazepine Sodium valproate Topiramate	Clobazam Gabapentin Levetiracetam Phenytoin Tiagabine	Acetazolamide Clonazepam Phenobarbital Primidone	

Based on the NICE Clinical Guidelines (4).

Table 6. Drug options by epilepsy syndrome

Epilepsy syndrome	First-line drugs	Second-line drugs	Other drugs	Drugs to be avoided (may worsen seizures)
Childhood absence epilepsy	Ethosuximide Lamotrigine Sodium valproate	Levetiracetam Topiramate		Carbamazepine Oxcarbazepine Phenytoin Tiagabine Vigabatrin
				Gabapentin/Pregabalin
Juvenile absence epilepsy	Lamotrigine Sodium valproate	Levetiracetam Topiramate		Carbamazepine Oxcarbazepine Phenytoin Tiagabine Gabapentin/Pregabalin Vigabatrin
Juvenile myoclonic epilepsy	Lamotrigine Sodium valproate	Clobazam Clonazepam Topiramate Levetiracetam	Acetazolamide	Carbamazepine Oxcarbazepine Phenytoin Gabapentin/Pregabalin Tiagabine Vigabatrin
Generalised tonic–clonic seizures only	Carbamazepine Lamotrigine Sodium valproate Topiramate	Levetiracetam	Acetazolamide Clobazam Clonazepam Oxcarbazepine Phenobarbital Phenytoin Primidone	Tiagabine Vigabatrin Gabapentin/Pregabalin
Lennox–Gastaut syndrome	Lamotrigine Sodium valproate Topiramate	Clobazam Clonazepam Ethosuximide Levetiracetam	Felbamate	Carbamazepine Oxcarbazepine
Infantile spasms (West syndrome)	Steroids Vigabatrin	Clobazam Clonazepam Sodium valproate Topiramate	Nitrazepam	Carbamazepine Oxcarbazepine
Focal epilepsies (symptomatic)	Carbamazepine Lamotrigine Oxcarbazepine Sodium valproate Topiramate	Clobazam Gabapentin Levetiracetam Phenytoin Tiagabine	Acetazolamide Clonazepam Phenobarbital Primidone	
Benign epilepsy with centrotemporal spikes	Carbamazepine Lamotrigine Oxcarbazepine Sodium valproate	Levetiracetam Topiramate	Sulthiame	

Based on the NICE Clinical Guidelines (4).

Tonic or atonic seizures: Tonic or atonic seizures typically indicate clinically significant diffuse brain injury. The Lennox-Gastaut syndrome is a common example of tonic seizures and best treated with broad-spectrum AEDs such as sodium valproate, lamotrigine, topiramate or felbamate as final-line. Clinical trials of levetiracetam and zonisamide are being conducted. Other modalities include the use of vagal nerve stimulation (VNS).

Myoclonic seizures: Myoclonic seizures have a bimodal distribution, occurring in infants and late childhood/adolescence. Infants with myoclonic epilepsies usually have a poor prognosis. After late childhood, JME is often the cause of myoclonic seizures, which is a typically benign disease that is relatively easy to treat, but with high recurrence rates after AED cessation. The most effective medications for JME and myoclonic seizures are sodium valproate, lamotrigine and topiramate. Benzodiazepines such as clonazepam and clobazam are also often very effective.

Primary generalised tonic-clonic seizures: Sodium valproate is the agent of first choice, as it treats a broad spectrum of seizure types. Lamotrigine, topiramate and phenytoin are reasonable second options. Levetiracetam has also gained recent FDA approval as adjunctive therapy. Carbamazepine should be avoided if there is any concern about concurrent myoclonic and absence seizures, as it may aggravate these seizure types.

Partial-onset seizures: Carbamazepine is considered first-line therapy. However, oxcarbazepine, lamotrigine, topiramate and sodium valproate may be considered. Partial-onset seizures can be difficult to control, and may require a trial of a number of different drugs as monotherapy first, then combination therapy if this fails. Adjunctive therapy with levetiracetam, tiagabine, gabapentin or pregabalin are all possible options.

Monitoring

There is often controversy about the need to monitor levels of AEDs. Regular blood testing of drug levels is rarely recommended as routine. The main anticonvulsant that may require measurement levels is phenytoin, as when its system of hepatic clearance becomes saturated, its metabolism changes from first-order to zero-order kinetics. Thus, a moderate increase in dose can cause a disproportionately large rise in plasma concentration to potentially toxic levels. Thus, phenytoin levels may be measured after dose increases, with steady-state concentrations reached in around 5-10 days [15]. Measurement of lamotrigine levels during pregnancy is indicated due to increased hepatic clearance that is induced by physiological changes during pregnancy. Drug levels may also need to be measured at the discretion of the clinician for documenting compliance in certain situations, or if there are concerns about overdosing. The target-dose ranges for each AED correspond to the average blood levels required for tolerability and seizure control. They may not correspond to that of an individual requires. Dosages should primarily be adjusted according to the patient's level of seizure control and side effects, rather than targeting levels within a pre-defined range [11].

Other laboratory tests (e.g. full blood count, electrolyte levels and liver function tests), may need to be performed due to potential metabolic derangements that AEDs can cause. This is more the case for the older agents (e.g. phenytoin, phenobarbital, carbamazepine and sodium valproate), where yearly monitoring is sufficient after more frequent monitoring in the first six months [11].

Table 7. Side effects of antiepileptic drugs [11,15]

Drug	Common side effects	Serious side effects (rarer)
Carbamazepine	dizziness, diplopia, ataxia, sedation, weight gain, mild leukopaenia, mild hyponatraemia	agranulocytosis, aplastic anaemia, Stevens-Johnson syndrome, anticonvulsant hypersensitivity syndrome,severe hyponatraemia
Oxcarbazepine	dizziness, ataxia, diplopia, nausea, vomiting, headache, mild hyponatraemia	Stevens-Johnson syndrome, severe hyponatraemia, anticonvulsant hypersensitivity syndrome
Gabapentin	sedation, dizziness, ataxia, weight gain	
Pregabalin	fatigue, dizziness, ataxia, diplopia, peripheral oedema, weight gain, constipation	
Lamotrigine	somnolence, dizziness, tremor, skin reactions	Stevens-Johnson syndrome
Levetiracetam	somnolence, dizziness, emotional lability	severe aggression, psychosis
Phenytoin	dizziness, ataxia, diplopia, gum hypertrophy, hirsutism, acne, fatigue	Stevens-Johnson syndrome, anticonvulsant hypersensitivity syndrome, blood dyscrasias, Osteoporosis
Phenobarbital	dizziness, ataxia, diplopia, mood and behavioural Disturbance	Stevens-Johnson syndrome, anticonvulsant hypersensitivity syndrome,blood dyscrasias
Sodium valproate	weight gain, sedation, tremor, mild thrombocytopaenia, Alopecia	hepatic toxicity, hyperammonaemia, severe thrombocytopaenia, pancreatitis, polycystic ovarian syndrome
Tiagabine	dizziness, ataxia, somnolence, nervousness, weakness	spike-wave status epilepticus
Topiramate	weight loss, ataxia, tremor, word finding difficulty, poor concentration, Peripheral paraesthesias	renal calculi, metabolic acidosis, acute angle closure glaucoma
Zonisamide	weight loss, drowsiness, ataxia, anorexia, nausea	renal calculi, metabolic acidosis, aplastic anaemia

Adverse Effects of AEDs

There is a wide range of various side-effect profiles from each of the AEDs. They are both dose and patient-dependent, and should be tailored to each individual's situation. The patient's co-morbidities and concurrent medications, as well as psychosocial situation must be considered in order to select the most appropriate therapy. See Table 7 for a list of common and important adverse effects.

Loss of bone density has been implicated by chronic treatment with phenytoin, and possibly other hepatic enzyme inducing agents (phenobarbital, carbamazepine and oxcarbazepine) as well as sodium valproate. It is recommended by some that both men and women taking these medications should receive supplemental calcium and vitamin D, as well as have periodic bone-density measurements [16]. However, this practice is not widespread.

Anticonvulsant hypersensitivity syndrome is a rare, but serious syndrome associated with carbamazepine, oxcarbazepine, phenytoin and phenobarbital. It usually occurs within four weeks of commencing therapy, and is characterised by fever, rash and multiple organ involvement (hepatitis, myocarditis, pneumonitis, lymphadenopathy, myositis). Drug cessation is essential when this syndrome is diagnosed [15].

Prognosis after Withdrawal of Treatment

After a patient has been seizure free for typically 2-5 years, physicians consider withdrawal of medications. However, the prognosis and relapse rates differ according to epilepsy syndrome, seizure type and patient factors such as age. In many epilepsies of childhood, such as benign childhood epilepsy with centrotemporal spikes (an idiopathic, partial-onset epilepsy), most children outgrow their disease and are seizure-free by early adolescence. This is in contrast to epilepsies such as JME, in which seizures can persist throughout life. In general, however, after the patient has been seizure-free for at least two years, a discussion should take place with the patient to discuss the risk and benefits of continuing or withdrawing AED therapy [4].

When AED treatment is being withdrawn, it should be carried out slowly (over several months), and only one drug should be withdrawn at a time if the patient is on multiple agents. Some medications such as benzodiazepines and phenobarbital should be withdrawn even more gradually. Should seizures return, the last dose reduction should be reversed and the patient should seek medical advice.

Table 8. Factors associated with an increased risk of seizure recurrence after AED discontinuation (1)

Abnormal EEG
Abnormal brain MRI (especially in cortical and limbic regions)
Several seizure types (especially if tonic or atonic seizures are present)
High number and frequency of seizures
Long duration of epilepsy before the seizures are controlled
Short duration of seizure freedom

Many neurologists use the same risk factors that assess prognosis for new-onset seizures to guide the decision to discontinue anticonvulsants. A normal sleep-deprived EEG and normal brain MRI lower the risk of relapse after discontinuation. Epileptiform or focal abnormalities on EEG and/or focal cortical abnormalities on MRI significantly increase the risk of seizure relapse following drug cessation [1]. See Table 8 for other factors associated with an increased risk of seizure recurrence. At least 50% of patients who have a seizure relapse do so in the first three months, with 75% of relapses occurring in the first year.

Surgery and Other Devices

There are two major categories of neurosurgical intervention for epilepsy: palliative and potentially curative. Several years ago, the most common palliative surgery was anterior callosotomy. This surgery was indicated for patients with intractable atonic seizures, who often had facial and neck injuries due to falls. However, the surgery is rarely performed today.

Surgery for focal structural pathologies may be very effective. The outcome depends on the exact location and extent of the underlying pathology, and surgical removal of a specific lesion may be limited by the proximity of eloquent brain regions that control movement, vision and speech. The most common surgery performed for epilepsy is removal of part of the temporal lobe, and outcomes of this surgery is better than lobectomy of other areas. For assessing the outcome after surgery for epilepsy, the Engel Class can be used, with a score from Class I to IV (Engel Class I defined as seizure free except for auras only or seizures related to medication withdrawal, Engel Class IV defined as no worthwhile reduction in seizures) [17]. If a patient has unilateral temporal lobe seizures confirmed by video-EEG, and corresponding unilateral hippocampal sclerosis on MRI, the likelihood of an Engel Class I outcome at two years is 85% (1).

Vagal nerve stimulation (VNS) can be used as an adjunctive therapy in reducing the frequency and severity of seizures in patients who are refractory to antiepileptic medication, but who are not suitable for surgical resection. It is useful for both partial-onset and generalised-onset epilepsies [18]. The use of VNS has reduced the need for anterior callosotomy.

Assessment of Seizure Control

There is no accepted standardised method for assessing control of seizures in patients who have not had surgical treatment. Patients and family members should be asked to record seizures and AED doses on a calendar. Any identifiable seizure triggers (e.g. sleep deprivation, alcohol, menses, concurrent illness, stress) should also be documented. A well-designed, comprehensive disease management program, including a seizure diary can improve patient empowerment and coordination of care between the patient and provider ([9]. An ongoing dialogue between the clinician and patient is essential.

Psychosocial Considerations

People with seizures experience psychosocial adjustments after their diagnosis such that social and/or vocational rehabilitation may be needed. Many clinicians underestimate the consequences that epilepsy may have on a patient, as many live in fear of experiencing their next seizure. Up to 55% of patients with uncontrolled epilepsy suffer from depression, and even patients with well-controlled seizures have higher rates of depression than the general population. In addition, suicide rates are tripled in the six months after diagnosis [11]. All patients with epilepsy should have regular reviews, and be specifically assessed for signs of depression as part of this.

On review, patients should have access to written and visual information, counselling services, information about voluntary organisations and epilepsy specialist nurses. The expertise of multidisciplinary teams is required to manage more complicated cases of epilepsy and should include neuropsychology, neuropsychiatry, social work, occupational therapy, neuroradiology and neurophysiology services in addition to the above. MRI and video telemetry facilities should be available.

Driving and Other Restrictions

Most people with epilepsy can work normally. The main problem for patients with seizures is the unpredictability of the next seizure. Some patients have exclusively nocturnal seizures, and this is less of an issue. It is important to balance the risk of subsequent seizure with the psychosocial implications of placing restrictions on the patient's work and lifestyle.

Laws and regulations regarding driving and epilepsy vary widely between different countries, and even between states in countries such as the United States [20, 21]. In general, guidelines suggest a seizure-free period between 1-2 years before passing a person as fit to drive, but some countries, including Australia, permit shortening of this period on the recommendation by an experienced neurologist that seizure control is adequate [22]. Holding a commercial licence to drive requires a much longer seizure-free period.

Other limitations placed on people with epilepsy include restrictions from working from heights or operating heavy machinery. If power tools are to be used, supervision may be needed, with the use of safety devices such as automatic shut-off switches recommended. Swimming or bathing may also require supervision if there is ongoing risk of seizure recurrence.

REFERENCES

[1] Cavazos, Jose E. Seizures and Epilepsy, Overview and Classification. [Online] 2007. http://emedicine.medscape.com/article/1184846-overview.

[2] Wolf P. Basic principles of the ILAE syndrome classification. *Epilepsy Res.* 2006;70 (Suppl 1): S20-6.

[3] Luders, H., et al., Semiological seizure classification. *Epilepsia,* 1998. 39(9): p. 1006-13.

[4] National Insititute for Clinical Excellence, *Clinical Guideline 20: The epilepsies: the diagnosis and management of the epilepsies in adults and children in primary and secondary care.* 2004, National Institute for Clinical Excellence: York, UK.

[5] Ko D. *Tonic-Clonic Seizures.* 2007 [cited 17 Dec 2008]; Available from: HYPERLINK http://emedicine.medscape.com/article/1184608-overview .

[6] Ko D. *Temporal Lobe Epilepsy*. 2006 [cited 18 December 2008]; Available from: HYPERLINK http://emedicine.medscape.com/article/1184509-overview.

[7] Segan S. *Absence Seizures*. 2005 [cited; Available from: HYPERLINK "http://emedicine.medscape.com/article/1183858-overview"

[8] Walczak, T.S. Incidence and risk factors in sudden unexpected death in epilepsy: a prospective cohort study. *Neurology*, 2001. 56(4): p. 519-25.

[9] Ko D. *Temporal Lobe Epilepsy*. 2006 [cited 18 December 2008]; Available from: HYPERLINK http://emedicine.medscape.com/article/1184509-overview.

[10] Radhakrishnan K; So EL; Silbert PL; Jack CR Jr; Cascino GD; Sharbrough FW; O'Brien PC. Predictors of outcome of anterior temporal lobectomy for intractable epilepsy: a multivariate study. *Neurology* 1998 Aug;51(2):465-71.

[11] French, Jacqueline A and Pedley, Timothy. A *Initial management of epilepsy*.. 2, 2008, Vol. 359.

[12] Randomized clinical trial on the efficacy of antiepileptic drugs in reducing the risk of relapse after a first unprovoked tonic-clonic seizure. First Seizure Trial Group (FIR.S.T. Group). *Neurology*, 1993. 43(3 Pt 1): p. 478-83.

[13] Marson, A, Jacoby A, Johnson A et al et al Immediate versus deferred antiepileptic drug treatment for early epilepsy and single seizures; a randomised controlled trial. *Lancet;* 2005, Vol. 365(9476), 2007-13.

[14] Lander, Cecilie M. Antiepileptic drugs in pregnancy and lactation. *Australia Prescriber* 2008; Vol. 31, pp. 70-2.

[15] Group, Neurology Expert. *Therapeutic Guidelines: Neurology*. 3rd. Melbourne : Therapeutic guideline limited, 2007.

[16] Drezner, MK Treatment of anticonvulsant drug-induced bone diseaes. *Epilepsy Behaviour*, 2004; Suppl 2, Vol. 5, pp. S41-47.

[17] Engel, Jerome. *Surgical treatment of the epilepsies*. 2 Sub edition. s.l. : Lippincott Williams and Wilkins, 1993.

[18] Labar, D, Murphy, J and Tecoma, E Vagus nerve stimulation for medication-resistant generalized epilepsy. *Neurology*; 7, 1999, Vol. 52, pp. 1510-2.

[19] Gunter, Margaret J, Brixner D, Von Worley A et al. Impact of a seizure disorder disease management program on patient-reported quality of life. *Disease Management;* 4, 2004, Vol. 7 (4) 333-47.

[20] Fisher RS, Parsonage M, Beaussart M, Bladin P, Masland R, Sonnen AE, Rémillard G (Joint Commission on Drivers' Licensing of the International Bureau for Epilepsy and the International League Against Epilepsy). Epilepsy and Driving: An International Perspective. *Epilepsia* 1994;35(3):675-84.

[21] Krumholz A. Driving and Epilepsy: A Historical Perspective and Review of Current Regulations. *Epilepsia* 1994;35(3):668-74.

[22] Austroads. *Assessing fitness to drive - commercial and private vehicle drivers: medical standards for licensing and clinical management guidelines*. Sydney : Austroads and National Road Transport Commission, 2006.

In: Social Epileptology
Editors: J. Pinikahana and C. Walker

ISBN 978-1-60876-228-6

Chapter 2

BELIEFS AND PERCEPTIONS OF EPILEPSY IN DIFFERENT CULTURES

Jaya Pinikahana*
The Epilepsy Foundation of Victoria and Monash University,
Victoria, Australia

ABSTRACT

This chapter discusses how epilepsy is perceived in different cultures, not as a 'neurological condition' but as a 'social condition'. Throughout a greater part of human history, epilepsy prevailed as a mysterious condition that at times provoked feelings of fear or ambivalence in people who witnessed major seizure attacks (tonic-clonic seizures). The mysterious and frightening aspects of epilepsy have led people to produce distinctive explanations within their belief systems, ranging from punishment for sins, to bewitchment, to disease. Not surprisingly, the remnants of these beliefs and perceptions have persisted despite scientific and technological advances in the 19th and 20th centuries.

These various ethno-cultural explanations demonstrate how epilepsy remains a profound social condition compounded by historical and socio-cultural interpretations. From ancient to modern times, epilepsy has carried with it an undesirable amount of stigma together with widespread ignorance, fear and misunderstanding. Social stigma affects people with epilepsy in varying degrees across different cultural and social settings, through hampering care, negatively affecting quality of life, and contributing to severe social disadvantages.

The management of epilepsy in different cultural settings requires knowledge and understanding of ethno-cultural interpretations of epilepsy coupled with an understanding of the barriers due to social stigma, thus moving beyond the usual practice of western medicine.

* Correspondence: Dr Jaya Pinikahana, Principal Social Researcher/Head, Research Division, The Epilepsy Foundation of Victoria, No 818 Burke Road, Camberwell, Victoria, 3124 Australia. Tel: 03 9805 9125; Fax: 03 9882 7159. Email: jpinikahana@epilepsy.asn.au

INTRODUCTION

The word 'epilepsy' is derived from Latin and Greek words for 'seizure'. It is an ancient disorder that can be traced through all civilizations. Epilepsy is the most common serious brain disorder apart from migraine (Betts, 1992), affecting approximately 50 million people worldwide, of whom 40 million are estimated to live in developing countries (WHO, 2004). It is perhaps one of the most universal of all medical disorders (JECA, 2006), and one of the world's most prevalent non- communicable diseases (WHO, 2001).

Epilepsy has no racial, geographical or social class boundaries; it includes both sexes, and affects people of all ages, races and levels of social status, though not equally. Epilepsy has a similar prevalence to diabetes and also requires long term drug treatment and monitoring (Couldridge, 2001). The incidence of epilepsy ranges from 23 to 190 per 100,000 population per year, with those from lower socio-economic backgrounds (particularly in developing countries) reflecting higher incidence levels (Beghi, 2007). In Europe and North America, the incidence ranges from 24 and 53 per 100, 000 per year (Kotsopoulos et al., 2002; MacDonald et al., 2000).

As with socio-economic background, the incidence of epilepsy is not uniform across the lifespan. The incidence in children is variable ranging from 25 to 840 per 100,000 per year (Beghi, 2007), mostly affecting children in the first decade of life, a period during which children undergo a critical part of their development. In addition to disproportionately affecting infants, epilepsy also affects the 80 years and over age group (Oun et al., 2003). The incidence of epilepsy has also been reported to be higher in men than in women in both developed and developing countries (Cockerell et al., 1995; Rwiza et al., 1992). The overall prevalence ranges from 2.7 to 41 per 1,000 population, and the rate of active epilepsy varies from 4 to 8 per 1,000 (Beghi, 2007). Similar to the incidence, the prevalence of epilepsy is generally lower in industrialised countries than in developing countries.

Epilepsy is not purely a 'neurological phenomenon' and it requires a juxtaposition of neurological, sociological, and anthropological components to elucidate the 'unexplored' dimensions of this 'disorder'. Although clinical, neurological, biological, psychiatric and even therapeutic aspects of epilepsy have been consistently reviewed, relatively little is known about sociological, anthropological and cultural aspects of this condition.

HISTORY OF EPILEPSY

The history of epilepsy has been described as '4000 years of ignorance, superstition and stigma, followed by 100 years of knowledge, superstition and stigma' (Kale, 1997). The earliest detailed account of epilepsy is contained in the 'Sakikku', a Babylonian medical text compiled between 1067 BC and 1046 BC (Wilson and Reynolds, 1990). The Sakikku comprises a few descriptions of various patterns of epileptic seizures, including probable simple and complex partial seizures. In the 'Charaka Samhita', a great Indian compendium compiled by Atreya in the 6th century BC, four different types of epilepsy were described (Pirkner, 1929). In ancient Chinese writings, the Huang Di Nei Chig (770 BC and 221 BC), a convulsive seizure was described under the heading of 'Dian- Kuang' (Lai and Lai, 1991). The Hippocratic writings, 'On the Sacred Disease' (400 BC), remain the oldest medical writings on epilepsy. Hippocrates held the view that epileptic disorder was not sacred or supernatural in its origin, but was a physical disease (Temkin, 1933). As Hippocrates put it:

> "I do not believe that the Sacred Disease is any more divine than any other disease but, on the contrary, has specific characteristics and a definite cause"...The brain is the seat of this disease, as it is of other very violent diseases".

In the book 'Celsus' De Medicina' (30 AD), there is a description of convulsion under the designation of 'Comitialis'. Galen (130 -210 AD) in his writing on seizure even gave a definition of epilepsy: *"If there is not only convulsion of the whole body, but also interruption of the leading function, then this is called epilepsy"* (Siegel, 1968). According to Lai and Lai (1991), the ancient Chinese text 'Zhu Bing Yuan Hou Lun', written by Cao Yuan Fang (610 AD), contained a classification of epileptic seizures. He seemed to have identified five types of epilepsy based on clinical factors: Yang epilepsy, Yin epilepsy, Wind epilepsy, Wet epilepsy, and Labour epilepsy (Eadie and Bladin, 2001). Strong and ambivalent emotions around a tonic-clonic epileptic seizure have existed throughout human history. As Louise Jilek-Aall puts it:

> "Witnessing a tonic-clonic epileptic seizure has throughout human history provoked strong and ambivalent emotions, reflected in a variety of names for this affliction: morbus sacer, morbus maior, morbus daemoniacus, lues deifica, the Holy Sickness, the Divine Disease, the Falling Evil, the Rod of Christ, and many more".

According to Tenkin (1971), the name *morbus maior* became 'grand mal' in medieval France. In medieval times, the understanding of epilepsy was further broadened by the writings of Arnold of Villanova (1234-1311), Bernard of Gordon (1305) and John of Gaddesden (1280-1360) (Lennox, 1941).

The understanding of epilepsy was also enhanced by the establishment of the science of neurology. In the 17th century, Thomas Wills (1621-1675), the founding father of the science of neurology published two main works, Cerebri Anatome (1664) and De Anima Brutorum (1672) (Feindel, 1965). In Wills' famous text, 'Pathology of the brain and nervous stock: On convulsive diseases (1684)', he began to develop the Hippocratic concept of epilepsy as a brain disorder for the first time in Europe. The first six decades of the 19th century witnessed the publication of a number of books containing various types of seizures, sub-types and their neurological and biological bases.

In the 19th century, neuropathology began to establish as a new discipline, followed by new developments in the areas of functional localisation in the brain, the motor cortex, and the concept of 'epileptiform' (Reynolds, 2005). By the middle of the 20th century it was well established that seizures were the result of electrical discharges in the brain. In the second half of the 20th century, remarkable progress was made in diagnostic facilities and possibilities through structural and functional neuroimaging including CAT and MRI, as well as in video-telemetry and magnetoencephalography (Reynolds, 2005).

Anthropological Approaches to Disease and Society

In all cultures, illness is associated with culturally specificaspects of belief systems and the people in these social contexts are more concerned with that particularity of illness. For instance, the question arises why some individuals in a given community suffer more misfortunes and illnesses than do others (Pritchard, 1937). Personalistic and naturalistic theories of disease causation were predominant prior to the introduction of modern 'scientific' medicine (Forster and Anderson, 1978). Personalistic theorists view sickness as the object of aggression or punishment against man and the agent causing illness may be a supernatural being (e.g. god, ancestor), or a human being (e.g. sorcerer). In contrast, naturalistic theorists recognised the natural causes of diseases such as burns, overeating and falls. The scientific paradigm of specific aetiology of disease which views diseases as having identifiable causes that can be treated was introduced from the early 19th century (Morgan et al., 1985).

Knowledge, attitudes and beliefs are derived from the social milieu in which people are born and live. Even though human beings are biologically similar, different life experiences and social experiences make them very different. Indeed, the cause and effect of individual behaviours can be linked to the social structure in which the individual is born. Brown (1952) defines the social structure as the complex network of actually existing relationships in any society. Fundamental social relations give the basic form of the social structure, and peoples' existence within the social structure consists of these social relationships (Armstrong, 1983; Firth, 1951). However, the structural system is actually more abstract in nature, and the formal aspects of society persist through 'social relations' that are beyond the level of individual interaction (i.e. social relationships; Brown, 1952).

Stacey (1976) stated that the perceptions of illness and disease are necessarily related to the institutional response to illness. He also described how the beliefs and knowledge which prevail in society influence the ways in which people perceive illness and misfortunes. That is, the culture in which a person lives will also influence the way in which they perceive and respond to signs and symptoms of the body. It is also clear that cultural perceptions of illness cannot be directly equated with biomedical perceptions. As Tyler (1969) notes, each person has a unique system of perceiving and organising material phenomena so that even though the same phenomena are objectively present, they are culturally perceived and organised in different ways. The prime objective of an ethnographer is to scrutinize the material phenomena (objects) through the conceptual system of the people which might reveal how they culturally perceive the world and life events. One can not understand how people perceive or react to illness without an understanding of the culture in which they live. It is necessary to perceive and interpret the world through the same 'lens' as the people growing up in that culture (Helman, 1986).

Epilepsy has been known throughout human history. In ancient times, it was referred to as the 'sacred disease'. Over many centuries, there have been two major explanations on why epileptic seizures occur in the human brain. Until recently, people in many parts of the world held the view that epileptic seizures were caused by supernatural powers. Remnants of supernatural beliefs still prevail even in the most advanced societies. The more recent alternative explanation of epilepsy places more emphasis on neurological and biological understanding of seizures, and is the preferred model at the present time. Jilek and Jilek (1989) identified four major categories of theories about the causes of epilepsy: epilepsy as a punishment for sin, epilepsy as bewitchment or possession, epilepsy as a contagious disease and the biological approach.

A Punishment for Sin

Epilepsy is seen as punishment for incest among the Navajo Indians in North America (Jilek, 1979; Levy et al 1979). Similarly, an association between epilepsy in children and parent's wrongdoing (e.g. adultery during pregnancy) is seen in many traditional African communities in Tanzania, Zimbabwe, South Africa, and Madagascar (Jilek, 1999; Gelfand, 1964; Laubscher, 1934; Terranova and Ratsifandribamanana, 1970). The Andean Indians of Peru believe that if someone breaks a taboo, the ancestral spirits send a strong wind causing a seizure to the person (Sally Rosas, 1965). In rural Ecuador, epilepsy is believed to be caused by 'trouble and woe' and by brooding and thinking too much about problems (Andermann, 1994).

Bewitchment or Spirit Possession

In many parts of the world, particularly in Africa and Asia, spirit possession is believed to be the main cause of a seizure and is manifested through violent tremors and shaking of the possessed person's body. Among the Moslem people in West and North Africa, people with epilepsy are believed to be possessed by the *jinn,* which are airy beings with transparent bodies. In Morocco, people with epilepsy are called *mejnun,* that is, afflicted with a *jinni* (Collomb et al., 1970)Among the Baganda in Uganda, epilepsy or *ensimbu* is one of the four diseases of the brain. *Ensimbu* is believed to be a major illness caused by witchcraft among the Baganda people and it is not curable by western medicine (Orley, 1970). In line with their beliefs, the Baganda people espouse spiritual remedies for people with epilepsy [*ensimbu*]. Among the Bamileke in Cameroon, epilepsy is believed to be the work of witches as well a contagious illness. In Nigeria, a seizure episode can be the revenge of aggrieved ancestors or the sign of visitation by the devil (Gelfand, 1973; Osuntokum, 1977).In Swaziland, epilepsy known as *sifosekuwa* or falling disease is seen as an illness caused by sorcery (Reis, 1994). During the process, an animal spirit (*tilwane*) is sent to the human body causing a seizure. Partial seizures are usually classified as madness (*buhlanya*) or hysteria (*lihabiya*) in Swazi culture (Reis, 1994). In Iraq, some people regarded epilepsy as an illness caused by supernatural powers, the ghost or the evil eye (Hamdi et al., 1977). In Papua New Guinea, the cause of epilepsy is seen as the possession of evil spirits (Hoskins et al, 1969). In Native North American Tewa, epilepsy is thought to be caused by object intrusion or contagious magic and witchcraft.

A Contagious Disease

Contagion as a cause of epilepsy can be traced in many places in Africa, such as Madagascar, Tanzania (Jilek-Aall, et al., 1979) and Nigeria (Awaritife et al., 1985). In a

Nigerian study, it was found that 40% of medical students were convinced that epilepsy is a contagious disease (Awaritefe, 1983). The Bini people in Nigeria believe epilepsy to be an illness in a person's heart. When foam is blocked in the heart, the circulation through the heart is stoped, causing a seizure (Andermann, 1994). Tekle-Haimanot et al., (1991) conducted a study in Ethiopia and found that 45% of respondents believed that epilepsy can be contagious through physical contact during an attack. Jilek (1979) suggests that the notion of epilepsy as a contagious illness originates from a historical and transcultural likening of epilepsy to rabies; the convulsions and frothing at the mouth in rabies could be mistaken for epilepsy. A study by Peltzer (2001) in South Africa found that although the majority of the students in his study had a positive attitude towards people with epilepsy through sharing a meal or room and willingness to marry a person with epilepsy, 17% thought that they could infect others with their saliva during a seizure, 12% felt that a person with epilepsy was a witch or wizard, and about 10% said a person with epilepsy must be isolated (Peltzer, 2001). In Nigeria too, Osuntokun and Odeku (1970) noted that epilepsy is believed to be transmitted via the patients' saliva.

Imbalance of Humours

In Ayurvedic medicine in India, epilepsy (*apasmara*) is thought to be caused when the *dosas* or *humours* have become aggravated and equilibrium is lost. Ayurveda includes five basic elements of the universe (*bhutas*), three humours (*tridosas*) and seven components of the body (*dhatus*). Ether (*akasa*), wind (*vayu*), water (*ap*), earth (*prthri*), and fire (*agni*) are the five elements of Ayurvedic doctrine (Filliozal, 1964; Obesekere, 1976). Good physical health is maintained by harmonic balance of three humours called wind (*vayu*), bile (pitta) and phlegm (*sema*) and any imbalance of a humour causes troubles (*dosa*) within the organism. When the equilibrium is lost in the body because of bad food or unhealthy regimens, humours enter the heart and create an overstimulation of emotions causing a seizure.

In traditional Chinese medicine, the illness was originally associated with 'wind' but it was described by a concept involving mucus or phlegm blocking the cardiac system (Andermann, 1995). Mental illness and mania are also attributed to similar causes of humour imbalance, indicating a link between epilepsy and insanity (Lai et al., 1990). In both rural and urban areas, people with epilepsy consult traditional Chinese medical practitioners in addition to western medicine practioners (Lai et al., 1990). Lai and his associates (Lai et al., 1990) found that 25% of respondents chose herbal medicine, 14% preferred acupuncture and 15% used Chinese folk medicine (*Dan Fang).* Although traditional Chinese medicine has explained epilepsy as having physical causes, some studies found that supernatural powers were still mentioned as a cause of a seizure (Kleinmann et al., 1995). In Pakistan, Shafig et al., (2008) found in a recent study that 25% of 487 adult residents of a slum area in Karachi believed that epilepsy was caused by evil spirits, black magic and envy by others.

Other Explanations

In Malawi, epilepsy is thought to be caused by an insect moving inside the belly (Watts, 1989). As Reis (1994) described, there are a number of causes of epilepsy cited by traditional healers in Swaziland which include heredity, difficult birth, skull trauma, and worries during pregnancy. In rural Ecuador, about 50% of cases of epilepsy are due to infection by pork tapeworm, the larvae which invade the brain causing seizures (Desjarlais et al., 1995). In Turkey, epileptic seizure (*sara*) is described as 'fainting', with fright, shock and major losses believed to possibly trigger seizures (Good and Good, 1993). Some believe in spirits (*jinn*) in the development of epilepsy and they receive treatment from religious healers (*hoca).* Epilepsy or '*nwaa'* in Cameroon means 'throwing a person on the ground'. They believe that people *die and resurrect* in epilepsy. Traore et al., (1998) found that seizure is attributed to excessive eating by Mauritanian Moorish populations. Baganda people in Uganda also believe that a lizard living in the head is making some disturbances from time to time making the person dizzy, and even causing seizures (Orley, 1970)

Traditional Therapies for Epilepsy

In many traditional societies, where ancestral spirits, magic or witchcraft are believed to cause epilepsy, people are very reluctant to accept anti epileptic medication. Until recently, and even now in many parts of the world, the treatment for any spirit possession including seizures, has been major exorcism. In Cameroon where epilepsy is thought to be caused by witchcraft, the first treatment is sought from a traditional healer followed by dietary restrictions to prevent the production of foam in the belly (Nkwi and Ndonko, 1989). In Malawi, traditional healers prescribe a mixture of roots to induce vomiting and purge the stomach for people with epilepsy (Watts, 1989). In Swaziland, traditional therapies include inhaling medicinal fumes, vomiting, sneezing and exorcism to get rid of epilepsy from the body (Reis, 1994). In many traditional African societies, patients prefer to visit traditional healers for epilepsy. In Ecuador, patients use traditional healers and home remedies such as pulling the sufferer's middle finger or rubbing them with cologne (Shorvon and Farmer, 1988). Many healers in Ecuador admitted that they could not do much to cure epilepsy and prescribed cold baths, a quiet life, and valerian (a sedative herb) (Temkin, 1971). In Ethiopia, epilepsy therapies include visits to holy waters, faith healing, exorcism, sacrifices, charms and local remedies (Tekle-Haimanot et al., 1991).

The Incas, Aztecs and the Guarani peoples in Latin America, used a large number of botanical medicines apart from magic treatments for epilepsy (Carod-Artal and Vazquez-Cabrera, 2007). In North America, several plants were used by native Americans to treat seizures (Herrick, 1977; Turner et al., 1990). Epilepsy treatments and therapists in China include Chinese herbal medicine, secret family herbal prescriptions, Taoist priests, Buddhist adepts and Muslim imams (Lai and Lai., 1991).

The study of knowledge, attitudes and practices of epilepsy in rural Sri Lanka by Seneviratne et al., (2002) indicated that traditional modes of treatment have been tried by 45.9% of 207 patients attending an epilepsy clinic.

Beliefs, Perceptions and Stigma

From ancient to modern times, epilepsy has carried with it an '*undesirable*' amount of social stigma that affects people with epilepsy in varying degrees in diverse cultural settings. In many parts of Africa, epilepsy is regarded as supernatural and is often associated with stigma; even the pronunciation of the word 'epilepsy' is a taboo (Carod-Artal and Vazquez-Cabrera, 2007). Even in industrial nations like America, epilepsy carries a stigma that dates back to ancient civilisations. Some argue that stigma related to epilepsy is worse than the stigma of cancer or HIV/AIDS. Misunderstanding, fear, and anxiety, resulting from stigma, hampers care and public recognition and results in social and even legal discrimination against those living with epilepsy. In a WHO (2001) document 'Epilepsy: social consequences and economic aspects', some misunderstandings about epilepsy from around the world have been summarised: in Cameroon, it is believed that people with epilepsy are inhabited by the devil; in China, epilepsy diminishes the prospects of marriage, especially for women; in some parts of India, attempts are made to exorcise evil spirits from people with epilepsy by tying them to trees, bearing them, and cutting a portion of hair from their head; in Indonesia, epilepsy is often considered as punishment from unknown dark forces; in Liberia, the cause of epilepsy is perceived as related to witchcraft or evil spirits; in Nepal, epilepsy is associated with weakness, possession by an evil spirit; in Swaziland, many traditional healers mention sorcery as the cause of epilepsy; in Uganda, epilepsy is thought to be contagious and so people with epilepsy are not allowed to join the communal food pot. Research shows that people with epilepsy in developing countries particularly in Africa, suffer substantially from stigma and social exclusion and they are more likely to be unemployed, and are less likely to be educated or married.

A recent study by Fernandes et al. (2007) in Brazil found that the magnitude of stigma differs within segments of the local society, highlighting that those socio-cultural factors such as gender, religion and level of education may be important predictors of stigma. In a Korean study involving 400 adults with epilepsy, Lee et al., (2005) found that 31% of them felt stigmatised by their condition. Dilorio et al. (2003) reported that people reporting higher levels of stigma were those who had their first seizure before the age of 50. In an Estonian study, Ratsepp and his colleagues (2000) found that overall, 55% of people with epilepsy believed that they had been treated unfairly at work or when trying to get a job, 51% of respondents felt stigmatised by epilepsy, and 14% of them highly so. Baker et al.'s (2000) review, 'Stigma of epilepsy: A European perspective', involving more than 5000 people with epilepsy in 15 countries across Europe found that 51% of respondents reported feeling stigmatised, with 18% reporting feeling highly stigmatised. Paradoxically, one British study found no evidence that stigma affects the lives of those whose epilepsy was not complicated by other pathologies (Britten et al., 1984).

Research shows that stigma has a negative affect on the quality of life (QOL) of people with epilepsy (Jacoby, et al., 1996; Baker et al., 1997). Hermann et al. (1990) found that stigma is one of seven key predictor variables for psychopathology. Perceived stigma was ranked fourth in importance in predicting quality of life, after psychological stress, loneliness and adjustment (Surmaijer et al., 2001). Stigma is also associated with reduced self-esteem, anxiety, depression, and helplessness (Jacoby, 1994; Dilorio et al., 2003; Westbrook et al., 1992).

Conclusion

Traditional ethno-cultural explanations of epilepsy being caused by divine punishment, spirit possession, or witchcraft contributes to the stigmatisation of people with epilepsy. A certain amount of higher social status and spiritual power is given to the person who is believed to be possessed by the spirit and gets seizures from time to time, no matter whether the spirit is god, demon or ancestor. In contrast, the belief that epilepsy is caused by divine punishment for sins, induces shame and guilt in the epilepsy sufferer. This might cause severe resentment, anger, and rejection of the sufferer from the family. The belief that epilepsy is contagious leads to severe consequences for the sufferer which might include complete isolation and segregation from the family and even from the whole community. All three sets of beliefs lead to discrimination and prejudice, separating individuals from one another based on a socially conferred judgement that these people are 'less than' the others. Despite all the medical efforts to explain the basic neurological, biological and clinical parameters of epilepsy, it is still seen as caused by supernatural powers in some societies. Research shows that many rural communities across the world have very poor knowledge of the causes and nature of epilepsy, resulting in discrimination, prejudice, and at times, a total rejection of the sufferers. The management of epilepsy in different cultural settings requires knowledge and understanding of ethno-cultural interpretations of epilepsy coupled with understanding barriers due to social stigma, thus moving beyond the usual practice of Western medicine.

References

Andermann L (1994) Traditional beliefs about epilepsy in rural and urban Ethiopia. Unpublished manuscript, Montreal.

Armstrong D (1983) *An outline of sociology as applied to medicine*. Wright, Bristol.

Awaritefe A, Longe AC, and Awaritefe M (1985) Epilepsy and psychosis: A comparison of societal attitudes, *Epilepsia,* 1, 1-9.

Awaritefe A (1983) Epilepsy: The myth of a contagious disease. *Culture Medicine and Psychiatry,* 13, 449-456.

Baker GA, Jacoby A, Buck D et al., (1997) Quality of life of people with epilepsy; European study. *Epilepsia*, 38, 353-62.

Baker GA, Jacoby A, et al., (1997) Quality of life of people with epilepsy; An European study. *Epilepsia*, 38(3), 353-62.

Baker GA. Brooks J. Buck D. Jacoby A. (2000)The stigma of epilepsy: a European perspective. *Epilepsia.* 41(1):98-104.

Baker GA, Brooks J, Buck D, Jacoby A (2000) The stigma of epilepsy: a European perspective. *Epilepsia*, 41(1), 98-104.

Beghi E (2007) Epilepsy, In *Handbook of Clinical Neuroepidemiology*, Nova Science Publishers (eds) VL Feigin and DA Bennett.

Betts T (1992) Epilepsy services, what people need, what they want, what they get. *Acta Neurologica Scandinavica*, 2, 95-101.

Britten N, Wadsworth ME, Fenwick PB (1984) Stigma inpatients with early epilepsy; a national longitudinal study. *Journal of Epidemiology and Community Health*, 38(4) 291-5.

Brown RAR (1952) *Structure and function in primitive society*. Free press, London.

Carol-Artal F and Vazgrez-Cabree CB (2007) An anthropological study about epilepsy in Native Tribes from central and South America. *Epilepsia*, 48(5), 886-893.

Cockerell OC, Eckle I, Goodridge DM (1995) Epilepsy in a population of 6000 re-examined: secular trends in first attendance rates, prevalence and prognosis. *Journal of Neurology Neurosurgery and Psychiatry*, 58, 570-76.

Collomb H, Dumas M, Ayats H, Virieu R, Simon M, Roger J (1970). Epidemiologie de l'epilepsie au Senegal. *Afr. J. Med. Sci.*, 1, 125-48.

Couldridge L, Kendall, S, March, A (2001) A systematic review: A decade of research; The information and counselling needs of people with epilepsy. *Seizure, 10*(8), 605-14.

Desjarlais R, Eisenberg L, Good B and Kleinman A (eds) (1995) *World mental health: Problems and priorities in developing countries*. NY, Oxford University Press.

Dilorio C , Obborne SP, Letz R et al (2003) The association of stigma with self management and perceptions of health care among adults with epilepsy. *Epilepsy and Behaviour*, 4(3) 259-267.

Eadie MJ and Bladin PF (2001) *A disease once sacred: A history of the understanding of epilepsy*. Eastleigh.

Feindel W (1965) The origin and significance of cerebri Anatome. In Feindel W(eds) *The anatomy of the brain and nerves*. McGill Press, Montreal.

Fernandes PT. Salgado PC. Noronha AL. de Boer HM. Prilipko L. Sander JW. Li LM (2007) Epilepsy stigma perception in an urban area of a limited-resource country. *Epilepsy and Behaviour*. 11(1):25-32.

Filliozal J (1964) The classical doctrine of Indian medicine, Delhi. Firth R (1951) *Elements of social organisation*. London.

Forster G and Anderson B (1978) *Medical anthropology*. John Wiley and Sons. London.

Gelfand M (1964) Epilepsy in the African central. *African Journal of Medicine*, 3, 1102.

Goffman E (1969) Stigma: notes on the management of spoiled identity. New Jersey, Prentice Hall.

Good B and Delvecchio Good M 1993) (1994) In the subjunctive mode: Epilepsy narratives in Turkey. *Social Science and Medicine*, 38(6), 835-842.

Good B and Delvecchio Good M (1993) Au mode subjonctif-La construction narrative des crises d'epilepsie en Turquie. *Anthropologie et sociétés*. 17(1-2), 21-42.

Hamdi HI, Al-Husaini AA, All-Hadithi F (1977) The epilepsies: Clinical and epidemiological aspects and desirability of services. In: Penry JK (eds) *Epilepsy: The Eighth International Symposium*. New York, Ravan Press, 393-9.

Helman CC (1986) *Culture, Health and Illness*. John Wright and Sons Ltd, Bristol.

Hermann BP, Whiteman, S et al (1990) Psycho-social predictors of psychopathology in epilepsy. *B. J. of Psychiatry*, 156, 98-105.

Herrick JW (1997) *Iroquois medical botany*. PhD thesis, State University of NY, Albany.

Hippocrates (1985). The sacred disease. In: The genuine works of Hippocrates. Birmingham AL. The Classics of Medicine Library, Gryphon Edition.

Hoskins JO, Kiloh LG, Cawte JE (1969) Epilepsy and guria : The shaking syndromes of New Guinea. *Social Science and Medicine*, 3, 39-48.

Jacoby A (1996) Assessing the quality of life in patients with epilepsy. *Pharmacoeconomics*, 9(5), 399-416.

Jacoby A (1994) Felt vs enacted stigma: A concept revisited; Evidence from a study of people with epilepsy in remission. *Social Science and Medicine*, 38, 269-74.

Jacoby A (1994) Felt versua enacted stigma: a concept revisited. Evidence from a study of people with epilepsy in remission. *Social Science and Medicine*, 38(2), 269-74.

Jacoby A, Baker GA, Steen N, Potts P, Chadwick D (1996) The clinical course of epilepsy and its psychosocial correlates; findings from a UK community study, *Epilepsia,* 37, 148-61.

Joint Epilepsy Council of Australia (2006) A national strategy for epilepsy in Australia, Epilepsy Foundation of Victoria, Melbourne.

Jilek-Aall and Jilek WG (1989) Epilepsy and its psychosocial implications in Africa. In Pelzer and P. Ebigbo (eds). *Textbook of clinical psychology in Africa*, University of Nigeria, Enugu Campus.

Jilek WG (1979) The epileptic outcast role and its background: A contribution to the social psychiatry of seizure disorders. *Journal of Operational Psychiatry*, 10(2), 128-32.

Jilek-Aall, JIlek L, and Miller JR (1979) Clinical and genetic aspects of seizure disorders prevalent in an isolated African population. *Epilepsia,* 20, 613-622.

Jilek-AAll L (1999) Morbus Sacer in Africa: Some religious aspects of epilepsy in traditional cultures. *Epilepsia,* 40(3), 382-386.

Kale, R (1997) Bringing epilepsy out of shadows: Wide treatment gap needs to be reduced. *BMJ,* 315(7099) 2-3.

Lee SA, Young Joo N (2005) Perceived self control of seizures in patients with uncontrolled partial epilepsy. *Seizure,* 14(2) 100-105.

Kleinman A, Wang, W, Li S, Cheng X, et al (1995) The social course of epilepsy: Chronic illness as social experience in interio China. *Social Science and Medicine*. 40(10), 1319-1330.

Kotsopoulos LAW, van Merode, T, Kessels FGH et al (2002) Systematic review and meta analysis of incidence studies of epilepsy and unprovoked seizures. *Epilepsy*, 43, 1402-1409.

Lai CW and Lai HC (1991) History of epilepsy in Chinese traditional medicine. *Epilepsia*, 32, 299-302.

Lai C, Huang X, Lai Y, Zhang Z, Liu G and Yang M (1990) Survey of public awareness, understanding and attitudes towards epilepsy in Henan Province, China. *Epilepsia,* 31(2), 182-187.

Laubscher BJF (1934) Sex, custom and psychopathology. London, Routledge and Kegan Paul Lee SA, Yoo HJ, Lee BJ, (2005) Factors contributing to the stigma of epilepsy. *Seizure,* 14(3), 157-163.

Lennox WG (1941) Bernard of Gordon on epilepsy. *Annals of Medical History*. 3, 372-383.

Levy JE, Neutra R and Parker D (1979) Life careers of Navajo epileptics and convulsive hysterics. *Social Science and Medicine*, 13B, 53-60.

MacDonald BK, Johnson AL, Goodridge DM et al (2000) Factors predicting progonosis of epilepsy after presentation with seizures. *Annals of Neurology*, 48, 833-841.

Morgan M, Calnan M and Manning N (1985) *Sociological approaches to health and medicine*. Groom Helm, London.

Nkwi PN and Ndouko FT (1989) The epileptic among the Bamileke of Maham in the Nde Division, *West Province of Cameroon, Culture, Medicine and Psychiatry*, 13, 437-448.

Obesekere G (1976) The impact of Ayurvedic ideas on the culture and the individual in Sri Lanka. In Leslie C (eds) *Asian Medical Systems*, Berkeley University Press.

Orley JH (1970) Culture and mental illness. Nairobi: Makerere Institute of Social Research. East African Publishing Press.

Osuntokum BO (1977) *Epilepsy in Africa. Tropical and Geographical Medicine*, 30, 23-32.

Osuntokun BO and Odekn EL (1970) Epilepsy in Ibadan, Nigeria. A Study of 522 cases. *African Journal of Medicine*. 1, 185-200.

Oun A. Haldre S.(2003) Magi M. Prevalence of adult epilepsy in Estonia. *Epilepsy Research*. 52(3):233-42.

Peltzer K (2001) Perceptions of epilepsy among black students at a University in South Africa. 62-67.

Pirkner EH (1929) Epilepsy in the light of history. *Annals of Medical History*, 1, 453-80.

Pritchard E (1937) *Witchcraft, Oracles and Magic Among the Azande*. Oxford University Press.

Ratsepp M, Oun A et al., (2000) Felt stigma and impact of epilepsy on the employment status among Estonian people. *Seizure*, 9(6), 394-401.

Rwiza HT, Kilonzo, GP, Haule J et al (1992) Prevalence and incidence of epilepsy in Ulanga, a rural Tanzanian district; a community based study. *Epilepsia*, 33, 1051-1056.

Reis (1994) Evil in the body, disorder of the brain. Tropical and Geographical Medicine, Vol 46, no 3, 40-43.

Reynolds H (2005) Epilepsy; the disorder. *Epilepsy Atlas*, WHO, 2005.

Sally Rosas (1965) Conception magic de la epilepsia en los indigenous Peruanos. *Rev. Psiquiatr Psychol Med Eur Am La*tin, 7, 109-31.

Seigel RE (1968) *Galen's system of physiology and medicine*, Karger, NY.

Seneviratne U, Rajapakkse P, Pathirana R and Seeta T (2002) Knowledge, attitude and practice of epilepsy in rural Sri Lanka. *Seizure*, 11, 40-43.

Shafig M, Mansoor T, Asma T, et al (2008) Myths and fallacies about epilepsy among residents of a Karachi slum area. *Tropical Doctor*, 38 (1) 32-3.

Shorvon SD and Farmer, PJ (1988) Epilepsy in developing countries: A review of epidemiological, socio cultural and treatment aspects. *Epilepsia*, 29, S36-s54.

Stacey M (1976) The biology of the national health. *Sociological Review Monograph*, 13, 45-56.

Suurmeijer TPBM, Reuvekamp MF Aldenkamp BP (2001) Social functioning, psychological functioning and quality of life in epilepsy, *Epilepsia*, 42, 1160-68.

Tekle-Haimanot R, Abebe M, Forsgren, L, Gebre-Mariam, A, Heijbel, J et al (1991) Attitudes of rural people in central Ethiopia toward epilepsy. *Social Science and Medicine*, 32, 203-209.

Temkin O (1933) The doctrine of epilepsy in the Hippocratic writings: *Bulletin of the History of Medicine*. 8, 277-322.

Temkin O (1971) *The falling sickness. Baltimore*: The John Hopkins Press.

Terranova R and Ratsifandribamanana B (1970) Aspects psychopathlogiques et psychosociaux de l'epilepsie dans un milieu transculturel. *Af. J. med. Sci.*, 1, 213-9.

Traore H, Diagana M, Debrock C et al., (1998) Sociocultural approach to epilepsy in Mauritania. *Medecine tropicale revue du Corps de sante colonial*, 58, 365-368.

Turner NJ, Thompson LC, Thompson MT (1990) Thompson Ethnography: Knowledge and usage of plants by the Thompson Indians of BC. Royal British Museum Memoirs, BC.

Tyler SA (1969) *Cognitive anthropology*. Holt Renehart and Winston, London.

Watts AE (1989) A model for managing epilepsy in a rural community in Africa. *British Medical Journal*, 298, 805-7.

Westbrook CE (1995) Adolescents with epilepsy: A psychological and social predictors. *Pediatric and Adolescent Medicine*, 6, 179-186.

Wills T. Pathology of the brain and nervous stock; on convulsive diseases (1684). In: Pordage S (eds) *The remaining medical works of that famous and renowned physician Dr Thomas Wills of Christ Church in Oxford and Sidley professor of Natural Philosophy in that famous university*, London, 1-89.

Wilson JVK and Reynolds EH (1990) Translation and analysis of a cuneiform text forming part of a Babylonian treatise on epilepsy. *Medical History*, 34, 185-98.

World Health Organisation (2001) Epilepsy' Social consequences and economic aspects, *Fact Sheet,* 166, Geneva.

World Health Organisation (2004) *Epilepsy in the WHO Africa region, bridging the gap: the global campaign against epilepsy, 'out of shadows'*, Geneva.

In: Social Epileptology
Editors: J. Pinikahana and C. Walker

ISBN 978-1-60876-228-6

Chapter 3

EPILEPSY, STIGMA AND SOCIETY

Graham Scambler*
University College of London

ABSTRACT

After a preliminary account of the nature and extent of the biomedical phenomenon of epilepsy, this chapter addresses its social ramifications. The pursuant discussion ranges over the impact of the diagnostic label itself to a wider consideration of the various disadvantages typically associated with living with epilepsy. The concepts of enacted and felt stigma play a pivotal role here. A review of the literature is followed by the commendation of a six-point research programme for a future sociology of epilepsy. Allowing fully for the vital relevance of both biological (including genetic) and psychological research, this programme accords a significant role also for the analysis of the social contexts in which people experience and 'live out' their identities as 'epileptics'.

INTRODUCTION

A paragraph or two about the nature of epilepsy - as defined by modern, western medicine - might usefully open this contribution to our understanding of epilepsy's varying significance by time and place. Within the biomedical paradigm an epileptic seizure is the product of an abnormal paroxysmal discharge of cerebral neurones. Epilepsy itself is often defined as a continuing tendency to epileptic seizures. The form taken by the seizure depends on the site of the neuronal discharge in the brain. There are as many causes of epilepsy as there are seizure types. Genetic disorders like Tay-Sachs disease, congenital malformations, anoxia, trauma, brain tumours, infectious diseases, acquired metabolic diseases, degenerative disorders and chronic alcoholism can all lead to epilepsy. There is evidence too that a low

* Correspondence: Graham Scambler, Professor of Medical Sociology, Research Department of Infection and Population Health, UCL Medical School, Mortimer Market Centre, London WC1E 6JB. Tel: +44(0) 845 1555000 (x8186). Fax: +44(0) 20 7380 9681f1. Email: rmhagns@ucl.ac.uk

convulsion threshold can be inherited. Epilepsy, in short, can be regarded as an umbrella term covering a heterogeneous set of symptoms of a wide range of pathologies.

If the neuronal discharge remains confined to one part of the brain, the seizure is described as 'partial'. If the discharge begins in one part but subsequently spreads to all parts, it is said to be 'partial with secondary generalization'. Not uncommonly the discharge has its genesis in the mesodiencephalic system and spreads more or less simultaneously to all parts of the brain, in which case reference is made to a 'primary generalized' seizure. Since it is generally accepted that all partial seizures arise from some focal area of structural abnormality in the brain, all partial seizures, together with those seizures which are secondarily generalized from some focal onset, can be described as 'symptomatic epilepsy'. Primary generalized epilepsy is not symptomatic of underlying brain damage, and is thus often described as 'idiopathic epilepsy'.

Epilepsy is more common than many realize, although estimates of rates depend on definitions and case ascertainment. Prevalence is typically said to be between five and 10 cases per 1000 persons, and the overall incidence to be approximately 50 cases per 100,000 persons. Significantly for its impact on people's lives, the highest incidence is at the two extremes of the lifecourse, with about half of all cases being either under the age of one or over the age of 60. The prognosis varies with such factors as number of seizures at presentation, seizure type and use of antiepileptic drugs (AED). In one recent review of the evidence (Bell and Sanders, 2002), four prognostic classes were identified:

1. excellent prognosis (20-30%): usually only a few seizures occur and spontaneous remission is the norm;
2. good prognosis (30-40%): seizures are readily controlled by AED and once remission is achieved it is usually permanent;
3. AED-dependent prognosis (10-20%): AED suppress seizures and remission may be achieved, but relapse is probable if AED are stopped;
4. poor prognosis (up to 20%): AED are palliative rather than suppressive of seizures, with only a minority responding to novel AED or surgery.

The mortality rate is marginally increased in those with epilepsy. In newly diagnosed epilepsy death is frequently attributed to the underlying pathology, while in chronic epilepsy a familiar cause of death is 'Sudden Unexpected Death in Epilepsy' (SUDEP) (the rate of unexpected death being three times higher in those with epilepsy than in the general population). It should be noted here that susceptibility to epilepsy, as to most conditions, is exacerbated by social standing: the 'lower' one's social class the greater the liability, rendering theories of aetiology more complex than simple epidemiological calculations might suggest.

Social Science and Epilepsy

For the social scientist these introductory paragraphs raise innumerable issues. As Temkins' (1971) classic record of *The Falling Sickness* testifies, different times and places produce different concepts. The concept of epilepsy explicated here belongs within the science of the occident. This is not to espouse some form of epistemological relativism (that is, that truth and falsity are culture-specific). Drawing on Sayer (2000), we would commend the acceptance of three complementary theses:

1. a realist ontology: there exist natural and social worlds independent of our knowledge of them;
2. an acknowledgement of an epistemology of time and place: we can only draw on the stocks of knowledge that happen to be accessible to us;
3. an enduring sense of rationality: the fact that our stocks of knowledge are bounded by time and place does not preclude the rational assessment of one theory relative to another, which remains entirely viable.

These theses allow for recognition that contemporary, scientific concepts of epilepsy capture the activity of real, generative mechanisms – biological, psychological and social – articulated in ways that both have and will change, but which nevertheless allow for rational adjudication.

The focus of this contribution is on social mechanisms, or the interface between the individual with epilepsy and the wider society. This raises issues not only of the nature of public knowledge, opinion and behaviour in relation to epilepsy, together with their consequences, but also of how these are processed and/or anticipated by people with epilepsy themselves. Labels like 'epilepsy' and 'epileptic' can have powerful effects. In a quite literal sense, they can have lives independent of seizure activity or other biological or psychological correlates. It may seem counter-intuitive, especially to physicians, but it is possible to 'be epileptic' without 'having epilepsy'.

Labelling

It is pertinent to this contribution to explore this possibility from the outset. It arises with epilepsy's not altogether exceptional medical, and therefore socially and legally authoritative, *mis*diagnosis. If an individual is told he or she has epilepsy by a state-licensed expert there is a clear sense in which the 'label' sticks. The well-documented reluctance of patients to 'become epileptic' counts for little when set against the judgment of the generalist let alone the specialist physician. Labels carry their own weight and ramifications. This is perhaps best captured in the sociological notion of *secondary deviance*.

In the 1950s and '60s American sociologists like Lemert, Erikson and Becker distinguished between 'primary' and 'secondary deviance'. Primary deviance referred to patterns of behaviour attracting labels with connotations of deviance, ranging from culpable behaviour like alcohol or drug taking ('achieved' deviance) to symptoms like epileptic seizures entirely divorced from will or choice ('acquired' deviance). Secondary deviance denoted those unavoidable effects of authoritative labelling, whether delivered by judges sitting in courts or physicians conducting clinics, that often resulted in 'career deviance'. In other words a medical diagnosis or *mis*diagnosis and subsequent communication of a label of epilepsy confers a new and largely unwelcome identity for self and for others, culminating in pressures for compliance. Like it or not, a person so labelled effectively 'is' epileptic, with all its consequences for the future.

What this reference to the more or less inevitable, *and irresistible* (in a Kafkaesque sense), sequelae of the misdiagnosis of epilepsy affirms is that biological mechanisms are not the only ones in play when 'living with epilepsy' is considered. We are not suggesting that *mis*diagnosis is common, merely that it occurs and has its own momentum.

Public Attitudes

Recent studies suggest a decline in negative public attitudes to the label of epilepsy and to people with epilepsy, although knowledge levels have remained fairly constant (Jacoby, 2002). Still discernible in present thinking, however, are 'old' ideas (Jacoby and Austin, 2007). A recent Austrian study, for example, revealed that 15% of those questioned would object to their child marrying someone with epilepsy (Spatt et al, 2005). In the Czech Republic, 29% retain the notion that epilepsy is a form of insanity (Novotna and Rektor, 2002). Jacoby and colleagues (2004) report that in the UK over half of 1,600 randomly selected informants agreed that people with epilepsy are treated differently, encompassing social avoidance and exclusion, a tendency they attributed in part to fears about their 'unreliability' and 'nonnormality'. More than one in five agreed that people with epilepsy experience more personality problems than those without. This relatively high prevalence of negatively oriented attitudes suggests that the diagnostic label might be routinely harmful.

Dilario and colleagues (2004) discern four underlying dimensions to current American attitudes about epilepsy. First, negative stereotypes reflect beliefs held and attributed to the 'generalized other' about people with epilepsy (for example that they are unreliable or should not marry). Second, concerns about risk and safety reflect underlying anxieties about those with epilepsy engaging in certain activities. Third, expectations connected to work and other roles reflect beliefs about the abilities of persons with epilepsy to cope and prosper in those roles. And fourth, personal apprehension and avoidance reflect affective responses to thoughts of being alone with someone with epilepsy. Over a quarter (27%) of this sample believed that each seizure carries a high risk of death, and two-thirds (66%) that an object should be inserted into the mouth of an individual having a seizure. Lower levels of knowledge were associated with higher perceptions of stigma.

A US survey of 19,000 teenagers revealed widespread ignorance and negativity (Austin et al, 2002). More than a half (52%) had never heard of epilepsy; almost as many (46%) were unsure whether or not it is contagious; and 40% were not sure whether people with epilepsy are dangerous. Less than a third of the same sample said they would consider dating someone with epilepsy, and three-quarters (75%) thought teenagers with epilepsy are more prone to be bullied or picked on than their peers without epilepsy. A UK study has suggested that social avoidance of teenagers with epilepsy might be a function of not knowing what to do in the event of a seizure (Robson, 2006).

Studies of beliefs and attitudes like those cited here bear testimony to the threat that the 'epileptic identity' associated and triggered by the communication of a diagnostic label can present. It does not follow, however, either that people without epilepsy act in ways consistent with the beliefs or attitudes they articulate when confronted by survey questions, or that what was earlier called secondary deviance automatically follows the labelling process.

Adjustment and 'Self-Labelling'

Studies indicating patterns in coping with or adjusting to epilepsy, against this backcloth of public misunderstanding and antipathy, began to take shape in the 1970s. One pioneering investigation was conducted in the USA by Schneider and Conrad (1983). They noted the potential for 'allies' of children with epilepsy, numbered among Goffman's (1968) 'wise', to act as 'stigma coaches'. In other words, one unintended by-product of well-intentioned but over-protective or solicitous parents or doctors was the introduction and propagation of the idea that epilepsy signals an undesirable and threatening identity best tidied away or kept 'in the closet' (Schneider and Conrad, 1981). These authors went on to draw a distinction between 'adjusted' and 'unadjusted' adaptations to life with epilepsy.

They identified three sub-types of adjusted adaptation. The first of these they termed the *pragmatic* type. Pragmatists seek to reduce the salience of, or 'minimize', their epilepsy, personally and with regard to others. This does not lead invariably to attempts to 'pass' (as normal) or to 'cover' for their epilepsy, but rather a policy of selective disclosure to those who 'need to know' is pursued. By combining selective disclosure with scepticism about the possibility of others' negative judgements were they to know, the pragmatist effects a relatively normal life. The second category is the *secret* type. Epilepsy is managed in this case by more or less steadfast attempts to conceal what is perceived as a stigmatizing, negative and 'bad' quality of self. To the extent to which the strategy is effective, cautious participation in most walks of life is accomplished. The final sub-type is found more rarely and named the *quasi-liberated* type. Individuals comprising this group straightforwardly acknowledge their epilepsy, and unlike the pragmatists broadcast the news far and wide to educate others and to tackle head-on any threat of stigmatization. As Jobling (1977: 83) put it in relation to (his) psoriasis, 'deviance is shown to be no more than difference and discredit is denied'.

Any sense of agency and control is missing in the ranks of the unadjusted. Those in this category, characterized by an absence of strategy, are 'overwhelmed' by their epilepsy. Among the unadjusted are those falling into an extreme sub-set of the *debilitated.* For these, epilepsy is a dominant or 'master status' that floods identity and behaviour, leading to 'a constipation of the social self'. Schneider and Conrad wisely add that some individuals adopt different strategies at different points of the lifecourse.

In the wake of this American study Scambler and Hopkins (1986) conducted an interview-based community survey in London. They reported that non-disclosure or concealment was the first-choice strategy for the great majority of people with epilepsy across their various social roles. Independently of its efficacy, however, it rarely brought the requisite peace of mind, which led the authors to distinguish between *felt* and *enacted stigma.* While enacted stigma refers to actual discrimination based on a sense of unacceptable difference, felt stigma refers to (1) a sense of shame attached to 'being epileptic', and (2) a fear of encountering enacted stigma. Felt stigma was the social strategy that stood in the way of peace of mind.

Concealment was not the only strategy found in Scambler and Hopkins' sample. Some opted for pragmatism by occasionally volunteering disclosure. Unlike in Schneider and Conrad's sample, however, pragmatism was almost always a back-up or second-choice strategy: they opted for openness only when the pursuit of concealment seemed counter-productive. Finally, a mere handful (2%) fell into the US category of quasi-liberated.

Scambler and Hopkins rejected an orthodox stance within the labelling perspective – namely, that the communication of the diagnostic label by a licensed practitioner leads inexorably to secondary deviance and a deviant career as 'an epileptic' – in favour of a *hidden distress model of epilepsy* (Scambler, 1989). It was a model epitomized in three propositions:

1. When people are given the diagnosis of epilepsy they more often than not adopt what Stebbins (1970) calls a 'special view of the world', at the core of which is felt stigma, which predisposes to a strategy of non-disclosure or concealment (children generally have this strategy chosen for them by parents, doctors etc *qua* stigma coaches);
2. This strategy of non-disclosure and concealment means that opportunities for enacted stigma tend to be quite rare;
3. As a result of (1) and (2), felt stigma is typically far more disruptive of the lives of people with epilepsy than enacted stigma.

In the London study people's epilepsy did not always have high salience for them: it was only intermittently intrusive. Most people most of the time felt 'like everyone else'. Their epilepsy only featured in circumstances that prompted them to engage with or retreat into their special view of the world (for example, a witnessed seizure or attendance at a wedding). Once under the influence of this special view of their world they were predisposed to certain stereotyped behaviours, namely, depending on whether they were discreditable or discredited, to pass or cover respectively (Goffman, 1968). Significantly, only 36% of those interviewed had experienced a seizure in the month prior to interview, and 31% had been seizure-free for two years or more.

It was apparent in this same study that people's epilepsy had more salience for them in some roles than others. Often, for example, individuals were content and well supported in their families but, due to an increase in seizure frequency for example, suffering from severe felt stigma in connection with his or her discreditable position at work. From time to time, however, some admitted to bouts of profound pessimism, even despair, when their epileptic status became a felt (or enacted) master status and they thought themselves 'cursed' (candidates for Schneider and Conrad's debilitated sub-type of unadjusted adaptation).

Disadvantage

It is foolhardy to infer rates of enacted or felt stigma, or of what might be termed 'legitimate discrimination' (for example, temporary driving bans), from data on public beliefs and attitudes towards epilepsy and people with epilepsy. A putative improvement in the latter need not signify a decline in the former. So what is known about the overall social disadvantage experienced by people with epilepsy? And how much of what disadvantage is documented is explicable via felt stigma, that is, socially generated but individually inflicted?

People with epilepsy are up to twice as likely as their counterparts without it to be at risk of unemployment (Jacoby at al, 1998; Fisher et al, 2000). This disadvantage in the labour market extends too to underemployment relative to skill level and experience (Scambler et al, 1980; Chaplin et al, 1998). Employment difficulties can translate into financial and psychological distress. Seizure frequency and type, as well as age at onset, duration of epilepsy and the cognitive effects of AED, are associated with work problems, as are psychological factors like lowered self-esteem and reduced expectation. An additional factor, unsurprisingly, is employer attitude.

Jacoby and colleagues (2005) conducted a mail survey of a random sample of UK companies selected as representative of the 14 UK economic regions and proportional to the number of employees. Twenty-six per cent of those who replied (41%) reported having experience of employees with epilepsy; 16% judged there to be no jobs suitable for people with epilepsy in their companies; and 21% thought employing people with epilepsy would be 'a major issue'. Employees were uniformly of the view that people with epilepsy should disclose their condition to prospective employers. Seizure severity, frequency and controllability were all considered salient to employability. About half of employers nevertheless expressed high concern, some linking epilepsy to the likelihood of a work-related accident. More positively, some employers indicated a willingness to be flexible with employees with epilepsy, this being more likely in larger firms and firms with past experience.

What these and other studies suggest is that:

1. people with epilepsy tend to experience more disadvantage in the labour market than those without epilepsy;
2. this may be due in part to employer beliefs and attitudes (although negative deeds do not automatically follow from negative words);
3. because epilepsy is a 'hidden disease', felt stigma might contribute as much or more to disadvantage than enacted stigma.

To fully test 1-3, and 3 in particular, qualitative studies are as important as quantitative, and these need to move beyond the 'personal tragedy' orientation found in the early work of Schneider and Conrad and Scambler and Hopkins (Scambler, 2004).

Stigma Reduction Programmes

The stigma associated with epilepsy has long been recognized and held responsible for disadvantage experienced in the workplace and elsewhere. Up to the 1960s in Britain this was in part diminished by the removal of patients from the community and their incarceration in 'epileptic colonies'. While there are many examples of stigma reduction strategies from around the world, few of these report outcome data (Birbeck, 2006). They tend to focus too on either people with epilepsy themselves or on the public. As Schneider and Conrad's coining of the term 'stigma coaching' indicates, family members can perpetuate epilepsy related stigma without intending to, as well as themselves being on the receiving end of what Goffman (1968) calls 'courtesy stigma' (or stigma by association). Birbeck reports no stigma reduction programmes aimed at families.

Morell (2002) suggests that the effects of enacted and felt stigma on the lives of people with epilepsy be countered by: optimum access to medical information, treatment and care, especially in the early years – 'stigma must be addressed early in life'; legislation against prejudicial and unacceptable discrimination against people with epilepsy on the part of employers and other third parties; and programmes to foster self-advocacy and to raise self-esteem.

What worthy strategies like these understandably fail to address is how stigmatization typically echoes deeper social divisions, like those of class, command, gender, ethnicity and so on (Scambler, 2006), and may in consequence be more obdurate and resistant to challenge than commonly thought.

Future Research Agendas

The point was made at the start of this chapter that sociology is only one discipline with a bearing on epilepsy-related quality of life: biological and psychological mechanisms are also at play. Scambler and colleagues (In Press) have argued that because biological, psychological and social mechanisms are likely to be simultaneously active (as it were 'beneath the surface'), separating out their effects ('above the surface') is very difficult. We have seen that epilepsy can have injurious consequences even in the absence of biological mechanisms - through *mis*diagnosis – but clearly biological mechanisms, embracing here epilepsy genetics, typically *matter*. Further, biological mechanisms can, given severe underlying pathology, simply overwhelm the contributions of psychological and social mechanisms. For their part, psychological mechanisms, stretching from neuropsychology to social psychology, typically *condition* people's handling of their biologically-induced impairment. They do so, and here is sociology's role, in socially-induced *contexts*. It is contexts we have dwelt on in this chapter.

We end this brief consideration with a specification of six areas of sociological enquiry as yet underdeveloped. Clearly a sociology of epilepsy does not begin and end with individual 'impairment effects' (Thomas, 2007) and coping, or even the social contexts in which embodied coping occurs. As Temkin's (1971) historical research shows, the authoritative categorization and labelling of epileptic phenomena by healers is subject to continuing change. Thus the 'taken-for-granted' diagnosis referred to in this contribution is historically recent and had its genesis in Occidential science and medicine. It will mutate in the future. A first series of sociological questions therefore concerns how social mechanisms influence the social construction of the biological sciences and the use to which they are put in theory and practice by professions of medicine. This extends also to the social construction of the psychology of the individual and its purchase on epilepsy.

A second topic is the extent to which people's social positions and the contexts in which they live and work contribute to the aetiology of epilepsy (epilepsy as primary deviance, as it were). It is a commonplace among social epidemiologists that those in more lowly positions in social hierarchies like those of class and status tend to experience weaker – biological, psychological and social – cultural, spatial and material asset flows known to be conducive to health and longevity (Scambler, 2007). A child from a low-income household, for example, is more likely than his or her counterpart in a moderate to high-income household to grow up in an environment where early illness and accidents in the home or neighbourhood are not uncommon, this increasing the likelihood of epilepsy of early onset.

A third series of issues has to do with the tensions between not-always-overlapping professional and lay or patient constructions of epilepsy. Professional knowledge feeds into but rarely encompasses what might be called 'experiential knowledge'. Moreover it is experiential knowledge that typically shapes 'illness behaviour', that is, how people come to see themselves as ill and what they do about it. Social mechanisms, in short, are pivotal for grasping the 'whys' and 'hows' of peoples' use of the 'popular', 'folk' and 'professional' sectors of what Kleinman (1985) usefully calls their 'local health care systems'. Those with medically-defined epilepsy who do not reach the professional sector not only miss out on the costs and benefits of treatment, probably with AED, but remain immune from medical labelling.

A fourth area of study focuses on the encounters between people with epilepsy *as patients* and their doctors. Once in Kleinman's professional sector, whether via a general practitioner or epilepsy nurse consultation, leading to a referral to a neurology out-patient clinic, or an ambulance pick-up to a hospital accident and emergency department, patients become involved in novel definitions of their situations. Such definitions are rarely cut-and-dried and always involve negotiation. Patients require numerous working definitions for-self and for-others: their roles, reference groups and the particular contexts in which they find themselves can all call for re-negotiation.

Social aspects of coping comprise a fifth dimension. Published work on what Bury (1982) terms the 'biographical disruption' often occasioned by chronic illness has been profuse, as it has on Charmaz's (1983) related notion of a 'loss of self' and Williams' (1983) discernment of the need for 'narrative reconstruction'. The diagnosis of epilepsy transmits more than information: it calls for a revised sense of who one is and one's future projects.

A sixth and as yet under-investigated domain involves the embedding of norms of shame in the structures and institutions of the wider society. As intimated previously, it is not possible to fully grasp relations of stigma in a societal vacuum. Any taint attached to epilepsy has roots also in the 'layering' of society: it reflects the multiplicity of ways in which people are valued and consequently classified and processed. As a topic requiring investigation, this sixth branch of a potential research programme on the sociology of epilepsy is perhaps the one furthest removed from biomedical thinking. It also points beyond the more limited – Occidental *and global* – fields of enquiry currently favoured.

REFERENCES

Austin,J, Shafer,P and Deering,J (2002) Epilepsy familiarity, knowledge and perceptions of stigma: report from a survey of adolescents in the general population. *Epilepsy Behaviour* 3 368-375.

Bell,G and Sanders,I (2002) The epidemiology of epilepsy: the size of the problem. *Seizure* 11 Suppl A, 306-16.

Birbeck,G (2006) Interventions to reduce epilepsy-associated stigma. *Psychology, Health and Medicine* 364-366.

Bury,M (1982) Chronic illness as biographical disruption. *Sociology of Health and Illness* 4 167-182.

Chaplin,J, Wester,A and Tomson,T (1998) Factors associated with employment problems of people with established epilepsy. *Seizure* 7 299-303.

Charmaz,K (2003) Loss of self: a fundamental form of suffering in the chronically ill. *Sociology of Health and Illness* 5 168-195.

Dilorio,C, Kabau,R, Holden,E, Berkowitz,J, Kamin,S, Antonak,R, Austin,J, Baker,G, Bauman,I, Gilliam,F, Thurman,D, Price,P (2004) Developing a measure to assess attitudes towards epilepsy in the US population. *Epilepsy Behaviour* 5 965-975.

Fisher,R, Vickrey,B, Gibson,P et al (2000) The impact of epilepsy from the patient's perspective. 1 – Descriptions and subjective perceptions. *Epilepsy Research* 41 39-51.

Goffman,E (1968) Stigma: Notes on the Management of Spoiled Identity. Harmondsworth; Penguin.

Jacoby,A (2002) Stigma, epilepsy and quality of life. *Epilepsy Behaviour* 3 S10-S20.

Jacoby,A and Austin,J (2007) Social stigma for adults and children with epilepsy. *Epilepsia* 48 (Suppl.9) 6-9.

Jacoby,A, Buck,D, Baker,G et al (1998) Uptake and costs of care for epilepsy: findings from a UK regional study. *Epilepsia* 39 776-786.

Jacoby,A, Gorry,J, Gamble,C and Baker,G (2004) Public knowledge, private grief: a study of public attitudes to epilepsy in the UK and implications for stigma. *Epilepsia* 45 1405-1415.

Jacoby,A, Gorry,J and Baker,G (2005) Employers' attitudes to employment of people with epilepsy: still the same old story. *Epilepsia* 1978-1987.

Jobling,R (1977) Learning to live with it: an account of a career of chronic dermatological illness and patienthood. In Eds Davis,A and Horobin,G: Medical Encounters: The Experience of Illness and Treatment. London; Croom Helm.

Kleinman,A (1985) Indigenous systems of healing: questions for professional, popular and folk care. In Ed Salmon,J: Alternative Medicines: Popular and Lay Perspectives. London; Tavistock.

Morrell,M (2002) Stigma and epilepsy. *Epilepsy and Behaviour* 3 21-35.

Novotna,I and Rektor,I (2002) The trend in public attitudes in the Czech Republic towards persons with epilepsy. *European Journal of Neurology* 9 535-540.

Robson,C (2006) *Examining the social stigma of epilepsy: a qualitative analysis of attitudes, perceptions and understanding towards epilepsy and people with epilepsy among young adults in the undergraduate population.* M.Sc Thesis, Department of Health Sciences, University of York.

Sayer,D (2000) Realism and Social Science. London; Sage.

Scambler,G (1989) Epilepsy. London; Tavistock.

Scambler,G (2004) Re-framing stigma: felt and enacted stigma and challenges to the sociology of chronic and disabling conditions. *Social Theory and Health* 2 29-46.

Scambler,G (2006) Jigsaws, models and the sociology of stigma. *Journal of Critical Realism* 5 273-289.

Scambler,G and Hopkins,A (1980) Social class, epileptic activity and disadvantage at work. *Journal of Epidemiology and Community Health* 34 129-133.

Scambler,G and Hopkins,A (1986) 'Being epileptic': coming to terms with stigma. *Sociology of Health and Illness* 8 26-43.

Scambler,G, Afentouli,P and Selai,C (In Press) *Discerning biological, psychological and social mechanisms in the impact of epilepsy on the individual: a framework and exploration.* In Eds Scambler,G and Scambler,S: The Sociology of Chronic and Disabling Conditions: Assaults on the Lifeworld. London; Palgrave.

Schneider,J and Conrad,P (1981) Medical and sociological typologies: the case of epilepsy. *Social Science and Medicine* 15A 211-219.

Schneider,J and Conrad,P (1983) Having Epilepsy: The Experience and Control of Illness. Philadelphia; Temple University Press.

Spatt,J, Bauer,G, Baumgartner,C, Feucht,M, Graf,M Mamoli,B and Trinka,T (2005) Predictors for negative attitudes towards subjects with epilepsy: a representative survey in the general public in Austria. *Epilepsia* 46 736-742.

Stebbins,R (1970) Career: the subjective approach. *Sociological Quarterly* 11 32-49.

Temkin,O (1971) The Falling Sickness. Baltimore; Johns Hopkins Press.

Thomas,C 2007) Sociologies of Disability and Illness. London; Palgrave.

Williams,G (1983) The genesis of chronic illness: narrative reconstruction. *Sociology of Health and Illness* 21 797-819.

In: Social Epileptology
Editors: J. Pinikahana and C. Walker

ISBN 978-1-60876-228-6

Chapter 4

WHO GETS TREATMENT FOR EPILEPSY? THE POLITICAL ECONOMY OF THE TREATMENT GAP

Christine Walker*
Chronic Illness Alliance Inc

ABSTRACT

In this chapter I explore some of the inequalities the studies of the 'treatment gap' have exposed to the public view; I examine some of the inadequacies of the analyses around the treatment gap and suggest that a broader political economy of health approach which includes an understanding of the place of epilepsy in global health inequalities will yield another direction to address both the gross and relative inadequacies in the care of people with epilepsy in both developing and developed economies.

INTRODUCTION

In 1997 the World Health Organisation, International League against Epilepsy and the International Bureau for Epilepsy established the 'Global Campaign Against Epilepsy: Out of the Shadows' (WHO 1997). This was in recognition that the burden of epilepsy throughout the world was underestimated and epilepsy itself was under-treated. The campaign also recognised that people with epilepsy suffered a low quality of life throughout the world due to stigma and discrimination.

This campaign has brought together data from across countries and regions, establishing that there are indeed deficits in treatment and care for epilepsy throughout the world and that treatment and care varies both between countries and within countries (WHO 2004a; WHO 2004b). Epilepsy is estimated to affect some 50 million people in the world, of whom four fifths live in developing countries (Mbuba et al 2008). In developing countries there are estimates that 90% of those with epilepsy receive either inappropriate or no treatment or are

* Correspondence: Dr Christine Walker, Chronic Illness Alliance Inc. 818 Burke Rd. Camberwell. Victoria, Australia 3124. .61 3 9882 4654 Email: cwalker@chronicillness.org.au

under-treated (WHO 1997; Meinardi et al 2001; Cruz 2005). This has become known amongst epilepsy researchers as the 'treatment gap'.

THE TREATMENT GAP IN EPILEPSY

The treatment gap is defined as the number of people with active epilepsy not on treatment or on inadequate treatment expressed as a percentage of all people in a population with active epilepsy. Active epilepsy is variously defined as: 'two or more unprovoked seizures on different days in the previous year' (Meinardi et al 2001) and having had one unprovoked seizure in the previous five years (Mbuba et al 2008). Meinardi et al (3) observe that the treatment gap also includes care in terms of quality of life. Following epidemiological estimations based on varying definitions in 2002 the Global Campaign on Epilepsy moved into a new phase where demonstration projects to address the treatment gap were implemented.

Epilepsy in the Western Pacific Region: A Call to Action (WHO 2004a) explores the prevalence and incidence of epilepsy in the region including China, Japan, Philippines and New Zealand and Australia. In all, there are 37 countries in the region with varying economies, cultures, political systems and health needs. The report concludes that there are insufficient epidemiological data in the countries in this region, no public education campaigns, poor distribution of neurologists and lack of access to Anti-Epileptic Drugs (AEDs). One of the first demonstration projects carried out in this region took place in five Chinese provinces. The project identified that the prevalence of active epilepsy was 4.6 per 1000 and that 63% of those with active epilepsy did not receive treatment in the week prior to the survey (WHO 2004a). Following this there was an intervention project where primary care doctors were trained in epilepsy care by neurologists.

A survey of epilepsy resources was also conducted in the region (WHO 2004a). This survey was completed by 25 of the 37 countries and demonstrated that only 9 of those 25 countries in the region had medical specialists in epilepsy. The 25 respondents identified that there were difficulties in all their countries regarding diagnosing and treating epilepsy including compliance and access to AEDs; suitable treatment infrastructure such as diagnostic tools and hospitals; lack of government funding and high levels of stigma and discrimination against people with epilepsy. Causes of epilepsy varied across the region from parasitic infection to head injuries, to unknown causes.

More specifically countries such as the Marshall Islands, Niue, Fiji and Micronesia reported having no epilepsy professionals, while some countries including Mongolia and Laos reported two and one respectively. Many countries listed the costs of medications in terms of the cost to the consumer with only Australia declaring its Pharmaceutical Benefits Scheme as a government subsidised source of access to AEDs.

Mbuba et al (2008) reviewed articles written on the treatment gap in other regions including the African region, where similar findings were reported. Poor health service infrastructure, cost and availability of AEDs, lack of access to medical services including distances to travel and cultural beliefs were all found to contribute to the treatment gap. Projects which aimed to reduce the treatment gap were also reviewed. These projects were generally short-term, the longest being a project which delivered education programs to some

200 health workers and neurologists in an Indian state. The shortest was a 2 month education program for 30 people with epilepsy in Nigeria. Mbuba et al (2008) conclude their review of these projects by cautioning that such projects may not reach those who most need them. They base this caution on the results on similar programs for other diseases where the supply of drugs and education programs have been implemented have not produced the anticipated good results. HIV/AIDS is one example of this where the supply of antiretrovirals in developing countries does not reach those who need them while the need to educate people who are HIV positive about drugs and their health care is elusive since many people in developing countries are not aware they are HIV positive (Furber et al 2004; Geberding 2004).

LIMITATIONS TO THE TREATMENT GAP

While Mbuba et al (2008) have a basis for their caution around such well intentioned projects, a more seminal reason that projects may not produce the desired outcomes is that they are based on the concept of the treatment gap which has internal limitations. The treatment gap is essentially a clinically oriented concept. It relates to improving treatment including access to drugs, education about drugs and educating health professionals and consumers about compliance to treatment regimes. The concept recognises that poverty related to poor income and poor health infrastructure creates barriers to treatment. As with HIV/AIDS, the stigma of epilepsy is a barrier to care of people with epilepsy since people with epilepsy may eschew treatment as a means to avoid identification with epilepsy. However the concept assumes that clinical treatment and medication for people with epilepsy will solve this. In addition, programs are largely designed and delivered by neurologists and other health professionals, as well as consumer organisations whose mission is closely identified with improving clinical outcomes. Terms of reference and methodologies for projects to identify the treatment gap and address the treatment gap are therefore closely identified with clinical outcomes. As a moral imperative or a visionary principle there is little wrong with this; the problem lies in that it is a teleological or self-confirmatory approach where the populations most in need of treatment remain under-identified and the barriers to improved clinical outcomes are barely analysed.

Some of these limitations show up in the surveys undertaken in the Western Pacific Region (2004a) and the African Region (2004b) to establish the extent of the treatment gap in the countries of each region. The items surveyed were essentially related to clinical outcomes including incidence and prevalence of epilepsy, costs of AEDs, number of health personnel including neurologists in each of the countries. Some other data were collected including access to drinking water and sanitation. Data were collected by neurologists or consumer organisation from neurologists or consumer organisations whose sources are mainly clinical lists. Epidemiological data are limited and unreliable and largely collected in these surveys from hospital and practice data of individual practitioners providing a skewed view towards those who receive some treatment but not providing a complete picture of epilepsy in the community, where there may be people receiving no treatment or no diagnosis.

Most problematical however is that the surveys and the consequent projects are conducted in isolation from the social, cultural, political and economic structures in which epilepsy is experienced, diagnosed and treated. The powerful interplay between these social factors, the health system and the health of individuals, their families and carers has implications for the treatment gap as it is experienced by people with epilepsy within countries, as well as between countries. The interplay of these factors also has relevance to whether programs can successfully target and address treatment gaps.

HEALTH INEQUALITIES AND ACCESS TO TREATMENT

Closing the treatment gap in epilepsy means access to treatment including AEDs for the world's poor. The variations in access to medical care and anti-epileptic drugs for groups of people with epilepsy apply to other health conditions and equate with unequal access to health and healthcare that have been observed to operate at the broadest levels throughout the world. Improving the health of the world's poor is not simply a case of providing them with access to drugs and healthcare. Neither is it simply a case of improving incomes for poor people so they have access to drugs and healthcare. Were that the case many conditions would have been eradicated decades ago.

The Global Burden of Disease 2004 Update (WHO 2008) provides the data to compare the state of health across the WHO regions of the world. Globally twenty percent of deaths in the world are children under 5 years; one third of them dying in the neonatal period. More children under 5 die in the poorer countries (45% of deaths in Africa are children under 5 while some 2 % of children under 5 die in Europe.) Children in Africa are approximately five times more likely to die of perinatal conditions than those in high income regions. Diarrhoeal and respiratory conditions as well as malaria all contribute to childhood deaths in African and South East Asian countries.

While cardiovascular diseases account for the majority of adult deaths, (27% of adult males die of cardiovascular disease) infectious and parasitic diseases account for some 17% of male adult deaths. These deaths are not evenly distributed across the world, with parasitic and infectious diseases including malaria, HIV/AIDS and TB accounting for the majority of deaths in low income countries and non-communicable diseases such as cancers, dementias, and heart disease accounting for more deaths in higher income countries.

In examining the burden of disease, WHO Global Burden of Disease 2004 Update (2008) claims that communicable diseases most burden the low income regions of Africa, South-East Asia and the Eastern Mediterranean. Non-communicable diseases in turn constitute a greater burden to low and middle income regions than they do in high income countries.

The report 'Closing the gap in a generation: health equity through action on the social determinants of health (CSDH 2008) says the message is clear; poverty and health are related. They are related in rich and poor countries alike. Few countries can demonstrate that health is evenly distributed amongst its total population.

The 'social gradient of health' (Marmot 2006) demonstrates that in countries such as the United Kingdom where the poor are far less deprived than those in Africa, people who are most disadvantaged have worse health as demonstrated by mortality rates, than those who are materially better off. (CSDH 2008:31). Mortality rates for 1999-2003 demonstrate that poorer males in the UK are 2.5 times more likely to die before retirement than are better off people (Marmot 2006). In the United States where income is increasingly unevenly distributed, in the early 1990s the United States had one of the highest rates of *absolute* (as well as relative) poverty amongst the developed countries and infant mortality rates amongst the worse off section of the population are higher than in better off sections of the American population, approaching rates closer to far poorer countries (Coburn 2004).

In Australia, despite an overall decline in Australian mortality rates between 1985-7 and 1995-7 the differences between socio-economic groups remain evident. Infant and perinatal mortality were highest in the most disadvantaged areas while mortality for both males and females between 25 and 64 was highest in the most disadvantaged areas (PHIDU 1999).

While poor income is related to poor health the relationship is not a simple one (Cruz 2005; Coburn 2004; Muntaner andLynch 2002). The social gradient of health provides evidence that unequal distribution of income rather than simply low income within a nation plays a role in health outcomes (Marmot 2006). Cuba, Sri Lanka, Kerala and Costa Rica all have relatively low incomes but good health outcomes (Marmot 2006; Deaton 2006). At the same time average income in South Africa would suggest the health of its whole population should be relatively good, but this income is unequally divided between the minority while population and a majority black population with the consequence that health is also unequally distributed (Marmot 2006).

Such anomalies as these suggest that underlying data on the relationship between income and health are complex social factors which influence access to treatment for many conditions including epilepsy, and also influence which groups of people globally will have poor health.

Political Economy and the Treatment Gap

As demonstrated by the anomalies above income in itself is not necessarily the main determinant of health. The unequal distribution of income rather than poor income has the greater impact on who receives treatment for epilepsy in all countries. It is however just one contributing factor to the strong relationship between the treatment gap and poverty.

The political economic structure of countries strongly influences who receives healthcare in a particular society, the quality of that healthcare and the design of its delivery as well as how a society pays for it.

> Poverty is not only lack of income. The implication, both of the social gradient in health and the poor health of the poorest of the poor, is that health inequity is caused by the unequal distribution of income, goods and services and of the consequent chance of leading a flourishing life. This unequal distribution is not in any sense a 'natural' phenomenon but is the result of policies that prize the interests of some over those of others-all too often a rich and powerful minority over the interests of a disempowered majority. (CSDH, 2008 p32)

The way a society organises its economy impacts on the distribution of income and wealth and this in turn influences the unequal distribution of health and health care. Stilwell (2008) argues that there is no single explanation of income inequality. The range of causal factors he identifies includes the labour-capital relationship, the power of corporate organisations in a society, the impact of globalisation, and the influences of public policy (neo-liberalism and distributive policies).

Stilwell (2008) continues that an economy based on capitalism creates income inequality. This is an internally driven process because capital is accumulated by a minority section of a society employing a larger workforce in the production of goods and services. Unequal power based on wealth rather than income results from this structure whereby those with capital (wealth) have control over the incomes as well as the quality of life of those who produce goods. It is important to acknowledge that capitalism has brought large-scale global improvements in health, largely through the consistent delivery of good nutrition, safe drinking water and improved sanitation. Deaton (2006) argues, as does Marmot (2006), that capitalism has improved health and levelled out health inequalities *up to a certain point:*

> For much of the last half century, there was a reduction in the contribution to compound inequality from the life expectancy component while life expectancies in the low life-expectancy countries grew closer to life expectancy in the high life-expectancy countries. But these gaps on longevity have opened up again in the past fifteen years…(Deaton 2006 p26)

Deaton's allusion to 'the past fifteen years' is an important one to which we will return. It is important to acknowledge beforehand that capitalist economies may be vastly differently organised throughout the world. Politics plays an important role in the structure and organisation of capitalist economies. This has important implications for the treatment gap for epilepsy.

Navarro and Shi (2002) demonstrate this point. The way a nation is governed influences its level of income inequality, its social inequalities and health indicators such as child mortality. Those countries where social democratic parties have been in power for long periods following World War II have had policies to redistribute wealth and ideologies that health care and education should be available to all citizens. The direct consequence has been lower child mortality. Where a nation has had liberal policies and less commitment to a redistribution of wealth the health indicators are worse.

To illustrate this point we may consider the following examples from Navarro and Shi (2002). Social democracies such as the Scandinavian countries of Denmark and Sweden favour high income taxes and have redistributive policies such as child welfare, services for elderly people, pensions and benefits and housing for low income families. Public expenditure on health care in social democracies is based on the view that all citizens should have equal access to health and health care. High expenditures are offset by the high employment rates (and hence, more taxes paid). Liberal countries such as the United States, and to some extent the United Kingdom are characterised by politics where the dominance of market forces are considered to be the better way to improve the quality of life, including health of the whole population. Navarro and Shi (2002) include the United Kingdom here as its welfare state is not universal with the exception of the National Health Service. In both the case of the United States and the United Kingdom benefits are means tested and often relate to workforce participation. Liberal governments spend far less than social democracies on their health care. Infant mortality (deaths per 1000 live births between 1960 and 1996) was 4.0 in Sweden, 5.2 in Denmark and 7.8 in the United States and 6.1 in the United Kingdom.

These examples suggest that the redistribution of wealth or 'social transfers' practiced by social democratic politics have a protective effect of health. In the United States where there are social transfers to the poor and elderly these transfers are conducted on an ideological basis relating to 'the deserving poor' (Rector and Hederman 2004). This does not produce as great a benefit as the universalistic approach of social democracies. Possibly it entrenches and emphasises the level of social and health inequality by discriminating between some poor people and other poor people. Despite the high percentage of GNP spent on health care in the United States, the United States ranks amongst the lowest of 25 industrialised countries in terms of life expectancy, infant mortality and other health indicators (Levins and Lopez 2002; Coburn 2004).

In the United States the treatment gap exists because health care is unevenly distributed in terms of class, race and regions. The uninsured poor of the United States experiences the treatment gap in delays in hospital care, and lack of access to appropriate care, including not being able to afford medicines and not receiving screening or diagnoses (Levins and Lopez 2002). In social democracies with universal health insurance systems and to a lesser extent those liberal countries with limited models of social health insurance such as Australia's, treatment gaps are considerably less for all people on lower incomes.

Capitalist economies may thus vary in terms of the levels of income and social inequality they foster according to the dominant political ideologies and policies. Deaton's reference to 'the past fifteen years' is important since it heralds two important social changes between 1985 and 2000, one ideological and the other health-related, that have produced greater social and health inequality in both advanced Western economies and developing economies. The ideological change is the spread of neo-liberalism while HIV/AIDS has become a major impediment to the growth of developing nation's economies and reduced any gains made previously in terms of life expectancy.

Neo-liberalism or economic rationalism began to dominate economic thought from the early 1980s through the policies of Reagan in the United States and Thatcher in the United Kingdom (Navarro 2002; Aspromourgos 2003). It precipitated the float of the Australian dollar in 1984 (Aspromourgos 2003; Quiggan 1999). This new ideology which is in fact old 'laissez faire' or mercantilist ideals in a new set of clothes, holds that state intervention, especially social welfare and state regulation of industry and finance is a hindrance to economic growth. When markets, neo-liberals maintain, are allowed to operate unfettered by anything but the limits of competition national economies will grow and all sectors of society will benefit, through higher employment rates, competitive products and the removal of dependence on welfare. Instead of receiving 'welfare handouts' individuals with no income or very low income will be 'incentivised' to seek work (Stilwell 2008). Individualism, noted by Doyal (1979) as early as 1979 is a hallmark of neo-liberalism. Individuals need to be responsible for their own welfare and their family's welfare. Successful individuals will benefit their society by creating work for others through employment and their own spending.

While neo-liberals claim success in reducing inflation, there is some evidence that this has been achieved through increased unemployment and lower wage increases. Unemployment grew in many OECD countries between 1980 and 1990, accompanied by increasing wage inequality due to labour market deregulation (Navarro 2002). Social expenditures also dropped in OECD countries while family debt increased. These indicators underlie regressive distribution which Stilwell (2008) describes as 'regressive social policy'. Quiggan (1999) argues that government policies aimed at reducing state regulation of the economy have produced greater economic inequality in Australia, as well as in other countries. Distribution of income has become more unequal in developed countries since the end of the 1970s. Income growth in the United States has accrued to the top 20% over the past 3 decades. Similar increases are reported in New Zealand and the United Kingdom

(Stilwell 2008; Deaton 2006; Quiggan 1999). In Australia there is mixed evidence regarding inequality, though an increase in inequality for wage-earners is evident since 1975. Greater polarity between income groups has emerged with the top 10% of workers earning greater income relative to median income and the lowest 10% having income falling even more sharply compared with the median. Wicks (2005) argues that official Australian government statistics demonstrate that assertions that inequality is moderating are based on averages that disguise the unequal growth of incomes in the lower income groups, which have worsened due to regressive tax policies such as the GST . Quiggan suggested in 1999 that this increasing income inequality was most likely due to neo-liberal policies that removed the buffering effects of welfare services or more specifically the redistribution of post-tax income, for the lower income groups. Further, inequality in labour markets has occurred where neo-liberal reforms have favoured higher skilled workers and removed the services that assisted lower skilled workers. Short-term contracts, competitive tendering and casualisation of the workforce have all led to increased inequality of both labour markets and incomes. Coburn (2004) argues that policies based on neo-liberal ideologies are associated with greater income inequalities, and greater health inequalities, within countries.

Neo-liberalism has made its mark on developing economies. In some cases developing economies such as the Eastern European and South East Asian ones have been seen as new markets while South East Asia, South and Central America have provided the basis for lowering the costs of production through cheap labour. In both cases, the local economies of these countries have been dislocated. For example large scale crops for trans-national companies have displaced the local crops which fed the local population (Tonkiss 2006). Women and children constitute sweated labour producing consumer goods for middle class consumers in developed economies (Tonkiss 2006; CSDG 2008).

Developing economies have been forced into a neo-liberal framework. Those developing economies that borrowed from the International Monetary fund for example, did so under certain conditions including developing export markets as a development strategy (Tonkiss 2006; Kolko 2002). This in fact increased indebtedness of developing economies. This strategy has important social and health related implications. The view that increased income for a country through its exports would improve the whole population's social and health outcomes has not eventuated in many instances. While the IMF reported improved spending on health and education in some developing countries these benefits were very unevenly spread. In some countries the wealthiest received the greatest education benefit while in other countries where health data are available, the wealthiest received the greatest share of the health allocation (Kolko 2002). Kolko (2002) provides an example from Vietnam where the wealthiest fifth of the population receives some 45% of public subsidies for health and education. In fact the IMF's own data show that the poorest three fifths of many countries receiving IMF assistance receive no benefit or their position has become worse (Kolko 2002). Deaton (2006) argues that where inequality exists income inequality will continue and reinforce health inequalities.

Deaton (2006) considers that the advent of HIV/AIDS in developing countries, most specifically African ones, has reduced life-expectancy and has widened international health inequalities. Because the data in developing countries are poorly and inconsistently collected estimates of mortality from AIDS are speculative. Booysen et al (2003) echo Deaton's concern about the impact of HIV/AIDS and the problem of reliable data. Both Deaton (2006) and Booysen et al (2003) agree that there are sufficient data to argue that HIV/AIDS operates in developing countries at epidemic levels and is changing the epidemiological and socioeconomic profile of these countries. The high prevalence of HIV/AIDS amongst adults estimated to be some 20% of 15-49 year-olds in South Africa means that economic growth, social life and poverty alleviation are all affected. The economic impact of HIV is experienced in terms of loss of labour, loss of household income, higher costs to employers in terms of the benefits they pay out to their employees, lower productivity and high government costs in health care. HIV/AIDS is estimated to reduce South Africa's Gross Domestic Product by some 13% to 17% by 2015 (Booysen et al 2003). Life expectancy in seven African countries where prevalence of HIV/AIDS is high has dropped from 62 years in 1999 to 49 years in 2003 (UN AIDS 2004).

Health and social inequalities will increase along the lines already entrenched in most developing countries. A direct consequence of this is the loss of the health gains such as the reduction of child and infant mortality and life expectancy made through economic growth in developing economies in the 1990s. That is, those already impoverished will be more impoverished, with women and children suffering the most (Booysen 2003; UN AIDS 2004). At the same time reductions in mortality in developed economies mean that health inequalities between countries has widened in the last fifteen years.

HIV/AIDS has cut a swathe through economic growth and social cohesion in developing countries. This has implications for the treatment gap in epilepsy in developing countries. Economies faltering through HIV/AIDS will have less time and ability to be concerned with epilepsy. Medical services and funds including those delivered by foreign aid will be concentrated on HIV/AIDS. The concentration of funding will also contribute to doctors specialising in HIV/AIDS rather than elsewhere. The social and economic effects of HIV/AIDS on families and communities in developing countries will leave little time for attention to family members with epilepsy. At the same time, one of the reasons that antiretrovirals cannot be accessed by those who most need them in developing countries is that there is a chronic shortage of health professionals to deliver them. Many trained health professionals have left developing countries to work in developed economies (Geberding 2004). There is less incentive for trained health professionals to stay to work with epilepsy.

To summarise, the economic organisation in all countries means inequalities in wealth and income between groups of people. This inequality may be ameliorated or worsened in a nation by the ideology or policies the government of each nation adopts. Entrenched inequalities in wealth and income have profound effects on the health of each nation's populations, with some groups having good health and good health care and other groups having relatively poor health.

Developing countries where absolute wealth and income may be lower than in developed countries also have greater inequalities in wealth and income and consequently both worse health in absolute terms and greater inequalities in health amongst their populations. However health inequalities in developing countries will also be ameliorated or worsened depending on the ideologies and policies of their governments. Developing countries have the additional problem of HIV/AIDS radically eroding their abilities to continue economic and social development.

Addressing the Treatment Gap in Epilepsy

Epilepsy is classified by the World Health Organisation as a neuropsychiatric disorder which accounts for some 2.2% of adult male deaths. This is similar to the prevalence of diabetes mellitus. Neuropsychiatric disorders constitute the most important causes of disability in all regions accounting for one third of 'Years Lost to Disability' (YLD) in adults over 15 years (WHO 2008). Consequently, addressing the treatment gap in epilepsy is as imperative as addressing the treatment gap in any other condition in the world.

The treatment gap however is in fact one small aspect of health care for all conditions. A gap in treatment exists where some groups are not able to access the health care they require for any health condition that reduces their quality of life. A treatment gap exists in all countries to some extent because of the above inequalities. In countries such as the United Kingdom, Denmark, Sweden and Australia the establishment of universal or near-universal systems of health care mean that treatment gaps are vastly smaller than in countries such as the United States, since all income groups are able to access health care including medications and specialist care.

But treatment gaps in developed economies are already smaller relative to developing economies. Access to education, information, clean water, sanitation, good nutrition and laws governing public safety are all part of the infrastructure to which most income groups in developed economies have access. In developing economies this infrastructure may not exist, may be less well developed or only available to the better off.

The treatment gap is also larger in developing economies because the causes of epilepsy in many of those countries remain unaddressed potentially allowing the numbers of people to develop epilepsy to grow. Cystercercosis, malaria, brain injuries due to traffic accidents and work accidents and birth trauma all contribute to epilepsy in developing countries, whereas in Western economies epilepsy is associated with childhood conditions and then ageing and cerebrovascular disease. These differences are important to addressing the treatment gap in epilepsy.

If the treatment gap in epilepsy is viewed in the context that treatment gaps exist for all conditions and that these gaps are part of the broader context of social and health inequalities which vary from economy to economy then some of the means to address those treatment gaps become apparent.

There are lessons to be learned from the literature on social and health inequalities. Kolko's (2002) example from Vietnam where the wealthiest fifth of the population receives some 45% of public subsidies for health and education demonstrates that simply supplying anti-epileptic drugs to a poor nation will not necessarily help those in that nation who need it most. Given the way health is organised they will assist those who least need the assistance. As Kolko (2002) pointed out because the poorest three fifths of many countries receiving IMF assistance receive no benefit or their position has become worse this will be replicated across many developing countries. Using broad epidemiological data on poverty and income for a country or region or even a small locality to decide where to provide treatment is no guarantee that the treatment gap will be addressed since the better off in those regions are those most likely to access the treatment. This unequal access is of course the basis for why projects in treating HIV/AIDS don't reach those who most need them. It will be the basis for failure in projects to narrow the treatment gap in epilepsy. Similarly, while cheaper medications are of relevance for both HIV/AIDS and epilepsy these may never reach those whom they would most benefit because of the above inequalities which includes the massive inequalities in the distribution of health care professionals to deliver care.

To address the treatment gap in epilepsy particularly in developing economies requires that the broader inequalities underlying health inequalities be addressed (CSDH 2008; Marmot 2006). These in general require economic remedies that are guided by the political will of governments to ensure that economic remedies do not selectively favour the better off in a society (Marmot 2006).

Economic remedies go far beyond improving individuals incomes. The political will to improve people's lives must include that governments undertake the tasks that provide an infrastructure for health. This includes the restoration of the role of the state in ensuring clean water, effective sanitation and adequate supplies of nutrition (CSDH 2008). In some countries the state must assume or resume the supply and regulation of utilities such as water, gas and electricity and the supply of education and health services rather than leaving them to the market. Additionally, state regulations such as road and traffic laws, labour protection laws, protection of women and children from exploitation are also important. They have a role to play in prevention of epilepsy as well as other conditions. This expanded state role implies that many governments must abandon ideologies that promote neo-liberal policies.

Where individuals' or households' incomes are concerned in both developed and developing economies, the use of social transfers to protect health for those whose incomes are low or non-existent must be instituted. These social transfers will range from providing free education, ensuring job retention, providing social security and pensions to providing childcare services. While incomes can never be equal in capitalist economies social transfers provide services to ensure those with lowest incomes still have access to a quality of life that is protective of their health (CSDH 2008).

Health care systems are part of this overall structure. A universal health system is more likely to provide better health care to people in the lower income groups in all economies than is a privatised health system. In developing countries, the focus must be on primary health care to ensure that health issues are dealt with at the local level. Primary health care also includes a preventive and public health component. Primary health care should also be a cheaper means of dealing with health issues in a developing economy than relying on expensive specialist care. Investment in primary health care systems in developing countries may also prevent the loss of trained health professionals to developed economies. This has implications for the treatment gap in epilepsy where there are not enough health professionals to deliver health care at either primary or specialist levels in developing countries. To that extent, building and retaining a health workforce is an imperative.

In developing countries, the social status and health of women requires special attention. While women carry the burdens of family and often are the breadwinners their lives are the most precarious. Health and violence, poor working conditions and low status reduce their capacities to maintain families. Poorer women in developing economies have little control over their health and reproduction. Treatment gaps in epilepsy are particularly wide for women and girls as part of their lower status.

Finally, but controversially perhaps the treatment gap in epilepsy in developing countries would be better addressed by addressing HIV/AIDS first. In many developing countries the impact of HIV/AIDS on adult men and women of working age has so reduced the capacity of economies that there is no means to bring about improvements in the health of people with epilepsy. At the same time many people with epilepsy are going to have HIV/AIDS as well as other conditions related to poverty and lower education. By addressing the needs of people with HIV/AIDS some of those conditions that create epilepsy in developing economies will also be addressed. The elimination of HIV/AIDS in developing countries will be done through addressing health inequalities through education and better living conditions and these are the foundations for improving the care of epilepsy as well.

Developing economies require assistance to establish infrastructures such as these. At present there are large amounts of foreign aid available for immunisation programs, to address AIDS, Tuberculosis and Malaria. These programs present something of a problem to creating a sustainable infrastructure. As short term aid programs they may not allow developing countries to set their own agendas or to plan on national scales. Funding for specific health programs means that many health professionals will follow this funding into specialist areas rather than committing to the development of a national primary health care system.

The International Monetary Fund through its Poverty Reduction Strategy Process has the ability to take the initiative in these areas by addressing the social determinants of health in each developing country and assisting governments to establish the necessary infrastructures to alleviate both poverty and social and health inequalities (CSDH 2008).

The role for national and international epilepsy bodies as well as other organisations and individuals concerned about the quality of life would appear to be restricted by this approach. In fact it is not. It is a changed role, but the aims still remain the same: improving the quality of the lives of people with epilepsy throughout the world and ensuring they have access to affordable treatment that works.

By taking into account that each country has a complex national structure where its ideologies, policies and economy are interrelated projects to alleviate the suffering of people with epilepsy can be specifically targeted. By partnering with projects working on poverty and health inequalities to reduce the effects of poverty, the lives of people with epilepsy will be improved. In developing countries, this would include working with HIV/AIDS, tuberculosis and malaria programs as the causes of epilepsy in those countries has the same basis as those diseases.

There are specific tasks to be addressed. Far better data are required about the incidence and prevalence of epilepsy in all countries. Without better and consistent epidemiological data it is impossible to have full pictures of the problem in local areas and to have comparable data. This means that there are no real measures of the changes that projects can make since there is no means to evaluate these projects properly. Problems of consistent definitions of epilepsy and classifications of epilepsy are also bound up with the problem of data collection. Work is required in these areas in order to properly implement projects to assist poor people in developing countries. Another specific problem related to improving the lives of people with epilepsy relates to access to AEDs. This requires political action in much the same way as HIV/AIDS activists demanded the manufacture and distribution of affordable antiretrovirals. Activists must be prepared to confront international pharmaceutical companies as well as governments.

Above all, the role of those people wanting to improve the lives of people with epilepsy requires political engagement before clinical services. Governments of all persuasions require the political will as well as a basis of understanding, to address the bases of poverty and inequalities that create the treatment gap in epilepsy as well as treatment gaps in other diseases.

Marmot (2006) argues for empowerment of people as one of the best means of improving their health. When people have control over their lives, including their communities, their working lives and have access to education and health services their health will improve. To achieve this in many countries whether developed or developing requires political action by leaders in order to demonstrate the value of empowerment and social inclusion.

The consequences of allowing such poverty and health inequalities to continue is that economies must falter and individuals, families and their communities must continue to suffer. People with epilepsy are amongst those who suffer most.

CONCLUSION

The treatment gap in epilepsy is particularly evident in developing economies. This was shown by the survey undertaken in the Western Pacific Region where developing economies had the least services or health care personnel available to care for people with epilepsy. A treatment gap exists in all developed economies as well. The treatment gap in epilepsy is however part of broader social and health inequalities.

Without an understanding of the relationship between poverty and health inequalities small, short-term clinically oriented projects aimed at reducing treatment gaps, conducted in regions where people those people with epilepsy who are amongst the poor are likely to replicate the health inequalities in that region so that projects produce outcomes for the better off with epilepsy while the poor continue to receive fewer services.

In order to address the needs of people with epilepsy and to reduce treatment gaps which exist in most economies throughout the world social and political actions are required. Poor people, including poor people with epilepsy in developing and developed countries require a level of social protection that comes from social transfers so that the wealth and income inequalities they face are reduced. Access through social transfers to education, health services, employment, welfare rights lead to improvements in health for all. Access to these services also introduces a level of empowerment for individuals and their families.

In developing countries, many of the conditions that foster HIV/AIDS, tuberculosis and malaria also foster higher levels of epilepsy in the community. Partnerships with programs to reduce these diseases will also influence the incidence and prevalence of epilepsy. As well, HIV/AIDS has reduced developing economies abilities to address the most basic needs of their populations. One means to address epilepsy might include working to eliminate HIV/AIDS.

Finally, the treatment gap in epilepsy requires that leaders in improving the quality of life of people with epilepsy need to influence governments at all levels to reduce health inequalities and so reduce the treatment gap in epilepsy.

REFERENCES

Aspromourgos T. (2003) Is zero government debt desirable? Evatt Foundation, Australia. Accessed June 2005. http://evatt.labor.net.au/publications/papers/64.html

Booysen F, Geldenhuys JP and Marinko M (2003) The impact of HIV/AIDS on the South African economy: a review of current evidence. Paper given to TIPS/DPRU conference 'The Challenge of Growthand Poverty: The South African Economy Since Democracy. 8-10 September 2003.

Coburn D (2004) Beyond the income inequality hypothesis: class, neoliberalism and health inequalities. *Social Science and Medicine,* 58 (1), 41-56.

Commission on Social Determinants of Health (2008) *Closing the gap in a generation: health equity through action on the social determinants of health. Final report of the Commission on Social Determinants of Health,* Geneva world Health Organisation

Cruz ME (2005) Epilepsy: the treatment gap in developing countries. Presentation made at Forum 9, Mumbai, India September 2005. www.globalforumhealth.org/filesupld/forum9/CD%20Forum%209/papers/Cruz%20M.pdf-

Deaton A (2006) Global patterns of income and health: facts, interpretations, and policies. Wider Annual Lecture, Helsinki October 2006.

Doyal L (1979) The political economy of health. Pluto Press, London.

Furber A, Hodgson I, Desclaux A and Mukasa D Barriers to better care for people with AIDS in developing countries *BMJ* 2004, 329, 1281-1283 (27 November), doi:10.1136/bmj.329.7477.1281

Gerberding J (2004) Steps on the Critical Path: Arresting HIV/AIDS in Developing Countries. *PLoS Med* 1(1): e10 doi:10.1371/journal.pmed.0010010.

Kolko G (2002) Ravaging the poor: The International Monetary Fund indicted by its own data in Navarro V (ed) The Political Economy of Social Inequalities in Health 2002, Baywood Publishing Co New York, 173-180.

Levins R and Lopez C (2002 Towards and ecosocial view of health in Navarro V (ed) The Political Economy of Social Inequalities in Health 2002, Baywood Publishing Co New York, 429-460.

Marmot M (2006) Health in an unequal world *Lancet,* 368, 2081-94.

Meinardi H, Scott RA, Reis R, Sander JW (2001) The treatment gap in epilepsy: the current situation and ways forward, *Epilepsia,* 42 (1),142-153.

Mbuba CK, Ngugi AK, Newton RN andCarter JA (2008) The epilepsy treatment gap in developing countries: Asystematic review of the magnitude, causes, and intervention strategies. *Epilepsia,* 49 (9), 1491-1503.

Muntaner C and Lynch J (2002) Income inequality, social cohesion, and class relations in Navarro V (ed) The Political Economy of Social Inequalities in Health , 2002, Baywood Publishing Co New York, 325-346.

Navarro V (2002) Neoliberalism, "globalization", unemployment, inequalities and the welfare state in Navarro V (ed) The Political Economy of Social Inequalities, 2002, Baywood Publishing Co New York, 33-108.

Navarro V and Shi L (2002) The political context of social inequalities in health in Navarro V (ed) The Political Economy of Social Inequalities, 2002, Baywood Publishing Co New York, 403-418.

Public Health Information Development Unit (1999) A Social Health Atlas of Australia [Second Edition] - Volume 1: Australia http://www.publichealth.gov.au/publications/a-social-health-atlas-of-australia-%5bsecond-edition%5d---volume-1%3a-australia.html

Quiggan J. (1999) Globalisation, neoliberalism and inequality in Australia. The *Economic and Labour Relations Review* 1999; 10: 240-59. Accessed January 2005 www.uq.edu/economics/johnquiggan/JournalArticles99/GlobalisELRR99.html.

Rector R and Hederman R (2004) Two Americas: One rich, one poor? Understanding income inequality in the United States. *The Heritage Foundation Backgrounder #1791.* http://www.heritage.org/research/taxes/bg1791.cfm

Stilwell F (2008) Driving inequality: Frank Stilwell asks should we accept the prevailing political economic arrangements that generate inequality. *Arena Magazine*, Feb-March 2008.

Tonkiss F (2006) Capitalism and globalisation in Contemporary Economic Sociology: globalisation, production, inequality. Routledge , London, 3-28.

UN AIDS Organisation (2004) 2004 Report on the global AIDS epidemic. 4th Global Report http://www.unaids.org/bangkok2004/GAR2004.pdf.

World Health Organisation (1997) *Global Campaign Against Epilepsy; Out of the Shadows.* Geneva.

World Health Organisation (2001) *Epilepsy' Social consequences and economic aspects*, Fact Sheet, 166, Geneva.

World Health Organisation (2004a) *Epilepsy in the Western Pacific Region: Call to action, Regional Office for the Western Pacific*, Philippines.

World Health Organisation (2004b) E*pilepsy in the WHO Africa region, bridging the gap: the global campaign against epilepsy, 'out of shadows',* Netherlands

WHO (2008) *Global Burden of Disease 2004* Update, Geneva.

Wicks J. (2005) The reality of income inequality in Australia Social Policy Issues Paper 1. St Vincent de Paul Society, Australia. Accessed June 2005 www.vinnies.org.au/files/QLD. Microsoft_word_-_SPIP1_doc.pdf

In: Social Epileptology
Editors: J. Pinikahana and C. Walker
ISBN 978-1-60876-228-6

Chapter 5

EPILEPSY AND WOMEN'S HEALTH ISSUES

Line Sveberg Røste* and Erik Taubøll
Department of Neurology, Division of Clinical Neuroscience,
Rikshospitalet University Hospital,
0027 Oslo, Norway

ABSTRACT

Awareness of gender related issues in medicine are increasing both among patients and physicians. For women with epilepsy in particular, topics related to gender specific stages throughout life need special attention.

These topics include epilepsy itself; the treatment of the epilepsy or other medical or psychosocial factors and have to be discussed. Sexual problems seem to be more frequent and fertility may be reduced. Cosmetic issues related to skin, hair or weight may cause signifcant worries not only in puberty. The use of antiepileptic drugs may interact with contraceptives leading to unplanned pregnancies and contraceptives may affect serum levels of antiepileptic drugs and precipitate seizures. Women with epilepsy are generally more reluctant to become pregnant. They need both reassurance and special care since most women with epilepsy experience normal pregnancies and deliveries, but there is a higher risk of birth defects among their children. The menopausal transition has received less attention, since the emphasis both clinically and scientifically has been on the child bearing years. There is, however, special attention required for menopausal women with epilepsy related to bone health and also to the relationship between menopause and seizures.

INTRODUCTION

A specific relationship between epilepsy and the female organs was already recognised in the times of Hippocrates around 400 BC [1], when the cause of seizures in women was thought to be due to migration of the uterus. Nowadays, female biology continues to be of

* Correspondence: Division of Clinical Neuroscience, Rikshospitalet University Hospital. 0027 Oslo, Norway. Tel: +4723073580; Fax: +4723073891. email: line.sveberg.roste@rikshospitalet.no

specific focus regarding epileptic seizures and their treatment, but it is recognised that other gender-related issues of psychosocial nature are also of importance.

Overall, women have a slightly lower incidence of epilepsy than men, and this has been attributed to higher exposure of men to risk factors for post-traumatic epilepsy and acute symptomatic seizures. Most data supporting this hypothesis are relatively old, and the lives led by the women of today may even out these epidemiological and risk exposure differences; nevertheless, differences in the ways that modern men and women live may still have an impact on their lives with epilepsy. Certain epilepsy syndromes however, are also more common in women than in men, and our knowledge supporting the differences between genders in the expression of some of the epilepsy syndromes is increasing.

The natural biological phases in life through which a woman passes need particular attention for a woman with epilepsy, and also for the therapists taking care of her. This is not only related to maternity issues, such as pregnancy and delivery, but also to puberty, menstruation, contraception, sexuality, and menopause, as well as the sex-specific effects of anti-epileptic drugs (AEDs).

A prospective epidemiological study from Iceland during 1995-1999 found no difference in the incidence of unprovoked seizures by sex [2], whereas retrospective and descriptive studies from 1935-84, 1964-1978, and 1993 showed a higher incidence of epilepsy in males [3,4]. Although these data may indicate that modern behavioural trends are of importance for epilepsy in women, inter-study comparisons are difficult due to differences in methodology.

Idiopathic generalised epilepsy (IGE) is more common in women than men, and there is also a trend towards cryptogenic localization-related epilepsies being more frequent in women [5, 6]. The female predominance of IGE was found to peak between the ages of 15 and 50 years, and this pattern, starting around puberty and then declining after menopause, suggests that sex hormones may be responsible for the difference in sex distribution. Two generalised epilepsy syndromes which begin at puberty, juvenile absence epilepsy and juvenile myoclonic epilepsy, are also more common in girls than boys.

In focal epilepsy, isolated auras and lateralised EEG seizure patterns occur more frequently in females more often than males, whereas men experience secondary generalised tonic-clonic seizures more frequently [7]. Sexual auras in particular have been shown to be more frequent in women with epilepsy [8].

Psychiatric disorders occur more often in people with epilepsy than in the general population, and anxiety has been recognized as the most common psychiatric comorbidity with epilepsy, particularly in women [9, 10, 11]. Women with epilepsy are also at increased risk of specific mood disorders, such as postnatal depression.

Life quality parameters for women with epilepsy differ from those in men, particularly with respect to factors related to independence. It has been noted that men with epilepsy are more likely to be employed or to possess a driver's licence than women with epilepsy [12].

Puberty and Menstruation

Navigating through the turbulent years of adolescence is a challenge for teenagers, both biologically and psychosocially. It is an epoch in life where standing out from the crowd is particularly difficult, independence is developing, and obtaining a driver's licence becomes important, where alcohol and late nights are introduced, hormones are changing, and sexuality is being explored. For a young woman with epilepsy all these areas may harbour specific challenges.

Some epilepsy syndromes, such as juvenile myoclonic epilepsy, are typically diagnosed in adolescents, [13] and are often precipitated by typical teenage activities such as sleep deprivation and excessive alcohol.

The onset of puberty is induced by changes in sexual hormones, which may be of importance for girls with epilepsy. The rise in follicle-stimulating hormone (FSH) and luteinizing hormone (LH) levels is followed by a gradual increase in oestrogen. Progesterone is produced by the onset of menarche, and the secretion of sex steroid hormones subsequently follows a cyclical pattern. Oestrogen is known to lower seizure threshold, thus increasing seizure susceptibility, whereas progesterone has the opposite effect [14]. The marked rise in oestrogen prior to ovulation might be of importance for changes in the seizure pattern of girls with epilepsy, as well as the debut of epilepsy in others.

From the opposite perspective, epileptic activity itself may affect the sex hormone balance. Regular LH pulsation is essential for induction of ovulation and thus also for menstruation. Epileptic activity has been shown to affect endocrine function at the hypothalamic level, including altering LH pulsatility [15].

A relationship between the onset of epilepsy and menarche has been reported to occur in between 20-30 % of all female patients with epilepsy [16]. However an increased incidence of epilepsy around puberty was not confirmed in the population-based Rochester study [4], but a study by Svalheim and co-workers [17] found an increase in epilepsy onset in adolescents as compared with children, although this increase was not directly related to menarche.

Menstrual disturbances are more often encountered in women with epilepsy. Irregular menstruation, anovulatory cycles and a greater likelihood of polycystic ovaries are the most frequent manifestations [15, 18, 19, 20]. The reasons for these disturbances are multifactoral. Firstly, the epilepsy itself may affect the hormonal balance; interictal epileptiform discharges in the temporal lobes, in particular, may affect the cyclic activity in the hypothalamus, and subsequently the pituitary, thereby disturbing the LH-pulsatility pattern. This, in turn, may result in anovulatory and irregular menstrual cycles [21]. Secondly, AEDs may disrupt this balance by affecting endocrine function (see below). Thirdly, psychosocial factors may indirectly cause menstrual problems.

GENDER -SPECIFIC SIDE-EFFECTS OF ANTI-EPILEPTIC DRUGS (AEDS)

Possible side effects of AEDs on the endocrine system have recently caused concern. Enzyme-inducing drugs, in particular phenytoin (PHT), phenobarbital (PHB) and carbamazepine (CBZ), may reduce the free fraction of the steroid hormones, primarily by increasing sex hormone binding globuline (SHBG) [20]. Use of valproate (VPA) has been associated with menstrual disturbances, hyperandrogenism and polycystic ovaries [22, 23]. The effect seems to be drug-specific, independent of the epileptic activity, as these findings have also been noted in women treated with VPA for bipolar depression [24,25,26], as well as in animal studies [27- 29]. Increased androgen levels are also found in prepubertal girls being treated with VPA for epilepsy [30, 31]. The valproate-induced endocrine effects seem, at least in part, to be reversible [32, 33]. The relative importance of epilepsy versus AEDs, especially VPA, for particular symptoms remains a topic of controversy [34-36]. Thus, until further research has been undertaken, the consequences of treatment of younger women with AEDs, in particular VPA, cannot be readily predicted. VPA is a widely-used drug and recognized as being very efficacious: for treatment of primary generalised epilepsies in particular, VPA may not be easily replaced. In younger women of fertile age, particularly if they are obese, have irregular menstruation, or have endocrine disturbances, a follow-up plan should be instituted for women on VPA, or those who are about to start VPA treatment. This includes endocrinological screening, ultrasound of the ovaries, height and weight measurements, and checking for fertility problems and menstrual disturbances.

With the exception of lamotrigine (LTG), newer AEDs have only rarely been investigated for endocrine effects. LTG does not seem to have any biologically relevant endocrine effects [27, 32, 37]. A few recent reports from animal studies may indicate a possible effect of levetiracetam (LEV) on endocrine function in females [38], but clinical studies are necessary to confirm this.

Cosmetic side-effects of AEDs are an issue for both men and women with epilepsy, and have a potentially significant impact on gender-related interactions [39]. Obesity is particularly associated with use of VPA, but can also be associated with CBZ and gabapentin use. It should be emphasised that obesity is more than a cosmetic problem, as it can evolve into a metabolic syndrome with major negative health effects [40]. Conversely, considerable weight-loss has been observed in association with use of topiramate and felbamate.

Regarding other cosmetic side-effects, VPA may cause hair-loss, whereas PHT may induce hirsutism. Acne, coarse facial structure, and gingival hyperplasia are also physical changes that have been reported after the use of PHT. As cosmetic problems may have a significant impact on a woman's medication compliance, they must be treated as important problems, and not dismissed as trivial difficulties.With the multitude of AEDs available, side-effects which the patient considers intolerable should be avoided when possible by choosing an alternative drug.

Catamenial Epilepsy

The cyclical nature of epilepsy related to the menstrual cycle was observed long ago by the ancient Greek physicians. Many women experience seizure clustering related to specific phases of the menstrual cycle, known as menstrual-related or catamenial epilepsy, for summary, see Herzog et al 08 [39]. Herzog and co-workers have described three different patterns of catamenial epilepsy. The most common variant is an increase in seizures immediately before, and in the beginning of, the menstrual cycle. A second pattern is a clustering of seizures at ovulation. The third variant is the occurrence of seizures throughout the follicular phase, and occurs primarily in women with anovulatory cycles. In the most frequent definition, the seizure count should be at least doubled in relation to menstruation or ovulation. Use of this definition has indicated that more than a third of women with epilepsy have catamenial epilepsy.

Cyclical fluctuations in oestrogen and progesterone concentrations during the menstrual cycle are thought to be the main inductors of catamenial epilepsy [15, 40, 41]: oestrogen concentrations increase prior to ovulation and menstruation, whereas progesterone levels are very low or decreasing. Other factors may also contribute to the establishment of this cyclical pattern. Alterations in the fluid balance may induce fluctuations in the serum concentrations of AEDs, and emotional changes related to pre-menstrual tension may also contribute. However, the lack of consistent definition in all studies means that many studies are difficult to interpret.

Several strategies have been used in the treatment of catamenial seizures, and with varying degrees of success. One strategy is altering the fluid and electrolyte balance by using diuretics or acetazolamide. It is not known whether this alteration is the actual mechanism of therapeutic effect, or whether it is due to its effect on pH or as a primary AED. Another theraputic approach is using cyclical alterations in the dose of the current AEDs, or adding benzodiazepines before menstruation. This strategy requires a cooperative and compliant patient, since the doses may need to be adjusted several times during a menstrual cycle. Finally, different hormonal treatment strategies can be used, and neuroactive steroid treatment is under development. To date, however, there has been no large, controlled, blinded trial of any of these treatment options [39].

CONTRACEPTION

Contraception counselling is very important in the follow-up of fertile women with epilepsy, because of the increased risk of pregnancy, and because of the interactions between AEDs and hormonal contraception. Although various studies have demonstrated associations between AEDs, reproductive risks, and contraception, women with epilepsy rarely consult for preconception planning or during the first week of pregnancy [42]. In a recent study from a US epilepsy clinic, 70% of the women were unaware that their prescribed AED might alter the efficacy of their oral contraception (OCP). They were also poorly informed about potential teratogenic effects and the consequences of unplanned pregnancy during AED use [43].

Studies from different countries have also shown that health care providers globally lack knowledge regarding reproductive risks and contraceptive interactions with AEDs [44-46]. Although awareness is increasing [47, 48], a high frequency of unplanned pregnancies has been shown in studies of women with epilepsy. Some AEDs accelerate the metabolic breakdown of hormones in contraceptives, due to enzyme induction in the liver. This is particularly applicable to the OCPs most frequently used at present, in which the oestrogen component is low. The concentration of oestrogen may fall below the level of anti-conceptional effect, and breakthrough bleeding is a sign of this. If this occurs, a change of medication to a contraceptive with higher oestrogen content is recommended. PHT, CBZ and PB are the AEDs most commonly associated with contraceptive failure, and it has been also noted with felbamate and high doses of topiramate and oxcarbazepine [49-52]. Higher oestrogen content (50μg oestrogen instead of 30μg) is recommended for women using enzyme-inducing drugs. LTG has not been found to affect oestrogen levels, but a decrease in levonorgestrel has recently been found [53]. The clinical importance of this finding has yet to be established.

As well as AEDs having an effect on the efficacy of OCPs, the effects of OCPs on AEDs must also be considered. Oral contraceptives have been found to reduce LTG plasma levels by up to 50% [54], so that women controlling their epilepsy with this AED become more susceptible to seizures. We would recommend that women taking this drug should have their serum concentrations of LTG measured 2 weeks after the initiation/cessation of OCP. Since the therapeutic range of LTG is not well established, an individual assessment of therapeutic range should be done in advance. Gestagens, however, do not seem to affect the metabolism of LTG [55]. As oestrogen and gestagens affect the excitability of the brain in different ways, it has been questioned whether seizure frequency alters due to use of hormonal contraception. Case studies have been published in which contraceptive pills have been found to affect seizure frequency in different ways, but most studies demonstrate seizure reduction. The effect of hormonal contraception on seizures is considered insignificant and is not part of the general counselling of patients.

Quarterly injections of depot medroxyprogesterone acetate (DMPA) represent an approach to birth control of greater convenience than oral contraception for many women. In addition, there are some indications that DMPA in doses that induce amenorrhea may reduce seizure frequency, particularly in women with catamenial epilepsy [55]. It is well known that this method of contraception often results in irregular bleedings, spot-bleeding, and a tendency for amenorrhea when the treatment is terminated, and that this applies to all women, not only those with epilepsy. Decreased bone mineral density has been associated with long-term use of DMPA, and this, although usually reversible, may be of significance for some women.

A frequently asked question regards the use of a gestagen-releasing intrauterine device (IUD) for contraception. The hormone-metabolising effect of AEDs also affects gestagens, but the changes on systemic hormonal levels are considered minimal. There is presently no reason to believe that a hormonal IUD should affect seizure frequency, but clinical experience is limited. Theoretically any effect should be beneficial, with a possible reduction of seizures in women with epilepsy, and therefore gestagen-releasing IUDs are generally considered a good contraceptive option for women with epilepsy [56].

An intravaginal ring that releases low-dose oestrogen (15μg estradiol/day) has recently been introduced. To date, no studies of women with epilepsy using this contraceptive have been published, but as the hormonal levels are very low the possibility of contraceptive failure in women using enzyme-inducing drugs cannot be excluded, and therefore we do not presently recommend the use of the intravaginal ring in these women. This also applies to the use of the contraceptive patch.

Contraceptive implants could be an attractive alternative for women with epilepsy, but use of subdermal levonorgesterl patches and single-rod etonogestrel implant have both induced contraceptive failures in women using enzyme-inducing AEDs [57, 58].

The emergency contraceptive pills releases a single high dose of gestagen and interaction with AEDs is therefore thought to be of minor importance. However UK guidelines from National Institute of Health and Clinical Excellence (NICE) recommend that the dose of levonorgestrel be increased to two doses of 1.5 mg and 0.75 mg taken 12 hours apart (advice for women taking enzymeinducing antiepileptic drugs) [59].

Pregnancy and Delivery

Epilepsy is one of the most common neurological diseases in fertile women. Although the majority of women with epilepsy have uncomplicated pregnancies and give birth to healthy children, various specific problems may occur. The subject of epilepsy and pregnancy has been discussed in national and international review articles, as well as consensus reports and books [59-62]. A summary of the practical advice derived from this literature, and based on our own experiences, is provided in the following table.

Before Pregnancy

- Is continued AED treatment necessary?
- Reduce the number and dosage of AEDs as much as possible without losing seizure control.
- Aim at an anticonvulsant with best effect for the particular epilepsy type.
- If possible, avoid use of VPA.
- Cautiousness in the use of new anticonvulsants without documentation in pregnancy.
- Give 0.4 mg folic acid to all. Prescribe 4-5 mg of folic acid/day to women using VPA or CBZ, and to women who previously have given birth to children with neural tube defects/have neural tube defects themselves, or have close relatives with such defects. The folic acid treatment should ideally start one month before pregnancy or as soon as pregnancy is recognised. If the highest dose is required (4-5 mg/day), the dose should be maintained throughout the first trimester after which the dose may be reduced to 0.4 mg/day.

In Pregnancy

- Consultations with the neurologist about once/trimester. This should, however, be individually evaluated.
- Serum concentration measurements every trimester. Additional monitoring in women using LTG and oxcarbazepine, after seizure occurrence and side-effects. Side-effects occurring in women using highly protein-bound AEDs (PHT, CBZ, PB, VPA) should be evaluated by free fraction measurements. Ultrasound investigations around 12th and 17th week of pregnancy.
- Use of VPA or CBZ: discuss the option of amniocentesis around week 15 (ultrasound and close clinical follow-up usually sufficient).
- Close observation of the growth of the foetus, especially in the third trimester.
- Vitamin-K, 10 mg/day during the last 4 weeks of pregnancy, in particular women using enzyme inducing AEDs.

At Delivery

- Do not forget to take AEDs at the same time as usual, also during the delivery.
- Avoid prolonged deliveries.
- Avoid hyperventilation.
- Show caution in the use of morphine, if necessary epidural anaesthesia is recommended.
- 1 mg vitamin-K to the child after birth.

After Birth

- Serum concentration measurements after 2-4 weeks, earlier when the dose is changed and in women using LTG and oxcarbazepine.
- Post partum consultation by neurologist after 6-8 weeks.
- Encourage breastfeeding.
- Ensure sufficient rest and sleep for the mother.
- Discuss safety issues concerning carrying, feeding etc. Nappy changing should be on the floor. Advice must be individualised.
- Home visit, possibly by epilepsy nurse if close follow-up is necessary.

Fertility

Fertility is reduced in women with epilepsy [63, 64], the reasons for which are multifactoral. Probably the main reason is the psychosocial aspects of living with epilepsy, but women with epilepsy may also have an increased frequency of anovulatory cycles, irregular menstrual cycles, and polycystic ovaries as previously described. Furthermore, epileptic discharges have been shown to affect the hypothalamus/hypophyseal function causing anovulation. The medication for epilepsy may theoretically also affect fertility, but there are no clinical data documenting the effects of specific AEDs on fertility. It is important to remember that epilepsy is a heterogeneous condition, and that the underlying structural cerebral changes may affect fertility via both organic and psychosocial mechanisms.

Preconceptional Counselling

Women with epilepsy should be offered preconceptional counselling, ideally in a co-ordinated consultation with both their neurologist and gynaecologist. At this consultation general information on epilepsy and pregnancy should be provided, and a plan, as suggested in above, should be discussed.

Effects of Epilepsy on Pregnancy

More than 90% of women with epilepsy have normal pregnancies, and the risk of major complications during pregnancy and delivery is small. Nevertheless, in women with epilepsy, vaginal bleedings in pregnancy occur more frequently, and several studies have found increased frequencies of hyperemesis gravidarum and pre-eclampsia in women with epilepsy [65, 66]. However, in recent years, the rate of pregnancy complications in women with epilepsy has been approaching those in the general population [67]. Premature birth and slightly reduced birth weight have also been described for women with epilepsy in some studies, but there is no significant difference in the frequency of spontaneous abortions.

Simple partial seizures are probably of no significance for the foetus, whereas it is less clear whether complex partial seizures or absence seizures have negative consequences. Generalised seizures will also rarely affect the foetus, but severe seizures in the first trimester may affect organogenesis and have teratogenic effects. The effects of seizures are difficult to differentiate from the effects of AEDs, as women with more severe epilepsy are often exposed to polytherapy and higher AED concentrations. However convulsive status epilepticus is regarded as dangerous both for foetus and mother [65]. Nevertheless, there is a lack of large prospective studies, and in the EURAP study, only one in 36 cases of status epilepticus ended in stillbirth, and none was associated with maternal death [67]. In general it has been considered that women with epilepsy who have uncontrolled seizures during pregnancy have increased morbidity in comparison with controls.

TERATOGENICITY

In any pregnancy, there is a 1-2 % risk of the child being born with malformations. However, the use of AEDs in pregnancy is associated with major congenital malformations (MCM) and may cause cognitive defects in children born to women with epilepsy. The precise risk has been difficult to estimate, and it is hoped that the prospective approach of the pregnancy registers willl shed more light on this important issue.

Currently it is established that VPA, both as monotherapy and as part of polytherapy, is associated with a higher risk of MCM, which seems to be dose dependent (Adab N et al 2004). Whether other AEDs pose a significant risk has not been definitely established; the risk for MCM during VPA treatment has been estimated to be 6.2 % whilst the risk for MCM in an untreated women with epilepsy (3.5 %), has been reported to be similar to that found if treated with other AEDs (CBZ, 2.2 %; LTG, 3.2%; PHT 3.7%). (Harden CL 08, Thomson T 08). Furthermore, VPA exposure *in utero* is associated with a risk of lower verbal intelligence in children. Results from ongoing long-term studies on neurodevelopmental effects of AEDs should provide further important information. In general, polytherapy is associated with a higher risk than monotherapy, both for MCM and other adverse cognitive outcomes (see Harden CL 2008 for further details). Identifying the AED with the optimum combination of high seizure protection and low teratogenicity is of obvious importance, and results from the pregnacy registers are anticipated to provide a valuable contribution to this quest.

Effects of Pregnancy on Epilepsy

The majority of women with epilepsy experience no changes in their seizure frequency upon becoming pregnant. Nevertheless, many of these women may experience a worsening in their seizures, while others may have fewer seizures [61]. The results from the prospective international pregnancy registers are expected to shed more light on this issue. Amongst a cohort of almost 2000 women in the EURAP study, 17.3 % had an increase in seizures during pregnancy, and 15.9 % a decrease. Increased occurrence of seizures was associated with localization-related epilepsy and polytherapy, and for tonic clonic seizures, with oxcarbazepine monotherapy [68]. It is also important to establish whether the seizures truly are epileptic, and not conditions that mimic epilepsy such as syncope and non-epileptic seizures.

A considerable problem seen in several pregnant women with epilepsy is sleep difficulty, and this may in itself precipitate seizures. Medication compliance is an important aspect to consider in pregnant women with epilepsy, as concerns about adverse effects on the foetus from the AEDs may prompt women to stop or reduce their AEDs without medical consultation.

Follow-up in Pregnancy

During pregnancy, major changes occur in the pharmacokinetics of AEDs [69]. Almost every physiological aspect that may influence drug-metabolism is altered in pregnancy from the non-pregnant situation. Gastrointestinal motility is altered, plasma volume is increased, total amount of body fluid is higher, and there are changes in liver function and in protein binding. These factors result in the total serum concentrations of most AEDs decreasing, gradually returning to normal after delivery.

The treatment of the pregnant woman with epilepsy should therefore be individually-tailored to the particular patient, with emphasis on the clinical situation and side-effects, rather than on serum concentration measurements (see, however, information on LTG and oxcarbazepine below). If there is a major change in the serum concentrations of the AED in use (i.e. more than 50% reduction), dose adjustments may be considered. For AEDs with high protein binding, such as PHT and VPA, it is important that free concentrations are measured before the dose is adjusted. Among the newer AEDs, the metabolism of LTG and oxcarbazepine appears to change significantly during pregnancy, and serum concentrations should be measured more frequently (i.e monthly/bimonthly) in patients using these drugs [70-72]. Pennell and coworkers have recently shown that the risk for seizure worsening occurred when the serum LTG concentration fell to less than 65 % of the target concentration (this should ideally be determined for each individual before pregnancy) [73]. Recent studies of LEV have also found a significant decline in serum concentrations of this AED during the last trimester [74, 75] indicating that awareness for seizure-breakthrough and measument of AED concentrations is also important for pregnant women using LEV.

Some women are afraid of using medication in pregnancy, and may reduce the dose without medical consultation. Thus, if an increase in seizures occurs, it is important to determine whether the medication is being taken as prescribed. If the dosage is increased during pregnancy, it is important to remember to reduce it post delivery. For LTG and oxcarbazepine, and probably also LEV, this should be done within 1-2 weeks post-partum, and serum concentrations should be monitored.

Prenatal Diagnostics

Prenatal diagnostics are important for women with epilepsy. In our clinic, all women with epilepsy are invited for an initial ultrasound at week 12, with follow-up in week 17-18, with particular focus on the possibility of congenital malformations, such as neural tube defects, cerebral malformations, and heart defects. Amniocentesis is discussed with women using VPA or CBZ, as well as women using newer AEDs for which knowledge is sparse. As ultrasound techniques have improved, an indication for amniocentesis in our clinic is now very infrequent.

Vitamin Supplementation

In the general population, low levels of folic acid in pregnant women are associated with a higher risk of neural tube defects in the unborn child. Several AEDs may result in reduced folic acid concentrations. In addition, a higher frequency of neural tube defects has been reported in babies whose mothers were taking VPA, and probably also CBZ, during pregnancy. It has therefore been recommended that all pregnant women using AEDs should have folic acid supplementation [76], particularly those women using VPA or CBZ, or who previously have had children with neural tube defects, who have neural tube defects themselves, or who have close relatives with neural tube defects. However, a recently published prospective study from the UK Epilepsy and Pregnancy Register did not find that per-conceptional folic acid supplementation had any effect, suggesting that the increased risk of MCM in this group occurs through mechanisms other than that of folic acid metabolism [77].

Coagulation disturbances are thought to be more frequently seen in children of women using enzyme-inducing AEDs, and also in the mothers themselves. Vitamin K supplementation (10 mg vitamin K /day) during the last month of the pregnancy has therefore been recommended. However different studies have provided conflicting results [78] and UK guidelines no longer recommend vitamin K supplementation in the last month of pregnancy. However 1 mg vitamin K should be administered to the baby immediately after birth.

In all pregnancies, the use of tobacco, alcohol, and illict drugs poses an increased risk of foetal malfomations, and women with epilepsy should be particularly aware of avoidable factors that may add to the risk of harming both themselves and their unborn child.

Delivery

Pregnancy in women with epilepsy is considered to be a risk, and women with epilepsy are found to be more anxious during pregnancy than women in the general population. Turner and coworkers recently found that although women with epilepsy experienced a significantly higher rate of fear of childbirth during pregnancy than healthy controls, following delivery the experiences and feelings about childbirth of women with epilepsy are very similar to those of women without epilepsy. In particular, women with epilepsy were more scared of the possibility of offspring malformations than of labour pain when compared with healthy controls [79]. Appropriate counseling is therefore necessary.

Complications are rarely seen during delivery in women with epilepsy. In the EURAP study, the risk of seizures during delivery was reported to be 3.5 % and occurred most commonly in women who had experienced seizures during pregnancy [67]. However, many women with epilepsy are anxious, and dread having seizures at delivery; for these patients counselling and planning of the delivery are of utmost importance.

It is also important that during the delivery, and afterwards, care is taken to ensure that AED intake is at a time as close as possible to their usual intake time. AEDs are often unavailable at the maternity ward, and the women should be encouraged to bring their own AEDs when they report to the maternity department for delivery. During delivery, exhaustion should be avoided if possible, and hyperventilation should be prevented. Decisions regarding use of epidural anaesthetics should be made after the usual obstetric considerations. In general, epilepsy is no indication for Caesarean section. Epileptic seizures at delivery should be handled as seizures in general. If treatment is necessary, benzodiazepines, including midazolam, are the first choice, administered rectally, by buccal administration, or intravenously. Seizures caused by pre-eclampsia may be a differential diagnosis. The patient's medical history must be studied, particularly with respect to blood pressure and proteins in the urine. Treatment of eclamptic seizures with magnesium sulphate is not known to be a risk to women with epilepsy. Women with epilepsy have been found to be at higher risk of post partum depression [80]. It is important to be aware of this, so that women at risk can be identified and treated as soon as possible.

Genetics and Epilepsy

Many parents with epilepsy are worried that their children will inherit their condition. The likelihood of this will mainly depend on the type of epilepsy. If one of the parents has partial epilepsy after a head trauma, it is obvious that the probability for inheritance is minimal. However, if a parent has generalised epilepsy, and several family members are affected, the risk of the child also having epilepsy will be greater. In general, it is estimated that when the mother is affected, the probability of the child having epilepsy is 4-5 %, and when the father has epilepsy, the probability of the child having epilepsy is approximately 2 % [81, 82]. The prevalence of epilepsy in the general population is about 0.7 %. Consequently for the majority of children of patients with epilepsy, the risk of inheritance is minor. Overall, generalised epilepsies are more frequently inherited than partial epilepsies. However, some specific epilepsy syndromes have considerably higher risks, necessitating individual counselling. (For a review, see Scheffer and Berkovic [3].

Breastfeeding

In general, all women should be encouraged to breastfeed, whether they have epilepsy or not, and irrespective of the AED that they use. However, AEDs may accumulate in the child, particularly after the use of barbiturates, such as PB and mysoline, as well as benzodiazepines. In these instances, the child may become drowsy, and withdrawal symptoms may be observed. Occasionally, some of these children may need short-term withdrawal therapy with barbiturates.

Our knowledge of newer drugs is limited, and therefore a generally cautious approach should be applied. Two of the newer AEDs which are being increasingly used, LTG and gabapentin, have been found to be transferred to the child in breastmilk, and may accumulate in the child in up to therapeutic concentrations. However data acquired to date have not demonstrated any harmful effects on the child [71, 84]. LEV has also been shown to transfer extensively from mother to foetus, and also into breastmilk, but serum concentrations in the breast-fed infants were minimal [85].

Sexual Function

Most women with epilepsy have a normal sex life [86]. However, a higher frequency of sexual problems has been reported in women with epilepsy than in the general population [87]. Problems with reductions in both libidio and arousal are most frequently reported. Morrell and co-workers have also demonstrated a higher frequency of dyspareuni, vaginism, and difficulties reaching orgasm [88] in women with epilepsy. From clinical experience, it has been noted that many women do not reach orgasm for fear of precipitating a seizure.

The aetiology for these sexual problems is multifactoral; psychological, social, cultural, neurophysiological, neuroendocrine, and drug-related factors might all contribute. One study from Egypt found sexual dysfunction in only 14 % of the women studied [89], in a Danish study, 29 % [90], and studies from USA, 36-50 % [91-93]. The difference in these figures emphasises the potential importance of psychosocial and cultural factors, as well as the need for proper controls in such investigations.

The epilepsy itself may affect sexual activity by activating cerebral regions of importance for sexual function and hormonal production. It has, for instance, been shown that patients with localization-related epilepsy have a higher frequency of sexual problems than patients with primary generalised epilepsy [92, 93]. Sexual ictal manifestations have also been found to predominate in women with temporal lobe epilepsy, suggesting sexual dimorphism in the human brain [8].

The extent to which AEDs affect sexual function has been investigated in several studies, but it is difficult to draw definitive conclusions [87]. Whilst it is known that some drugs affect hormonal levels by enzyme induction and changes in SHBG concentrations, there is no definitive evidence that these drugs have a significant effect on sexual function. When sexual problems do occur, they tend to appear at the onset of the epilepsy. This is no different when chemotherapy is not being used, and, additionally, is apparently not correlated to the number of AEDs in use. It is our personal impression that sexual problems improve when the seizures are under control, even if this has necessitated using higher doses of AEDs.

The sparse literature that exists from outpatient clinics on patients with epilepsy living in stable relationships indicates that this group of patients have no more sexual problems than control groups [90, 94]. Additionally, it is important to emphasise to both the patients and their partners that seizures related to sexual activity are very rare. Nevertheless, some women may require psychological and sexual counselling.

When women with epilepsy report sexual problems, they should be carefully and sympathetically questioned, and relevant gynaecological, endocrinological, and neurological examinations should be performed, before an epilepsy-related cause can be concluded.

Menopause

The research on women with epilepsy has mainly been directed towards women in their fertile years, and relatively little is known about the relationships between menopause and epilepsy. There are indications that epilepsy may affect the time of the menopause, as some studies have shown that women with epilepsy may reach menopause at an earlier age than women in the general population [95]. The effects of menopause on epilepsy are thought to be related to changes in levels of oestrogen and progesterone [96]. Few studies have been published, but the main findings in those available, are that seizure frequency seems to be higher in perimenopause than after established menopause [96-100]. However the studies are small and the conclusions uncertain. Reduced seizure rates in association with menopause are probably more probable if the seizure pattern has been catamenial, epilepsy debut was at a relatively older age, and seizures were well-regulated. Poor seizure control before menopause is probably a bad prognostic factor.

Oestrogen substitution (hormone replacement treatment, HRT) seems to have a variable effect on seizure frequency. One retrospective questionnaire showed that after hormone substitution the epilepsy of as many as 63% of respondents had worsened, while only 12 % of those without oestrogen substitution experienced the same [96]. In a smaller study [100], Abbasi and co-workers could not verify worsening of seizures after HRT. However a study by Harden and coworkers [101], also reported seizure exacerbation after HRT. It has been suggested that substitution with a combination of oestrogen and progesterone would overcome these problems [102], but this has presently not been confirmed by larger studies. As our knowledge in this field is currently limited, initiation of hormonal treatment must be carefully discussed between doctor and patient. A combination drug, together with detailed information of possible negative and positive effects, and subsequent evaluations of outcome and seizure frequency, may be the best available option at present.

Osteoporosis

Several AEDs are associated with disorders of bone metabolism, including osteoporosis, hypocalcemia, hypophosphatemia, reduced serum concentrations of vitamin D metabolites, secondary hyperparathyreoidism, and increase in markers of bone turnover [102]. Although these effects have been observed in both males and females, it is of particular importance for postmenopausal women with epilepsy who are especially at risk of developing osteoporosis and fractures because of their low estrogen levels [103-5]. Traditionally, these features have been attributed to AEDs that induce the cytochrome P450 enzyme (CBZ, PB, and PHT). However, other studies indicate that VPA, which is a cytochrome P450 inhibitor, could also affect bone metabolism [106]. Thus, the mechanisms by which AEDs affect bone health are not presently established.

An additional risk factor for bone fractures in menopausal women with epilepsy is the increased risk of trauma due to seizures and AED-induced dizziness and ataxia. A particular awareness of risk factors for osteoporosis should therefore be implemented in the treatment of women with epilepsy. Although no definitive guidelines exist, it has been recommended that bone density measurement (DXA) should be conducted 5 years after initiation of AEDs, and before treatment in postmenopausal women [107]. Women with epilepsy in particular should be given advice regarding life-style choices such as exercise, smoking, and alcohol consumption. Women using enzyme-inducing drugs should take calcium and vitamin D daily, and the use of biphosphonates should be evaluated if osteophenia/osteophorosis is found.

Conclusion

Women with epilepsy have a number of gender-specific problems related to the epilepsy itself, to the treatment of their disease, and also to the psychosocial consequences of their disease. Many of these problems may be solved, or at least diminished, by increased knowledge among healthcare workers and the patients, and better understanding and awareness of the relevant issues can relieve many of the specific problems. The goal for women with epilepsy, as for patients with epilepsy in general, is a treatment tailored to the specific needs of the individual.

References

[1] Betts T, Dutton N, Yarrow H. Epilepsy and the ovary (cutting out the hysteria). *Seizure* 2001: 10: 220-228.

[2] Olafsson E, Ludvigsson P, Gudmundsson G et al . Incidence of unprovoked seizures and epilepsy in Iceland and assessment of the epilepsy syndrome classification: a prospective study. *Lancet Neurology* 2005; 4: 627-34.

[3] Granieri E, Rosati G, Tola R, et al. A descriptive study of epilepsy in the district of Copparo, Italy, 1964-1978. *Epilepsia* 1983; 24: 502-14.

[4] Hauser WA, Annegers JF, Rocca WA. Descriptive epidemiology of epilepsy: Contrinutions of population -based studies from Rochester, Minnesota. *Mayo Clinic Proceedings* 1996; 71: 576-586.

[5] Christensen J, Kjeldsen MJ, Andersen H et al. Gender differences in epilepsy. *Epilepsia* 2005; 46. 956-960.

[6] Mullins GM, O´Sullivan SS, Neligan A, McCarthy A et al. A study of idiopathic generalised epilepsy in an Irish population. *Seizure* 2007; 16: 204-210.

[7] Janszky J, Schulz R, Janszky I et al. Medial temporal lobe epilepsy: gender differences. *Journal of Neurology, Neurosurgery and Psychiatry* 2004; 75: 773-775.

[8] Rémillard GM, Andermann F, Testa GF et al. Sexual ictal manifestations predominate in women with temporal lobe epilepsy: A finding suggesting sexual dimorphism in the human brain. *Neurology* 1983; 33: 323-30.
[9] Jacoby A, Baker GA, Steen N et al. The clinical course of epilepsy and its psychosocial correlates. Findings from a U.K. Community study. *Epilepsia* 1996; 37: 148-161.
[10] Beyenburg S, Mitchell AJ, Schmidt D et al. Anxiety in women with epilepsy: systematic review and suggestions for management. *Epilepsy and Behaviour* 2005; 2: 161-171.
[11] Mensah SA, Beavis JM, Thapar AK et al. A community study of the presence of anxiety disorders in people with epilepsy. *Epilepsy and Behaviour* 2007; 11: 118-24.
[12] Sillanpaa M and Shinnar S. Obtaining a driver's license and seizure relapse in patients with childhood-onset epilepsy. *Neurology* 2005; 64: 680-686.
[13] Wheless JW and Kim HL. Adolescent seizures and epilepsy syndromes. *Epilepsia* 2002; Suppl 3: 33-52.
[14] Stitt SL, Kinnard WJ. The effect of certain progestins and estrogens on the threshold of electrically induced seizure patterns. *Neurology* 1968; 18: 213-216.
[15] Herzog AG and Friedman MN. Menstrual cyclus interval and ovulation in women with localization-related epilepsy. *Neurology* 2001: 57: 2133-2135.
[16] Klein P, van Passel-Clark L, Pezzullo JC. Onset of epilepsy at the time of menarche. *Neurology* 2003; 60: 495-497.
[17] Svalheim S, Taubøll E, Bjørnenak T, Røste LS, Mørland T, Sætre ER, Gjerstad ER. Onset of epilepsy and menarche - is there any relationship? *Seizure* 2006; 15:571-575.
[18] Herzog AG, Seibel MM, Schomer DL, Veitukaitis JL, Geschwind N. Reproductive endocrine disorders in women with partial seizures of temporal lobe origin. *Arch. Neurol.* 1986; 43: 341-346.
[19] Herzog AG, Coleman AE, Jacobs AR et al. Interictal EEG discharges, reproductive hormones, and menstrual disorders in epilepsy. *Ann. Neurol.* 2003; 54: 625-537.
[20] Perucca E, Hedges A, Makki KA et al. A comparative study of the relative enzyme inducing properties of antiepileptic drugs in epileptic patients. *Br. J. Clin. Pharmacol.* 1984; 18: 401-410.
[21] Herzog AG. Is there a lateral assymmetry in the respons of the brain to hormones in epilepsy? *Epilepsy and Behaviour* 2007; 11: 157-9.
[22] Isojärvi JIT, Laatikainen TJ, Pakarinen AJ, Juntunen KTS, Myllylä VV. Polycystic ovaries and hyperandrogenism in women taking valproate for epilepsy. *N. Engl. J. Med.* 1993; 329: 1383-1388.
[23] Isojärvi JIT, Taubøll E, Pakarinen AJ, Van Parys J, Rättyä J, Flinstad Harbo H, et al. Altered ovarian function and cardiovascular risks in valproate treated women. *American Journal of Medicine,* 2001; 111:290-296.
[24] O'Donovan C, Kusumakar V, Graves G, Bird D. Menstrual abnormalities and polycystic ovary syndrome in women taking valproate for bipolar mood disorder. *J. Clin. Psychiatry* 2002; 64: 322-330.
[25] McIntyre RS, Mancini DA, McCann S, Srinivasan J, Kennedy SH. Valproate, bipolar disorder and polycystic ovarian syndrome. *Bipolar Disorders*; 5: 28-36.
[26] Joffe H, Cohen LS, Suppes T et al. Longitudinal follow-up of reproductive and metabolic features of valproate-associated polycystic ovarian syndrome features: a preliminary report. *Biological Psychiatry* 2006; 60: 1378-1381.

[27] Røste LS, Taubøll E, Berner A, Isojärvi JIT, Gjerstad L. Valproate, but not lamotrigine, induced ovarian morphological changes in Wistar rats. Exp *Toxicol. Patho*l 2001; 52; 545-552.

[28] Røste LS, Taubøll E, Isojärvi JIT, Pakarinen AJ, Huhtaniemi I, Gjerstad L. Effects of chronic valproate treatment on reproductive endocrine function in female and male Wistar rats. *Reprod. Toxicol.* 2002; 16; 767-773.

[29] Taubøll E, Gregoraszczuk EL, Kolodziej A, Kajta M, Ropstad E. Valproate inhibits conversion of testosterone to estradiol and acts as an apoptotic agent in growing porcine ovarian follicular cells.*Epilepsia* 2003; 44:1014-1021.

[30] Rättyä J, Vainonpää L, Knip M, Lanning P, Isojärvi JIT. The effects of valproate, carbamazepine, and oxcarbazepine on growth and sexual maturation in girls with epilepsy. *Pediatrics* 1999; 103: 588-593.

[31] Vainionpää LK, Rättyä J, Knip M, Tapanainen JS, Pakarinen AJ, Lanning P, et al. Valproate-induced hyperandrogenism during pubertal maturation in girls with epilepsy. *Ann. Neurol.* 1999; 45: 444-450.

[32] Isojärvi JIT, Rättyä J, Myllylä VV, Knip M, Koivunen R, Pakarinen AJ, et al. Valproate, lamotrigine, and insulin-mediated risks in women with epilepsy. *Ann. Neurol.* 1998; 43: 446-451.

[33] Lossius MI. Tauboll E. Mowinckel P et al. Reversible effects of antiepileptic drugs on reproductive endocrine function in men and women with epilepsy-a prospective randomized double-blind withdrawal study. *Epilepsia* 2007; 48:1875-82.

[34] Isojärvi JIT, Taubøll E, Tapanainen JS, Pakarinen AJ., Laatikainen TJ, Knip M, Myllylä VV. On the association between valproate and polycystic ovary syndrome: A response and an alternative view. *Epilepsia* 2001; 42:305-10.

[35] Genton P, Bauer J, Duncan S, Taylor AE, Balen AH, Eberle A, Pedersen B, Salas-Puig X, Sauer, MV. On the association between valproate and polycystic ovary syndrome. *Epilepsia* 2001; 42:295-304.

[36] Herzog AG, Schachter SC. Valproate and the polycystic ovarian syndrome: Final thoughts. *Epilepsia* 2001; 42: 311-15.

[37] Betts T, Yarrow H, Dutton N, Greenhill L, Rolfe T. A study of anticonvulsant medication on ovarian function in a group of women with epilepsy who have only ever taken one anticonvulsant compared with a group of women without epilepsy. *Seizure*, 2003 (S7); 12: 323-329.

[38] Svalheim S, Taubøll E, Surdova K, Ormel L, Dahl E, Aleksandersen M, McNeilly A, Gjerstad L, Ropstad E. Long term levetiracetam treatment affects reproductive endocrine function in female Wistar rats. *Seizure*. 2008;17:203-9.

[39] Herzog AG. Catamenial epilepsy: definition, prevalence, pathophysiology and treatment. *Seizure* 2008; 17:151-159.

[40] Logothesis J, Harner R, Morrell F et al. The role of estrogens in catamenial exacerbation of epilepsy. *Neurology* 1959; 9: 352-360.

[41] Herzog AG. Hormones and epilepsy. *Acta Neurol. Scand.* 2000; 102 (suppl 175): 29-31.

[42] Seale C, Morrell MJ, Nelson L et al. Analysis of prenatal and gestaional care given to women with epilepsy. *Neurology* 1998; 51: 1039-1045.

[43] Davis AR, Pack AM, Camus A Yoon A, Kritzer J, Patient knowledge of teratogenicity and contraceptive interactions of antiepileptic drugs. *Obstet. Gynecol.* 2007; 109, 60S.

[44] Russell A, Macpherson H, Cairnie V et al. The care of pregnant women with epilepsy- A survey of obstetricians in Scotland. *Seizure* 1996; 5: 271-277.

[45] Krauss GL, Brandt J, Campbell M et al. Antiepileptic medication and oral contraceptive interactions: A national survey of neurologists and obstetricians. *Neurology* 1996; 46: 1534-1539.

[46] Shorvon SD, Tallis RC and Wallace HK. Antiepileptic drugs: Coprescription of proconvulsant drugs and oral contraceptives: A national study of antiepileptic drug prescribing practice. *J. Neurol. Neurosurg Psychiatry* 2002; 72: 114-115.

[47] Foy R, Penney G and Greer I. The impact of national clinical guidelines on obstetricians in Scotland. *Health Bull.* 2001; 59: 364-372.

[48] Morrell M, Sarto GE, Shafer PO et al. Health issues for women with epilepsy: A descriptive survey to assess knowledge and awareness among healthcare providers. *J. Womens Health Gend. Based Med.* 2000; 9: 959-965.

[49] Crawford P, Chadwick DJ, Martin C et al. The interaction of phenytoin and carbaamzepine with combined contraceptive steroids. *British journal of clinical pharmacology* 1990; 30: 892-896.

[50] Saano V, Glue P, Banfeld CR et al. Effects of felbamate on the pharmacokinetics of a low-dose combination oral contraceptive. *Clinical Pharmacological therapy* 1995; 58: 523-531.

[51] Doose DR, Wang S-S, Padmanabhan M et al. Effect of topiramate or carbamazepine on the pharmacokinetics of an oral contraceptive containing norethindrone and ethinyl estradiol in healthy obese and non-obese female subjects. *Epilepsia* 2003; 44: 540-549.

[52] Fattore C, Cipolla G, Gatti G et al. Induction of ethinyl estradiol and levonorgestrel metabolism by oxcarbazepine in healthy women. *Epilepsia* 1999; 40: 783-787.

[53] Sidhu J, Job S, Singh S et al. The pharmacodynamic consequences of the co-administration of lamotrigine and a combined oral contraceptive in healthy female subjects. *British Journal of Clinical Pharmacology* 2005; 62: 191-199.

[54] Sabers A, Öhman I, Christensen J, Tomson T. Oral contraceptives reduce lamotrigine plasma levels. *Neurology* 2003; 61: 570-571.

[55] Reimers A, Helde G, Brodtkorb E. Ethinylestyradiol, but not gestagens reduces lamotrigine serum concentrations. *Epilepsia* 2005; 46: 1414-1417.

[56] Bounds W and Guillebaud J. Observational series on women using the contraceptive Mirena concurrently with anti-epileptic and other enzyme-inducing drugs. *J. Fam. Plann. Reprod Health Care*. 2002; 28: 78-80.

[57] Harrison-Woolrych M and Hill R. Unintended pregnancies with the etonogestrel implant (Implanon): A case series from postmarketing experience in Australia. *Contraception* 2005; 71: 306-308.

[58] Shane-McWhorter L, Cerveny JD, MacFarlane LL et al: Enhanced metabolism of levonogestrel during phenobarbital treatment and resultant pregnancy. *Pharmacotherapy* 1998; 18: 1360-1364.

[59] National Institute for Health and Clinical Excellence (NICE) 2004. *The diagnosis and management of epilepsy in adults and children in primary and secondary care.*

[60] Roste LS, Henriksen T, Gjerstad L, Husby H, Taubøll E et al. Retningslinjer for behandling av kvinner med epilepsi. *Konsensusrapport* 2006 http://www.legeforeningen.no/asset/33810/1/33810_1.pdf.

[61] International League Against Epilepsy. Guidelines for the care of women of childbearing age with epilepsy. Commission on genetics, pregnancy, and the child. *Epilepsia* 1993;34:588-589.

[62] Tettenborn B. Management of epilepsy in women of childbearing age. *CNS Drugs* 2006; 20: 373-387.

[63] Webber MP, Hauser WA, Ottman R, Annegers JF. Fertility in persons with epilepsy: 1935- 1974. *Epilepsia* 1986; 27: 746-752.

[64] Artama M, Isojärvi JIT, Raitanen J, Auvinen A. Birth rate among patients with epilepsy: A nationwide population-based cohort study in Finland. *Am. J. of Epidemiol* 2004; 159: 1057-1063.

[65] Teramo K, Hiilesmaa VK. Pregnancy and fetal complications in epileptic pregnancies. In: Janz D, Dam M, Bossi L et al eds. *Epilepsy, pregnancy, and the child.* New York: Raven Press, 1982; 53-59.

[66] Yerby MS, Leppik I. Epilepsy and the outcome of pregnancy. *J. Epilepsy* 1990; 3: 193-199.

[67] The EURAP Study Group. Seizure control and treatment in pregnancy: observations from the EURAP Epilepsy Pregnancy Registry. *Neurology* 2006; 66: 354-60.

[68] Harden CL. Antiepileptic drug teratogenesis: what are the risks for congenital malfomations and adverse cognitive outcomes? *International review of neurobiology* 2008; 83: 205-213.

[69] Pennell PB and Hovinga CA . Antiepileptic drug therapy in pregnancy I. Gestation-induced effects on AED pharmacokinetics. *Int. Rev. Neurobiol* 2008; 83: 227-240.

[70] Tran TA, Leppik IE, Blesi K, Sathanandan ST, Remmel R. Lamotrigine clearance during pregnancy. *Neurology* 2002; 59: 251-255.

[71] Ohman I, Vitols S, Tomson T. Lamotrigine in pregnancy: pharmacokinetics during delivery , in the neonate, and during lactation. *Epilepsia* 2000; 41: 709-713.

[72] Mazzucchelli I, Onat FY, Ozkara C et al. Changes in disposition of oxcarbazepine and its metabolites during pregnancy and puerperium. *Epilepsia* 2006; 47: 504-509.

[73] Pennell PB, peng L, Newport DJ et al. Lamotrigine in pregnancy, clearence, therapeutic drug monitoring, and seizure frequency. *Neurology* 2008; 70: 2130-6.

[74] Tomson T, palm R, Källen K et al. Pharmacokinetics of levetiracetam during pregnancy, delivery, the neonatal period and lacation. *Epilepsia* 2007; 48: 1111-6.

[75] Westin AA, Reimers A, Helde G et al. Serum concentration/dose ratio of levetiracetam before, during and after pregnancy. *Seizure* 2008; 17: 192-8.

[76] Morrell MJ. Folic acid and epilepsy. *Epilepsy Currents* 2002; 2: 31-34.

[77] Morrow JI, Hunt SJ, Russell et al. Folic acid use and major congenital malformations in offspring of women with epilepsy. A prospective study from the UK Epilepsy and Pregnancy Register. *J. Neurol. Neurosurg*. Psychiatry published online 31 Oct 2008;

[78] Kaaja E, Kaaja R, Matila R et al. Enzyme-inductive aeds in pregnancy and the risk of bleeding in the neonate. *Neurology* 2002; 58: 549-553.

[79] Turner K, Piazzini A, Franza A et al. Do women with epilepsy have more fear of childbirth during pregnancy compared with women without epilepsy? A case-control study. *Birth* 2008; 35: 147-152.

[80] Turner K, Piazzini A, Franza A et al. Postpartum depression in women with epilepsy versus women without epilepsy. *Epilepsy and Behavior* 2006; 293-297.

[81] Tsuboi T, Endo S. Incidence of seizures and EEG abnormalities among offspring of epileptic patients. *Hum. Genet.* 1977; 36: 173-189.
[82] Ottman R, Annegers JF, Hauser WA, Kurland LT. Higher risk of seizures in offspring of mothers than of fathers with epilepsy. *Am. J. Hum. Genet* 1988; 43: 257-264.
[83] Scheffe IE and Berkovic SF. The genetics of human epilepsy. *Trends in Pharmacol Sci* 2003; 428-433.
[84] Ohman I, Vitols S, Tomson T. Pharmacokinetics of gabapentin during delivery, in the neonatal period, and lactation: does a fetal accumulation occur during pregnancy? *Epilepsia* 2005; 46: 1621-1624.
[85] Johannesen SI, Helde G, Brodtkorb E. Levetiracetam concentrations in serum and in breast milk at birth and during lactation. *Epilepsia* 2005; 46: 775 -777.
[86] Lambert MV. Seizures, hormones and sexuality. *Seizure* 2001; 10: 319-340.
[87] Harden CL. Sexual dysfunction in women with epilepsy. *Seizure* 2008; 17: 131-135.
[88] Morrell MJ. Sexuality in epilepsy. I: Engel J, Pedley T red. *A Comprehensive textbook of Epilepsy*. Philadelphia: Lippincott-Raven, 1997: 2021-2026.
[89] Demerdash A, Shaalan M, Midani A, Kamel F, Bahri M. Sexual behavior of sample of females with epilepsy. *Epilepsia* 1991; 32: 82-85.
[90] Jensen P, Jensen SB, Sorensen PS et al. Sexual dysfunction in male and female patients with epilepsy: a study of 86 outpatients. *Arch. Sex Behav* 1990; 19: 1-14.
[91] Morrell MJ, Guldner G. Self reported sexual function and sexual arousability in women with epilepsy. *Epilepsia* 1996; 37: 1204-1210.
[92] Blumer D, Walker AE. Sexual behavior in temporal lobe epilepsy. *Arch. Neurol.* 1967; 16: 37-43.
[93] Taylor DC. Sexual behavior and temporal lobe epilepsy. *Arch Neurol* 1969; 21: 510-516.
[94] Duncan S, Blacklaw J, Beastall GH, Brodie MJ. Sexual function in women with epilepsy. *Epilepsia* 1997; 38: 1974-1981.
[95] Klein P, Serje A, Pezzullo JC. Premature ovarian failure in women with epilepsy. *Epilepsia* 2001; 42: 1584-1589.
[96] Harden CL, Nikolov BG, Koppel BS, et al. Seizure frequency and age of menopause in women with epilepsy. *Epilepsia* 2001; 42 (suppl 7): 291.
[97] Lee MA. Epilepsy in the menopause. *Neurology* 1999; 53 (suppl 1): 41.
[98] Harden CL, Pulver MC, Ravdin L, Jacobs AR. The effect of menopause and perimenopause on the course of epilepsy. *Epilepsia* 1997; 38 (suppl 8): 133-134.
[99] Harden CL, Pulver MC, Ravdin L, Jacobs AR. The effect of menopause and perimenopause on the course of epilepsy. *Epilepsia* 1999; 40:1402-1407.
[100] Abbasi F, Krumholz A, Kittner SJ, Langenberg P. Effects of menopause on seizures in women with epilepsy. *Epilepsia* 1999; 40: 205-210.
[101] Harden CL, Herzog AG, Nikolov BG et al. Hormone replacement therapy in women with epilepsy: A randomized double-blind, placebo-controlled study. *Epilepsia* 2006; 47: 1447-1451.
[102] Pack AM, Morrell MJ. Adverse effects of antiepileptic drugs on bone structure: epidemiology, mechanisms and therapeutic implications. *CNS Drugs* 2001; 15: 633-642.
[103] Stephen LS, McLellan AR, Harrison JH. Bone density and antiepileptic drugs: a case-controlled study. *Seizure* 1998; 339-342.

[104] Cummings SR, Nevitt MC, Genant HK et al. Risk factors for hip fracture in white women. Study of osteoporotic fractures research group. *New England Journal of Medicine* 1995; 332: 767-773.
[105] Ensrud KE, Walczak TS, Blackwell T et al. Antiepileptic drugs use increases rates of bone loss in older women: a prospective study. *Neurology* 2004: 62: 2051-2057.
[106] Kumandas S, Koklu E, Gumus H, Koklu S, Kurtoglu S, Karakukcu M, Keskin M. Effect of carbamazepine and valproic acid on bone mineral density, IGF-I and IGFBP-3. *J Pediatr Endocrinol Metab* 2006; 19: 529-534.
[107] Pack AM, Morrell M. Epilepsy and bone health in adults. *Epilepsy and Behaviour* 2004; S24-S29.

In: Social Epileptology
Editors: J. Pinikahana and C. Walker

ISBN 978-1-60876-228-6

Chapter 6

INJURIES IN EPILEPSY

Rita Nguyen and José F. Téllez Zenteno*
Division of Neurology, Department of Medicine,
University of Saskatchewan, Saskatoon, Canada

ABSTRACT

Currently, there is intense clinical research into various aspects of the medical risks relating to epilepsy, including total and cause-specific mortality, accidents and injuries in patients with epilepsy and mortality related with seizures. Seizures occurring in precarious situations and resulting in injuries are still an important concern for patients with epilepsy, their employers and their caregivers. Submersion injuries, motor vehicle accidents, burns, and head injuries are among the most feared epilepsy-related injuries. These concerns seem valid because the hallmark of epilepsy, episodic impairment of consciousness and motor control, may occur during interictal EEG epileptiform discharges, even in the absence of a clinical seizure. In addition, psychomotor comorbidity and side effects of antiepileptic drugs may contribute to the risk of injuries in patients with epilepsy. Published risk factors for injuries include the number of antiepileptic drugs, history of generalized seizures, and seizure frequency. In general, epidemiological information about incidence of injuries has been conflicting and sparse. In general, studies focusing on populations with more severe forms of epilepsy tend to report substantially higher risks of injuries than those involving less selected populations. On the other hand, studies based in non selected populations of people with epilepsy have not shown an increase frequency of injuries in people with epilepsy compared with the general population. Some studies have shown that patients with epilepsy are more frequently admitted to the hospital following an injury. Possible explanations include are more cautious attitudes of clinicians toward injuries occurring in the setting of seizures; hospitalization required because of seizures and not related to the injuries themselves; and hospitalization driven by other issues, such as comorbidities, which are highly prevalent in patients with epilepsy. Potentially the high rate of hospitalizations could be related to the severity of the injury. This chapter reviews the best available

* Correspondence: Dr. José Francisco Téllez-Zenteno. Division of Neurology. Department of Medicine. Royal University Hospital 103 Hospital Drive. Box 26, Room 1622. Saskatoon SK S7N OW8 Canada. Tel (306)9668011. Fax: (306)9668008. E mail: jft084@mail.usask.ca

epidemiological information about injuries, including incidence and risk factors. Also this chapter reviews information about specific type of injuries such as fractures, burns, concussions, dislocations, etc. Information about accidents in people with epilepsy is also discussed.

INTRODUCTION

Epilepsy is a clinical phenomenon diagnosed by the occurrence of two or more unprovoked seizures. It is estimated that approximately 0.5-2% of the population suffers from a seizure disorder (Zwimpfer, et al. 1997). People with epilepsy (PWE) are at increased risk for seizure-related injury, and it is reported that PWE also have higher incidences of home, street, and work accidents, even without a seizure (van den Broek, et al. 2004). These may be due to interictal EEG epileptiform discharges occurring in the absence of obvious clinical seizure activity (Aldenkamp and Arends. 2004, Tellez-Zenteno, et al. 2008). PWE are more likely to die as a result of an accident than non-epileptic patients, and a person with epilepsy has a 5% chance per annum of visiting an emergency department due to a seizure-related injury (Buck, et al. 1997, Spitz. 1998).

Fortunately, the majority of seizure-related injuries are nonfatal, with the most common injuries being burns, fractures, soft-tissue injuries, and submersion accidents. Risk factors for injuries associated with epilepsy include seizure frequency, type of seizure, and associated use of anti-epileptic drugs. PWE oftentimes also suffer from other comorbid conditions such as a learning disability, somatic and psychiatric comorbidity that puts them at an increased risk for accidental injury. Because of the increased risk of injury, PWE are subject to employment, recreational, and driving restrictions. These limitations have personal and social consequences, leading to inactivity, isolation, and dependency.

Although it is widely known that PWE are at increased risk for accidental injury as compared to the general population, there are conflicting reports in the literature and some of them have shown a similar risk of injuries. The contradictory results are due to a number of factors, including the population type in the study, the definition of epilepsy used in the study, accuracy of injury reporting, study design, and length of observation period.

This chapter reviews the best available epidemiological information about injuries, including epidemiological information such as incidence and risk factors, along with information about specific types of injuries such as fractures, burns, concussions, and dislocations.

EPIDEMIOLOGY OF SEIZURE-RELATED INJURIES

The literature provides conflicting data regarding the risk of accidental injury in PWE, with most studies overestimating the risk of injuries. The variation in data results from differences in the study population, with population-based samples providing a more accurate picture than referral patients, who oftentimes suffer from more severe disease. Conflicting results can also be due in part to differences in defining the disease (idiopathic, cryptogenic, or symptomatic), the accuracy of injury reporting (types of injury, circumstances, severity), the study design (retrospective versus prospective) and the length of the observation period.

Selection bias is the most important explanation for inconsistent results, as patients with symptomatic epilepsy and frequent seizures have a higher prevalence of accidents and injuries than those with milder symptoms (Beghi. 2005).

The largest study assessing the risk of accidents in PWE was performed by Beghi et. Al (Beghi, et al. 2002). The study involved 951 referral patients with idiopathic, cryptogenic, or remote symptomatic epilepsy, followed for 17, 484 person-months along with matched controls (relatives or friends). The majority of patients (55%) suffered from partial epilepsy, and 37% suffered from generalized epilepsy. 83% of subjects experienced a seizure within the last two years and in the majority of cases, seizure frequency was less than one per month. 270 accidents were reported by 199 epileptic patients, and 149 accidents by controls. The commonest injuries both in subjects with epilepsy and control subjects were contusions and wounds, followed by abrasions and fractures. PWE experienced a higher percentage of wounds, abrasions, and head concussions than controls, and this difference was significant. 24% of the accidents were seizure-related. Among the epileptic group, the relative risk (RR) of experiencing one accident was 1.2 (CI_{95}: 1.0-1.3), and the relative risk of experiencing two accidents was 1.4 (CI_{95}: 1.2-1.6). The cumulative probability of accidents in cases with epilepsy was 17% and 27% by 12 and 24 months, compared to 12% and 17% in controls ($p<0.0001$). The cumulative risk of accidents decreases significantly (14% and 22%) when seizure-related events are excluded. However, PWE were still found to have a higher rate of accidents than controls. The authors concluded that most epileptic patients suffer from trivial injuries, and although they do experience a higher incidence of injuries, the increased risk is modest, and is decreased significantly when seizure-related incidences are controlled for. Patients with epilepsy who are appropriately managed are not at any significantly higher risk of accidents than the general population.

In a recently published, retrospective, population-based study of 247 persons with epilepsy, conducted by Lawn et al (Lawn, et al. 2004), patients were followed for 2714 person-years. The majority of patients suffered from partial seizures, followed by generalized seizures. In the follow-up period, 16% of patients experienced at least one seizure-related injury. The majority of injuries were mild head injuries. 66% of the injuries were single injuries, and 34% were multiple injuries (limb contusions with mild head injury). 8% of injuries required hospital admissions. The cumulative risk of injury was 5.4% at one year (CI_{95}: 2.5-8.2), 12.7% at 5 years (CI_{95}: 8.0-17.0), 14.6% at 10 years (CI_{95}: 9.5-19.3) and 26.1% at 20 years (CI_{95}: 15.6-35.3). The authors of this study also concluded that the risk of seizure-related injury in persons with epilepsy is small, and most injuries are minor and do not carry any adverse social or occupational consequences.

The most recent population-based study on the prevalence of injuries in persons with epilepsy is a Canadian study presented by Tellez-Zenteno et al (Tellez-Zenteno, et al. 2008). The study analyzes the prevalence of injuries among people with self-reported epilepsy, with the data obtained by the Canadian Community Health Survey, a door-to-door, cross-sectional survey that collects data pertaining to health status, use of health resources, and determinants of health of the Canadian population. The weighted prevalence of epilepsy was determined to be 5.6 per 1000 (CI_{95}: 5-7). The relative risk of injuries causing limitation of normal activities was higher in persons with epilepsy; however, the difference from the general population was not significant. The most common injuries in both the general population and persons with epilepsy are orthopedic injuries (broken/fractured bones, dislocations, sprain/strain), followed by superficial injuries (cuts, scrapes, burns), and lastly concussions/internal injury.

PWE experienced a higher frequency of burns, scaldings, or poisonings than the general population; however, the sample sizes were too small to make any accurate analysis. There was no difference in rates of orthopedic injuries and superficial injuries between PWE and the general population. PWE have a higher frequency of falls than the general population; however, this difference was not statistically significant. PWE were also found to be admitted to the hospital three times more frequently than the general population following an injury. From the results of the population-based survey, the authors concluded that the prevalence of injuries overall and of most specific injuries did not differ between persons with epilepsy and the general population. The most significant difference between PWE and the general population was the higher rate of hospital admission following an injury in persons with epilepsy.

Thus, from the data found in the largest study on epilepsy and injuries (Beghi, et al. 2002, van den Broek, et al. 2004), and the two most recent population-based reports (Lawn, et al. 2004, Tellez-Zenteno, et al. 2008), it can be concluded that although the risk of injuries in PWE is higher than that of the general population, the difference is not extraordinary, and the majority of injuries are minor and do not cause significant disability or limitation from normal activities.

Fractures

One of the most common injuries persons with epilepsy suffer from is fractures. This may be due to the inability to activate protective reflexes during a seizure, resulting in falls and subsequent fracture. Seizures also cause an increased load on the skeleton due to muscle contractions during convulsions, leading to crush fractures of the spine or fractures of the humerus (Aboukasm and Smith. 1997, Kristiansen and Christensen. 1984). Some anti-epileptic drugs are also known to decrease bone mass density, which plays a role in increasing the fracture risk among epileptics. PWE are most likely to sustain a fracture within the first one to two years after diagnosis (Persson, et al. 2002).

In a recent meta-analysis of the literature on fracture risk in epilepsy, it was found that PWE are approximately twice as likely to sustain a fracture than normal controls (Vestergaard. 2005). Increase in hip fracture ranged from 2.3 – 12.1, with a pooled estimate relative risk of 5.25 ($p < 0.01$). The risk of forearm fractures ranged from 1.6 – 3.2, with a pooled estimate relative risk of 2.53 ($p < 0.02$). PWE were also at increased risk for spine fractures, with the relative risk ranging from 2.36-6.2, and a pooled estimate risk of 6.16 ($p<0.49$). These results agree with the population-based retrospective study of Souverein et al (Souverein, et al. 2005). This study reviewed 40, 000 patients with epilepsy, who were followed for a median of 3 years. It was determined that the risk of fractures among PWE was twofold higher compared with the general population patients not having epilepsy. PWE were at increased for all types of fractures. PWE were at highest risk for sustaining a hip fracture, with a relative risk of 2.79 (CI_{95}: 2.41-3.24).

These results conflict with some population based studies such as the studies of Beghi and Cornaggia (Beghi, et al. 2002) and Tellez-Zenteno et al (Tellez-Zenteno, et al. 2008), who found no significant difference in the risk of fractures among PWE and the general population. The explanations for discrepancy in results are many and have been aforementioned.

Risk factors for fracture injury among epileptics include recent diagnosis of epilepsy, age 45 years or older, male sex, occurrence of generalized seizures, AED polypharmacy, and institutionalization status (Nei and Bagla. 2007, Persson, et al. 2002, Vestergaard. 2005). The risk of fractures is highest in the first one to two years after diagnosis (Annegers, et al. 1989, Persson, et al. 2002, Vestergaard, et al. 1999). This may be due to the fact that risk of seizures in epilepsy declines over time (Cockerell, et al. 1995), and patients over the years learn to take precautions to avoid injury.

Anti-epileptic drugs increase fracture risk as they reduce bone mineral density by increasing vitamin D catabolism and decreasing calcium absorption through induction of liver enzymes (Vestergaard. 2005). AEDs that induce the cytochrome p450 system include phenobarbital, phenytoin, primidone, and carbamezepine. The evidence available for the use of non-inducing AEDs (i.e., lamotrigine, valproic acid) to reduce AED-related risk is conflicting (Sheth, et al. 1995, Stephen, et al. 1999).

DISLOCATIONS

Posterior shoulder dislocations are frequently described in textbooks as being associated with seizure events. During a seizure, the shoulder is in a position of adduction, internal rotation, and flexion. In this position, the humeral head is drawn cranially and posteriorly against the glenoid fossa by contraction of the shoulder muscles. The infraspinatus, teres minor, deltoid, latissimus dorsi, and teres major provide the force necessary to dislocate the humerus posteriorly. In the post-ictal period, the humerus is located behind the glenoid fossa, often with a large impression fracture of the head medial to the minor tubercle near the anatomical neck of the humerus (reversed Hill-Sachs lesion). If the seizure continues, the anatomical neck of the humerus is pulled towards the rim of the glenoid fossa, becomes impacted, and can eventually be fractured (Gosens, et al. 2000, Shaw. 1971).

Posterior shoulder dislocations are a rare occurrence, comprising 1.5-4.3% of all shoulder dislocations (Gosens, et al. 2000). Bilateral posterior shoulder dislocations are even rarer, and some authors have even suggested that such a presentation is pathognomonic of a convulsive disorder (Buhler and Gerber. 2002, Shaw. 1971, Silbergeld, et al. 1991). Although seizure disorders are commonly linked with posterior shoulder dislocations, anterior dislocations have also been reported. In one study of 26 patients with shoulder dislocations caused by an epileptic seizure, the frequency of anterior and posterior shoulder dislocations was equal (Buhler and Gerber. 2002). The same study also found that the dislocations in this group of patients were associated with a high number of Hill-Sachs lesions.

The suspicion of posterior shoulder dislocation should arise in PWE who presents with pain or stiffness of the shoulder after a seizure. The arm will be in a position of adduction and internal rotation, and the patient will not be able to abduct and externally rotate the arm. The diagnosis of posterior shoulder dislocation is often missed, but axillary x-ray or CT scan should aid in diagnosis. Surgical treatment is required for shoulder dislocations to obtain clinical stability, and anterior shoulder dislocations are noted to be more difficult to treat (Buhler and Gerber. 2002). Medical stabilization of epilepsy and compliance with medications will reduce the frequency of seizures and therefore help prevent shoulder dislocations in persons with epilepsy.

Thus, posterior shoulder dislocations are a rare event; however, one should be aware of their association with seizure disorders. Other dislocations that can occur in PWE include dislocations of the hip and dislocations of the temporomandibular joint (Gosens, et al. 2000).

MOTOR VEHICLE ACCIDENTS

Driving is a concerning issue among PWE and their physicians, as unprovoked seizures while driving undoubtedly puts the patient and the public at risk for accidents and injuries. Legislation regarding licensing PWE varies from country to country and state to state. In the United States, patients are required to be seizure-free for 3-12 months before driving (Krauss, et al. 2001, Sheth, et al. 2004), whereas the United Kingdom requires a one-year seizure free interval before granting or renewing a driving license, although most require a two year period (Beghi and Sander. 2005). In six American states, five Canadian provinces and several other countries, mandatory reporting is also required of physicians (Bird. 2005, McLachlan, et al. 2007)

In a retrospective analysis over two years of death certificates from the National Center for Health Statistics, Sheth et al. (Sheth, et al. 2004) compared annual totals and disease-specific risk for fatal crashes associated with seizures and other medical conditions. 0.2% of motor vehicle accidents in the United States between 1995-1997 were related to seizures. The rate for fatal seizure-related crashes among PWE was 8.6/100, 000. Fatal crashes in the general population were 2.6 times greater than for those with epilepsy. People with associated alcohol abuse had a fatal crash rate 8 times greater than patients with epilepsy. However, the relative risk for fatal crashes for patients with seizures is 2.3 times higher than for those with cardiovascular or hypertensive disease, and 4.6 higher than for patients with diabetes. Thus, although the rate of fatal motor vehicle accidents in PWE is low, having a seizure disorder increases the likelihood that a person will have an accident while driving. This agrees with other reports in the literature, which have found that road accidents due to epilepsy are few in number and there is only a moderate risk of driving accidents in PWE (Hansotia and Broste. 1991, Taylor, et al. 1996, van den Broek, et al. 2004).

In a 10-year historical cohort study of 159 subjects with epilepsy and 559 individually matched controls, it was found that there was a seven-fold increased risk of emergency department visits after a car accident involving PWE (Lings. 2001). These data should be taken cautiously as the sample size in the study was small.

Identified factors that reduce the risk of having a seizure-related driving accident include long seizure-free intervals, reliable auras, few prior nonseizure-related accidents, and good compliance with AEDs (Krauss, et al. 1999). In patients who had a ≥ 12-month seizure free interval, the risk of having a road accident was reduced by 93%. Having reliable auras reduces the risk of a driving accident as it allows patient to remove himself from the road before experiencing a seizure. 26% of patients will still have a motor vehicle accident despite having an aura, and this may be due to a short aura, traffic conditions that make it difficult for the driver to pull aside, and the belief that one can make it home before the seizure occurs. On a point of interest, female drivers with epilepsy have fewer accidents than male drivers with epilepsy (Masland. 1978, McLachlan, et al. 2007, Waller. 1965).

BURNS

The population-based epidemiological study of Tellez-Zenteno et al. (Tellez-Zenteno, et al. 2008) indicated that persons with epilepsy had a higher frequency of burns than the general population (6.9% vs. 3.9%) Unfortunately the small sample size did not allow for an accurate analysis of the increase in relative risk for burns in patients with epilepsy. Burns as a consequence of an epileptic seizure accounts for 1.6 – 10% of admissions to burns units (Bull, et al. 1964, Josty, et al. 2000, Maisels DO and Corps BVM. 1964, Richards EH. 1968, Tempest. 1956). The majority of burns in PWE occur while carrying out activities of daily living, such as cooking, ironing, blow-drying, or bathing. Domestic scalds have become the most common cause of admission in burned patients with epilepsy (Josty, et al. 2000).

In a retrospective review of a burn center registry, it was found that 72% of burns in PWE were full-thickness burns, compared to 68% in the general burn population (Rimmer, et al. 2007). These full-thickness burns require hospital admission and surgery to promote healing, retain function, and reduce scarring. In contrast to the findings of Josty et al (Josty, et al. 2000), this particular study found that the majority of burns in epileptic patients were due to fire/flame while cooking.

Identified risk factors for sustaining a burn injury as a person with epilepsy include number and type of seizure, female gender, and presence of neurological deficit. The more seizures individuals have, the more likely they are to suffer from a burn injury (Spitz, et al. 1994). Occurrence of a complex partial seizure also correlated with the likelihood of a burn during seizure (Hampton, et al. 1988). Women are twice as likely to sustain a burn injury due to epilepsy, and this is likely due to the fact that women more often carry out cooking duties and hair-styling tasks associated with epileptic burns. Spitz et al (Josty, et al. 2000) also found that having a neurological deficit was protective against burns, possibly because patients with a neurological deficit are less likely to perform dangerous tasks for themselves, or will do these tasks under supervision (Spitz, et al. 1994).

Several guidelines and prevention strategies have been developed in order to protect those with epilepsy from sustaining a burn injury. These strategies include use of the microwave instead of the stove, having the bath water temperature at 48.9°C, and having a shower instead of a bath (Rimmer, et al. 2007).

HOSPITALIZATIONS

It is a well-established fact that PWE have more hospital admissions than the general population. The Centre for Disease Control (CDC) estimated that approximately 93,000 hospitalizations each year are attributed to epilepsy (CDC). 1995), and in their population-based epidemiological study, Tellez-Zenteno et al (Tellez-Zenteno, et al. 2008) determined that among individuals who received care within 48 hours, hospital admissions following injuries were three times more frequent in persons with epilepsy as compared to the general population (24.2% vs. 8.1%, RR: 3.0, CI_{95}: 1.3-4.7). The injuries in PWE were no more severe than those sustained in the general population. Other studies have also noted the same trend in increased hospitalizations among persons with epilepsy although the difference is not as striking (3% of patients versus 1% of controls) (van den Broek, et al. 2004). In the study by van de Broek and Beghi (van den Broek, et al. 2004), fractures were the most common reason for hospital admission. Aside from hospitalizations due to injuries, it has also been found that PWE are more often hospitalized for general illnesses than controls (24% versus 6%; $p<0.0001$).

In a study of hospital records from the health district of South Glamorgan from 1991-1995 by Currie et al (Currie, et al. 1998), it was determined that PWE were responsible for 2.8% of hospital admissions. The rate of admissions with epilepsy as the primary diagnosis was 94/100,000 population per year, and the largest proportions of admissions was to pediatric neurology (53.4%), those due to mental handicap (25.1%) and to neurosurgery (9.1%). It was also found that the average length of stay was longer for those with epilepsy than for the general population (24.8 days versus 9.1 days). It was concluded that PWE comprise a significant portion of hospital admissions and occupy patient beds for a longer time than the general population. This serves as a drain on the healthcare resources. The authors suggested that there may be evidence for cost-containment by reducing multiple admissions.

Possible explanations for the higher incidence of hospital admissions in PWE include a more cautious attitude of clinicians towards injuries occurring in the setting of seizures, hospitalizations required because of seizures and not because of the injuries themselves, hospitalization driven by other issues, such as comorbidities, which are highly prevalent in patients with epilepsy, and possibly more severe injuries in PWE than in the general population (Tellez-Zenteno, et al. 2008).

Factors that contribute to a higher likelihood of hospital admission among epileptic patients include higher seizure frequency and lower quality of life. Age, marital status, race/ethnicity, educational level, and annual household income are not associated with higher rates of hospital admission (Bautista, et al. 2008).

Risk Factors

There are several risk factors that lead to increased risk of injury in PWE in general. Seizure type has the highest correlation with increased injury risk. Generalized tonic-clonic seizures, atonic seizures, and complex partial seizures are associated with the highest risk of injury because of the alteration in or loss of consciousness (Zwimpfer, et al. 1997). Patients having at least one seizure a month, and with more than three adverse effects due to antiepileptic drugs are also more likely to sustain an injury due to seizures. Epilepsy duration, sex, and age are not significant risk factors (Spitz. 1998).

Risk of injury in a person with epilepsy affects employability, insurance eligibility, education and recreational opportunities (Anonymous 1997, Davidson and Macdonald. 2002, Jones. 1998, Lawn, et al. 2004).

Table 1. Reported Injury Rates in Studies of Patients with Epilepsy

Author	Country/Population	Study Type	Number of Patients	Injury Rate
Nakken and Lossius (Nakken and Lossius. 1993)	Norway. Multihandicapped patients with intractable epilepsy	Prospective	62 cases	32.3% of patients had seizure related injuries in a 13-month period
Ziegler et al (Ziegler, et al. 1994)	Switzerland. Children with epilepsy without motor or mental handicap	Retrospective	198 cases	6 injuries during 1056 person-years.
Kirby and Sadler (Kirby and Sadler. 1995)	Canada. Adults with seizures presenting to the ER	Prospective	560 cases	Incidence of seizures resulting in injury was 29.5 in 100,000 population Incidence of seizures causing injury or death in the general population was 32.2 in 100,000 population 15% of seizures brought to medical attention resulted in injury or death
Wirrell et al (Wirrell, et al. 1996)	Canada. Young adults with a history of typical absence epilepsy. Controls were young adults with juvenile rheumatoid arthritis (JRA)	Retrospective chart review	59 patients/61 controls	24.6/100 person years injury rate for children with AE, compared to 18.7 for children with JRA ($p < 0.04$)
Buck et al (Buck, et al. 1997)	UK. Adults with active epilepsy without severe physical or learning disabilities	Retrospective population-based survey	696	35% sustained a seizure-related injury in the past year
Neufeld et al (Neufeld, et al. 1999)	Israel. Adults with epilepsy	Retrospective survey.	298	30% of patients reported seizure-related injury. This translates to one seizure-related injury every 21 patient-years, and a serious injury once every 64 patient-years
Kirsch and Wirrell (Kirsch and Wirrell. 2001)	Canada. Cases were cognitively normal children ages 5-16 with epilepsy attending a pediatric neurology clinic. Controls were the children's 'best friends'	Retrospective case-control study	25 cases/25 controls	Injuries in the past year not requiring medical treatment occurred at a median of 1 (25th-75th percentile 0, 4) for cases and at a median of 0 (0, 5) for controls ($P = .81$) 14% of cases had sustained at least 1 injury as a result of a seizure in their lifetime

Table (Continued)

Author	Country/Population	Study Type	Number of Patients	Injury Rate
Beghi and Cornaggia (Beghi, et al. 2002)	Italy, Germany, Holland, England, Portugal, Russia, Estonia, Slovenia. Children ≥ 5 years and adults, general hospital and university centers. Healthy controls	Prospective, case-control study	951 cases/909 controls	At 12 months: injury in 17% of cases and 12% of controls At 24 months: injury in 27% of cases and 17% of controls ($p<0.0001$)
Appleton (Appleton and Mersey Region Paediatric Epilepsy Interest,Group. 2002)	UK. Newly diagnosed children 1-16 years attending one of seven UK hospitals	Prospective	198 children	12.6% of children experienced a seizure-related injury before the diagnosis of epilepsy was established.
Lawn et al (Lawn, et al. 2004)	USA. Patients diagnosed with epilepsy between 1975 and 1984	Retrospective chart review.	247 adults	62 seizure-related injuries identified in 39 patients over 2714 patient-years of follow-up (16%, one injury in every 44 person-years)
Tellez-Zenteno et al (Tellez-Zenteno, et al. 2008)	Canada. Unselected patients with epilepsy in general population. Control was the general population	Retrospective survey	835 cases, 130 882 controls	14.9% of persons with epilepsy had an injury causing limitation of normal activities in the past 12 months compared to 13.34% of the general population ($p<0.05$). This yields an RR of 1.1 (CI_{95}: 0.8-1.4)

It is noted that patients with active epilepsy are at increased risk for injury (van den Broek, et al. 2004), and therefore it is important to keep epilepsy under pharmacological remission in order to reduce the risk of injury to the patient, thereby allowing the person to enjoy normally acceptable occupational and social privileges and thereby improving their quality of life.

PREVENTION

There are general guidelines in place to prevent injury in those with epilepsy. For all patients, epilepsy should be treated to reduce seizure frequency, drug-related balance problems should be minimized, swimming should be supervised, and regular exercise should be undertaken to maintain bone mass. Patients at higher risk (those with the risk factors as defined above) should avoid unsupervised bathing, minimize burn risks, and avoid high places (Spitz. 1998). The International League Against Epilepsy has laid out guidelines for prevention of injury in children (Anonymous 1997). The guidelines have few restrictions on activity, but there is the stipulation that children should be monitored while bathing, while using the stove or oven and during sports and recreational activities. These principles are time-limited. For example, restrictions to activity and supervision should be undertaken (a) for 2-3 months after a first untreated seizure; (b) after treatment is initiated and until it can be determined that further seizures are unlikely, and (c) for a few months after antiepileptic drugs (AEDs) have been discontinued. Restrictions may be required indefinitely in children who have persistent recurrent seizures uncontrolled by treatment.

By and large, the risk of injury to patients with controlled epilepsy is small, and these patients should be encouraged to enjoy as normal of a lifestyle as possible.

REFERENCES

ILAE commission report. restrictions for children with epilepsy. commission of pediatrics of the ILAE. international league against epilepsy. *Epilepsia* 1997; 38: 1054-6.

Aboukasm AG, Smith BJ. Nocturnal vertebral compression fracture. A presenting feature of unrecognized epileptic seizures. *Arch. Fam. Med.* 1997; 6: 185-7.

Aldenkamp A, Arends J. The relative influence of epileptic EEG discharges, short nonconvulsive seizures, and type of epilepsy on cognitive function. *Epilepsia* 2004; 45: 54-63.

Annegers JF, Melton LJ,3rd, Sun CA, Hauser WA. Risk of age-related fractures in patients with unprovoked seizures. *Epilepsia* 1989; 30: 348-55.

Appleton RE, Mersey Region Paediatric Epilepsy Interest,Group. Seizure-related injuries in children with newly diagnosed and untreated epilepsy. *Epilepsia* 2002; 43: 764-7.

Bautista RE, Glen ET, Wludyka PS, Shetty NK. Factors associated with utilization of healthcare resources among epilepsy patients. *Epilepsy Res* 2008; 79: 120-9.

Beghi E. Injuries in patients with epilepsy. *Lancet neurol* 2005; 4: 71-2.

Beghi E, Sander JW. Epilepsy and driving. *BMJ* 2005; 331: 60-1.

Beghi E, Cornaggia C, RESt-1 G. Morbidity and accidents in patients with epilepsy: Results of a european cohort study. *Epilepsia* 2002; 43: 1076-83.

Bird S. Epilepsy, driving and confidentiality. *Aust. Fam. Physician* 2005; 34: 1057-8.

Buck D, Baker GA, Jacoby A, Smith DF, Chadwick DW. Patients' experiences of injury as a result of epilepsy. *Epilepsia* 1997; 38: 439-44.

Buhler M, Gerber C. Shoulder instability related to epileptic seizures. *J. Shoulder Elbow Surg* 2002; 11: 339-44.

Bull J, Jackson DM, Walton C. Causes and prevention of domestic burning accidents. *Br. Med. J.* 1964; 2: 1421-7.

Centers for Disease Control and Prevention (CDC). Hospitalization for epilepsy--united states, 1988-1992. MMWR *Morb Mortal Wkly Rep* 1995; 44: 818-21.

Cockerell OC, Sander JW, Shorvon SD. Remission of epilepsy. the NGPS. national general practice study of epilepsy. *Lancet* 1995; 346: 1228.

Currie CJ, Morgan CL, Peters JR, Kerr M. The demand for hospital services for patients with epilepsy. *Epilepsia* 1998; 39: 537-44.

Davidson DL, Macdonald S. The costs of trauma caused by seizures: Can they be reduced?. *Seizure* 2002; 11: 344-7.

Gosens T, Poels PJ, Rondhuis JJ. Posterior dislocation fractures of the shoulder in seizure disorders--two case reports and a review of literature. *Seizure* 2000; 9: 446-8.

Hampton KK, Peatfield RC, Pullar T, Bodansky HJ, Walton C, Feely M. Burns because of epilepsy. *Br. Med. J. (Clin Res Ed)* 1988; 296: 1659-60.

Hansotia P, Broste SK. The effect of epilepsy or diabetes mellitus on the risk of automobile accidents. *N. Engl. J. Med.* 1991; 324: 22-6.

Jones MW. Consequences of epilepsy: Why do we treat seizures? *Can. J. Neurol. Sci.* 1998; 25: S24-6.

Josty IC, Narayanan V, Dickson WA. Burns in patients with epilepsy: Changes in epidemiology and implications for burn treatment and prevention. *Epilepsia* 2000; 41: 453-6.

Kirby S, Sadler RM. Injury and death as a result of seizures. *Epilepsia* 1995; 36: 25-8.

Kirsch R, Wirrell E. Do cognitively normal children with epilepsy have a higher rate of injury than their nonepileptic peers?. *J. Child Neurol.* 2001; 16: 100-4.

Krauss GL, Ampaw L, Krumholz A. Individual state driving restrictions for people with epilepsy in the US. *Neurology* 2001; 57: 1780-5.

Krauss GL, Krumholz A, Carter RC, Li G, Kaplan P. Risk factors for seizure-related motor vehicle crashes in patients with epilepsy. *Neurology* 1999; 52: 1324-9.

Kristiansen B, Christensen S. Fractures of the proximal end of the humerus caused by convulsive seizures. *Injury* 1984; 16: 108-9.

Lawn ND, Bamlet WR, Radhakrishnan K, O'Brien PC, So EL. Injuries due to seizures in persons with epilepsy: A population-based study. *Neurology* 2004; 63: 1565-70.

Lings S. Increased driving accident frequency in danish patients with epilepsy. *Neurology* 2001; 57: 435-9.

Maisels DO, Corps BVM. Burned epileptics. *Lancet* 1964; 1: 1298-301.

Masland RL. The physician's responsibility for epileptic drivers. *Ann. Neurol.* 1978; 4: 485-6.

McLachlan RS, Starreveld E, Lee MA. Impact of mandatory physician reporting on accident risk in epilepsy. *Epilepsia* 2007; 48: 1500-5.

Nakken KO, Lossius R. Seizure-related injuries in multihandicapped patients with therapy-resistant epilepsy. *Epilepsia* 1993; 34: 836-40.

Nei M, Bagla R. Seizure-related injury and death. *Curr. Neurol. Neurosci.* Rep. 2007; 7: 335-41.

Neufeld MY, Vishne T, Chistik V, Korczyn AD. Life-long history of injuries related to seizures. *Epilepsy Res* 1999; 34: 123-7.

Persson HB, Alberts KA, Farahmand BY, Tomson T. Risk of extremity fractures in adult outpatients with epilepsy. *Epilepsia* 2002; 43: 768-72.

Richards EH. Aspects of epilepsy and burns. *Epilepsia* 1968; 9: 127-35.

Rimmer RB, Bay RCR, Foster KN, Jones MACNA, Wadsworth M, Lessard C, et al. Thermal injury in patients with seizure disorders: An opportunity for prevention. *Journal of Burn Care and Research* 2007; 28: 318-23.

Shaw JL. Bilateral posterior fracture-dislocation of the shoulder and other trauma caused by convulsive seizures. J Bone Joint Surg Am 1971; 53: 1437-40.

Sheth RD, Wesolowski CA, Jacob JC, Penney S, Hobbs GR, Riggs JE, et al. Effect of carbamazepine and valproate on bone mineral density. *J. Pediatr.* 1995; 127: 256-62.

Sheth SG, Krauss G, Krumholz A, Li G. Mortality in epilepsy: Driving fatalities vs other causes of death in patients with epilepsy. *Neurology* 2004; 63: 1002-7.

Silbergeld DL, Harkness WF, Bell BA, Bircher MD. Posterior fracture dislocation of the shoulder secondary to epileptic seizures. *J. R Coll Surg. Edinb* 1991; 36: 139-40.

Souverein PC, Webb DJ, Petri H, Weil J, Van Staa TP, Egberts T. Incidence of fractures among epilepsy patients: A population-based retrospective cohort study in the general practice research database. *Epilepsia* 2005; 46: 304-10.

Spitz MC. Injuries and death as a consequence of seizures in people with epilepsy. *Epilepsia* 1998; 39: 904-7.

Spitz MC, Towbin JA, Shantz D, Adler LE. Risk factors for burns as a consequence of seizures in persons with epilepsy. *Epilepsia* 1994; 35: 764-7.

Stephen LJ, McLellan AR, Harrison JH, Shapiro D, Dominiczak MH, Sills GJ, et al. Bone density and antiepileptic drugs: A case-controlled study. *Seizure* 1999; 8: 339-42.

Taylor J, Chadwick D, Johnson T. Risk of accidents in drivers with epilepsy. *J Neurol Neurosurg Psychiatry* 1996; 60: 621-7.

Tellez-Zenteno JF, Hunter G, Wiebe S. Injuries in people with self-reported epilepsy: A population-based study. *Epilepsia* 2008; 49: 954-61.

Tempest M. A survey of domestic burns and scalds in wales during 1955. *Br. Med. J.* 1956; 1: 1387-92.

van den Broek M, Beghi E, RESt-1 G. Accidents in patients with epilepsy: Types, circumstances, and complications: A european cohort study. *Epilepsia* 2004; 45: 667-72.

Vestergaard P. Epilepsy, osteoporosis and fracture risk - a meta-analysis. *Acta Neurol Scand* 2005; 112: 277-86.

Vestergaard P, Tigaran S, Rejnmark L, Tigaran C, Dam M, Mosekilde L. Fracture risk is increased in epilepsy. *Acta Neurol Scand* 1999; 99: 269-75.

Waller JA. Chronic medical conditions and traffic safety: Review of the california experience. *N. Engl. J. Med.* 1965; 273: 1413-20.

Wirrell EC, Camfield PR, Camfield CS, Dooley JM, Gordon KE. Accidental injury is a serious risk in children with typical absence epilepsy. *Arch. Neurol.* 1996; 53: 929-32.

Ziegler AL, Reinberg O, Deonna T. [Epilepsy and accidents: What is the risk in children?]. *Arch. Pediatr.* 1994; 1: 801-5.

Zwimpfer TJ, Brown J, Sullivan I, Moulton RJ. Head injuries due to falls caused by seizures: A group at high risk for traumatic intracranial hematomas. *J. Neurosurg.* 1997; 86: 433-7.

In: Social Epileptology
Editors: J. Pinikahana and C. Walker
ISBN 978-1-60876-228-6

Chapter 7

EPILEPSY, DRIVING AND LAW

Roy G. Beran*
University of New South Wales,
School of Medicine at Griffith University,
Queensland, Australia

ABSTRACT

There exists the saying "The law is the law". This suggests application of the law is as simple as calculating a mathematical equation but were that true we could dismantle the very expensive legal industry devoted to creating, interpreting and administering the law and adopt a type of calculator or computer algorithm with a totally predictable outcome. Law is not a universal truth but rather man-made limitations governing behaviour, dependent upon jurisdiction, legal system (be it common law with an adversarial format, Roman (civil) law with an inquisitorial approach or religious law, imposed by clerics as is determined in Sharia law) and acceptance by those who are subject to the law. Understanding these concepts allows one to explore the relationship between epilepsy and the law with particular consideration of activities such as driving, employment or social interaction. The topic is far too broad to review in its entirety but examination of such set examples within a defined legal system, such as common law, as prevails in North America, United Kingdom or Australia, will allow an appreciation of how the law affects those who have epilepsy and how epilepsy may impact upon those expected to respect legal imposts when dealing with epilepsy.

INTRODUCTION

"Health law…is fluid and diverse. Just as health knowledge and interventions are changing fundamentally with advances such as the Human Genome Project, so too is health law in order to impose regulation and constraint upon quickly evolving clinical development…It needs to be adaptable and able to comply with human rights; to facilitate

* Correspondence: Prof. Roy G. Beran, Suite 5, 6th Floor. 12 Thomas Street, CHATSWOOD. NSW 2067, Australia. Email: roy@royberan.com

ethical practice by health practitioners; to satisfy the requirements of vested interests; to meet the challenges of fast-moving medical technologies; to address social policy development and principles of governance and regulation; as well as to enable resolution of disputes in a way that satisfies community expectations of fairness and justice…" (Freckleton and Petersen, 2006).

This quotation encapsulates the broad impact the law has on everyday life without going into the various legal systems that exist, be they: the Common Law, which is practiced in the adversarial legal system which devolved from Britain and the British colonies as exist in countries such as North America (USA and Canada), United Kingdom or Australia (Meek, 1999), Civil Law sometimes referred to as Roman Law which is based upon a codified inquisitorial system that is evident in most European countries and said to have four major strands namely, French, German, Scandinavian and Chinese (Wacks, 2008), or the Religious Legal system typified by Sharia Law (Van Hoorebeek Gale, 2008) based largely on the teachings of the Koran in which clerics impose strict Islamic Codes of acceptable behaviour based upon interpretation of the scriptures. Clearly any meaningful discussion of the law, and its impact upon those affected by it, must take into account the legal system in which it is being analysed and the jurisdiction governing such imposition. For the purposes of this analysis the discussion will focus on the Common Law system which is based upon precedence and judge-made law derived from judicial interpretation of cases consequent to an adversarial process (Wacks, 2008). In this system the parliament sets out the law by way of Acts of parliament (statutes) and the judiciary interprets the law based upon evidence, precedence and a legal hierarchy of levels of judicial opinion with appeals available at various stages up to a High or Supreme Court which represents the ultimate decision within this hierarchy (Meek, 1999)

Many non-legally trained people, who comment on the law, expect it to be quite straight forward and quote legal dogma as if it were axiomatic but this is less than correct. This is exemplified by the split decision in the New South Wales Supreme Court case of *Woods v Lowns* (Woods v Lowns, 1995). The majority decision in the Court of Appeal (Kirby P and Cole JA) supported the trial judge who found that Dr Lowns owed a duty of care to attend a boy who was not, and had never been, his patient but who was experiencing epileptic seizures and for whom the court was told his sister sought the doctor's assistance. Mahoney JA gave a dissenting opinion in which he indicated that he felt that it was inappropriate for the Court to impose a legal obligation that had "…not previously existed…" (Lowns v Woods, 1996). He acknowledged that his dissenting opinion would not alter the outcome of the case (based on the majority decision) which found against the doctor, thereby creating such legal 'duty of care' in the Australian State of New South Wales. He also recognised that prior to this case there was no legal obligation on a general practitioner to attend someone with whom he had no prior relationship and he differentiated between moral and legal obligations (Lowns v Woods, 1996), indicating that he felt that the duty to attend in such circumstances was moral rather than legal.

What this case demonstrates is that the outcome of litigation is never predictable and thus it is wise for someone who is contemplating litigation to seriously explore alternative forms of dispute resolution. Such alternatives offer greater certainty because the solution is governed by compromise between the parties to the dispute. In the *Woods* case, the Court redefined what amounts to legal obligation for New South Wales doctors, a situation that is not necessarily followed in any other Australian state. A similar conclusion might have emerged in the District Court case of *Gillett* in which a driver with nocturnal epilepsy falsely denied his epilepsy when applying for a driver's licence. He was involved in a fatal motor vehicle accident in which a family of three was killed and he was found guilty of dangerous driving causing death (Beran and Devereux, 2007). Medical expert evidence suggested that he had complied with medical advice (with therapeutic blood levels of the antiepileptic medication carbamazepine immediately after the accident) and the neurologists, giving expert testimony, indicated that he, Gillett, satisfied the conditions within the AUSTROADS guidelines, applicable to epilepsy, to be permitted to hold a licence had he declared his illness to the driving authorities. The guidelines were ruled as inadmissible into evidence by the trial judge in the lower court ((Beran and Devereux, 2007). This decision rendered the guidelines as irrelevant to the legal proceeding but, in the Criminal Court of Appeal, McClellan CJ in CL found that the trial judge had erred in refusing admission of the guidelines thereby reinstating their relevance (Gillett v Regina, 2006).

These two cases, both of which dealt with issues relating to epilepsy, highlight how unpredictable the legal process can be and the need to approach legal interpretation with respect for the system but also an anticipation that the unexpected may well happen. Thus, while the law provides the framework in which any particular society functions, one cannot pre-empt what the final decision will be in any case once litigation has been initiated. It follows that alternative methods of compromise, between parties to any dispute, may have a better chance of reaching an outcome in which both parties, within the adversarial system, feel that they have achieved a degree of satisfaction, although not necessarily perfect, rather than there being definite winners and losers.

What follows will examine just a few areas of the interface between epilepsy and the law to offer an overview of how the system functions and its potential to influence the social fabric of the life of the person with epilepsy.

Epilepsy, Driving and the Law

Having touched on *Gillett* it seems appropriate to open specific consideration of epilepsy and the law with a brief overview of epilepsy and driving. Driving is widely accepted as a means of gaining independence for people seeking mobility in a fast moving society but is denied to those who have active epilepsy, unless the seizures experienced have no impact on consciousness, such as simple partial seizures with 'aura' as their only manifestation, or those with purely nocturnal (sleep-related) seizures (NRTC, 2001; Beghi and Sander, 2005; Devereuz, 2002; Johnston, 2004). It is reasonable to accept that anything which might impair consciousness will also make driving dangerous for both the person with such impairment and other road users. What is less clear is who should be responsible for fulfilling the role of gatekeeper to monitor if, and when, a person with epilepsy should be afforded the privilege of being able to driving.

Some jurisdictions impose a mandatory, statutory responsibility on doctors to report patients who pose a risk if driving (Johnston, 2004; Black, 2003; Beran, 1998; Ooi and Gutrecht, 2000; McLachlan et al, 2007), thereby jeopardising the doctor-patient relationship with the potential for patients to conceal their true seizure rate from their attending physician (McLachlan et al, 2007). In most jurisdictions the doctor is indemnified from litigation if the reporting, of a patient to the driving authorities, is done in good faith with the ultimate goal being the respect of the greater 'duty of care' to the wider society (NRTC, 2001; Black, 2003; Fisher et al, 1994; Beran, 2005). Should the doctor choose to place his/her respect and loyalty for the patient above that wider 'duty of care' to the community, then the doctor may be the subject of litigation for failing to protect even the patient, or that patient's estate (Johnston, 2004), let alone other individuals who may be hurt by the foreseeable risk posed by that patient (Tarasoff v Regents, 1976). *Tarassof* was American case in which the therapist failed to warn an identifiable victim of impending danger and was found guilty of negligence for not protecting against a foreseeable risk. It can be argues that this situation is similar to that imposed by the uncontrolled patient with epilepsy who continues to drive against medical advice. This leaves the doctor with a conflict of interest when trying to balance the responsibilities to the patient against those for the community as a whole.

Some argue that the doctor should not be placed into the position of having to make this decision and demand that the Licensing Authorities accept their role, as the final arbiters, which should reflect the true legal position (Somerville, 2008) but, as was stated earlier, may not represent the final outcome of any contested litigation.

Doctors may well be found liable to third parties for injuries sustained, consequent to failing to report a patient or for certifying a patient as fit to drive, contrary to expectations set out in the guidelines (Johnston, 2004). While this has not been tested in the Australian courts, overseas experience has shown the lack of consistency in the courts with decisions going in either direction (Johnston, 2004; Harden v Dalrymple, 1995).

Of interest is the fact that studies have shown that Australian neurologists are far more lenient in their attitudes towards driving restrictions, for those with epilepsy, than is the stated requirement within the guidelines (Beran et al, 2007) and, while they endorse the concept of reporting recalcitrant patients, they rarely do so (Beral et al, 2007). Recent fear of possible criminal litigation, which did not eventuate but was widely publicised (Somerville et al, 2008), has seen a shift against even assessing patients as fit, or not, to be able to drive with the onus being forced back onto the Licensing Authorities. Neurologists are not alone in their attitudes to reporting patients to the Licensing Authorities and the intrusion into the doctor-patient relationship is a real issue that affects future management (Jang et al, 2007).

Not all jurisdictions impose identical restrictions upon those with epilepsy (Beghi and Sander, 2005; Devereux, 2002; Ooi and Gutrecht, 2000; Fisher et al, 1994; Krumholz et al, 1991; Krauss et al, 2001; Ben-Menachem, 2004) which means that the doctor will need to be familiar with the local rules and regulations which vary between countries and even between states within the same country. While doctors are often ignorant of the relevant guidelines (Shanahan et al, 2007; Beran, 2008), this does not provide legal protection if a harm has occurred. Thus doctors need to be cognisant of both their responsibilities and their personal risk for suit should they fail to live up to expectation (Hurley, 2007).

Similarly patients are also not exempt from serious consequences should they fail to report their epilepsy and injury, or even death, eventuates as was the case with *Gillett* (Beran and Devereu, 2007; Gillett v Regina, 2006).

ADVOCACY AND THE PERSON WITH EPILEPSY

Much of the discussion, thus far, has focused upon the therapeutic relationship between the doctor and patient and the way in which the legal imperative may adversely affect the doctor-patient relationship. Doctors also have a very special, positive role to play for their patients with regards to advocating for patients' rights, as do the patient self-help organisations which represent them (Beran et al, 2008; Finucane, 1999; Beran, 2008). People with epilepsy are often the subject of discrimination which is unjustifiable and which requires someone in authority to stand up and fight for them (Beran, 2008). Who better to do this than their doctor? The person with epilepsy may need a paraclete who is willing to represent the particular case when the person with epilepsy feels incapable of adequately defending themselves.

People with epilepsy do have the fall back position of relying on statutory protection as may be afforded by the various anti-discrimination laws (Disability Discrimination Act, 1992; Americans with Disabilities, 1990) but, as has already been discussed, reliance on litigation is not absolute and far from predictable. It follows that the medical profession has a duty to try to improve and lessen the stigma felt by those with epilepsy (Sutton and Beran, 1983). It is amazing that, in the 21st century, people can still be defined by their diagnosis rather than the people they are (Beran, 2008). People with epilepsy are still referred to as "epileptics" rather than individuals with epilepsy (Beran, 2008).

Reliance on statutory protection may well have the effect of forcing discrimination underground as it is impossible to legislate to change attitudes and consequently the discrimination that is practised will simply become more covert. Employers will still be selective regarding whom they employ and it behoves people with epilepsy to make themselves the most valuable employees possible, which is the best defence against such discrimination (West et al, 2006).

Advocacy is not restricted to employment or education and affects all types of daily activity. Even the concept of informed consent, not just for research involvement but for acceptance of treatment in general, is a form of patients' rights which require protection (Beran, 2003). Doctors have a 'duty of care' to empower patients to make informed decisions concerning their treatment. Failure to discuss 'material issues' the discussion of which is pivotal to the patient's decision to accept the type of the treatment being offered, may generate a successful action against the doctor (Beran, 2008).

Application of the Ipp Report (Review of the Law of Negligence, 2002) has gone some way, by employing statutory change to effect tort law reform, to redress what many doctors perceived as unacceptable legal bias and legal constraints on medical practice, with the passage of the *Civil Liability Act* 2002 (NSW). This protected doctors against some actions for negligence, consequent to the decision in *Whitaker* (Rogers v Whitaker, 1992), in which an ophthalmologist was found liable for not discussing a rare complication about which the patient had specifically asked but for which most ophthalmologists, up until that time, would have been fairly dismissive because of its very rare occurrence. The change provided protection for the doctor if it could be shown that what was done conformed to the practices of a respected body of that doctor's peers (referred to as the Bolam Principle (Bolam v Friern Hospital Management Committee, 1957). The pendulum is still swinging, regarding application of this Act (Halverson and Ors v Dobler, 2006) and its final resting place is still to be determined. As such it is imperative that doctors do consider their patients' attitudes and also there is a definite requirement for doctors to remain up-to-date with current medical practice and knowledge (Halverson and Ors v Dobler, 2006) which may prove very difficult in this age of ever changing knowledge and science. The upshot of these changes has been to better protect the patient against doctors who fail to keep up to date though there may be a tendency to judge doctors, especially general practitioners, not necessarily by their peers but by those who are more specialised (Halverson and Ors v Dobler, 2006), and hence it remains to be seen where the pendulum will stop. As with medicine, law is also a changing vista but it would appear, on surface evaluation, that patient protection remains at the forefront of legal consideration.

Advocacy for the patient may even transcend what amounts to the usually accepted issues of patient management and may involve considering novel approaches to patient care, such as not always discussing issues with patients when the identification of well recognised but unavoidable risks may adversely affect the patient's quality of life. This can only be considered if the issues to be discussed, or not discussed, do not have material consequences, in other words when one cannot change the outcome but the discussion itself might adversely affect the patient, such as discussion of Sudden Unexpected/Unexplained Death in Epilepsy (SUDEP) (Beran et al, 2004). It must be recognised that if the patient seeks the information, and asks the appropriate questions, it is then the doctor's duty to answer those questions honestly and with sufficient clarity for the patient to understand the matters discussed. In these circumstances the patient has clearly expressed a wish to know the facts and thus discussion of them no longer poses a risk of introducing information that the patient would prefer not to know or alternatively the doctor deems is in the patient's best interests not to be discussed at the given time. In all therapeutic relationships it is best, when creating a relationship of trust, to have an honest and open exchange of information if the patient has voiced a wish for this to happen.

Another area in which advocacy for the patient may mean challenging accepted values is when it is felt that these values are not in the patient's best interests and may usurp the patient's autonomy. Such a situation exists with the automatic exclusion of women who become pregnant during the course of clinical drug trials (Beran, 2006). There can be no argument that it is unethical to recruit women who want to become pregnant into such trials, as it poses an unacceptable risk for the foetus (Beran, 2006). Similarly it is unethical to recruit breastfeeding mothers into such trials due to the potential risks for the infant (Beran, 2006). The issue which flaunts the accepted practice is when a woman, who has accepted that pregnancy is contraindicated in a trial and who has agreed to practice acceptable methods of contraception as part of 'informed consent", becomes pregnant while participating in such a trial.

The argument is that, once pregnancy has been established, it is well into the first trimester which is the time when teratogenicity is most likely to have occurred. Hence the removal of the woman from the trial no longer protects anyone, be it the woman, the foetus or the sponsoring pharmaceutical company. What it does do is place the woman, and possibly the foetus, at increased risk, if the withdrawal of the experimental/trial antiepileptic medication is precipitous or the trial medication has been efficacious and its removal places the pregnant woman at greater risk of recurrence of seizures, or even status epilepticus (Beran, 2006). Thus proper advocacy for the patient would dictate that the patient has the right to be told all the options, including the unknown risk of teratogenicity, and the patient makes an informed decision regarding ongoing management, be it abortion, stopping the medication or continuing on the trial with the knowledge that the foetus is definitely at risk (Beran, 2006). It can be seen that advocacy for the patient can take many forms and the doctor has a real possibility of making a significant difference to the patent's life by being more that just a diagnostician and therapist but by being a true paraclete who fights for the rights of his or her patients.

SOCIAL CONSEQUENCES OF THE LAW

It is only fairly recently that the legal barriers which prevented people with epilepsy from marrying have been removed (Shostak and Ottman, 2006; Mani, 1997). Only relatively recently has there been a real appreciation of the need to encourage the integration of people with epilepsy into society and to break down the social barriers (Masia and Devinski, 2000).

Not only are marriage rates lower for those with epilepsy but rates of divorce are also higher (Dansky et al, 1980; Collins, 1990; Taylor and Falconer, 1968) making questions of family law and property settlements of greater importance. With better management of epilepsy, resulting in better seizure control, there can emerge a changed family dynamic which dictates that the carer is no longer required to be in control and the person with epilepsy may have greater self-control which can alter the family interactions and contribute to the increased divorce rates. Nowhere is this more apparent than in the context of epilepsy surgery where the changes can be most dramatic (Carran et al, 1999).

Personal insurance is something that most people take for granted, be it health insurance, life insurance or travel insurance. Epilepsy, if it is a pre-existing condition, may make it impossible to garner health or life insurance, with only those with well controlled epilepsy being able to achieve a degree of cover, possibly having to pay additional premiums (Beghi et al, 2000). Travel itself may be a difficulty for those with epilepsy, with patients deemed to be too much of a risk for the airline to accept, thereby forcing patients with epilepsy to accept conditions for travel that are demeaning, discriminatory and would be otherwise unacceptable, let alone being denied protection because travel insurance is unobtainable (Bera, 2008).

Many recreational pursuits are denied to the person with epilepsy, be it via regulation or direct law. These include competitive driving, diving, flying and many other activities that require a medical certificate to confirm a minimum standard of health (CAMS, 1989; Wilks, 2000; CASA, 2003).

Those occupations that require a uniform are usually legally off-limits for people with epilepsy, be it soldier, sailor, pilot or fireman (Beran, 2004; CASA, 2003; AFAC, 2006). Thus there is real legal impediment for some people with epilepsy to achieve their life's ambition with the consequence being that the person with epilepsy may become demoralised and accepting underemployment, possibly well below their true potentia (Chaplin et al, 1998).

These chosen topics, from within the plethora of potential legal constraints that affect people with epilepsy, and their social development, clearly demonstrate the vast capacity for the law to negatively impact upon the social fabric of life for the person with epilepsy. The scope of such discussion is so enormous that it is impossible to cover the topic exhaustively in a brief chapter such as this. The examples chosen have been provided to offer food for thought, to whet the appetite, and to encourage further exploration of a fascinating topic.

CONCLUSION

What has been provided within this chapter serves as an introduction to epilepsy and the law with a particular focus upon the social consequences thereof. It has identified that law, per se, is not a static set of rules or regulations but rather a continuingly evolving interface between the society and its values that govern the way it functions. The very fact that even the systems of law, that are practiced, differ between societies, nations and cultures demonstrates that the impact of law will vary depending upon the type of legal system is being followed and the attitudes of the citizens within the relevant society.

Epilepsy offers an example of a chronic illness to which is attached a real stigma and the health profession has an opportunity and an obligation to act as advocates for those affected by it. This allows doctors to step outside their usual role, of offering diagnosis and treatment, to offer holistic medicine that recognises the constraint faced by the patient. The doctor should not feel restricted by accepted standards and needs to explore the boundaries of how far they can help patients to achieve their maximal potential while always remaining within the law and its dictates. Loyalty to the patient may need to be secondary to 'duty of care' to the wider community, as is the case with recalcitrant patients who would drive against medical advice. At all times the doctor must evaluate the situation and offer the optimal care for the patient while also accepting that what is best for the patient may be at odds with what is usual practice, or even what the patient demands, as is the case with driving. Decisions in this domain require experience and appreciation of what is needed to provide the best outcome for the patient, who should always hold the position of absolute priority within the decision making process, when balanced within the wider picture of what is best for all concerned.

REFERENCES

Americans with Disabilities Act 42 U.S.C. 12101 et seq 1990 USA.

Australian Fire Authorities Council (AFAC) (2006) *Medical Guidelines for Fire Fighters. Summary Document* AFAC, at 4-12.

AUSTROADS and National Road Transport Commission (NRTC) (2001) *Assessing Fitness to Drive – Commercial and Private Vehicle Drivers: Medical Standards for Licensing and Clinical Management Guidelines.* AUSTROADS and NRTC, Sydney (reprinted September 2003 and 2006).

Beghi E, Brown S, Capurro D, Chadwick D, Cornaggia CM, De Boer H, Garattini L, Hauser A, Homsma SJ, Lazazzera M, Sillanpaa M, Sonnen AE, Thorbecke R (2000) IBE Commission Report @nd Workshop on Epilepsy, Risks and Insurance. *Epilepsia* 4; 110-12.

Beghi E, Sander JW (2005) Epilepsy and Driving – Regulations in the European Union need harmonisation as well as greater flexibility *Brit. Med. J.* 331:60-61.

Ben-Menachem E (2004) Towards a More Pragmatic View of Driving and Epilepsy. *Epilepsy Current* 4; 133-34.

Beran R. G. (2008) Medical aspects of fitness to drive. What do Public Hospital Doctors know and think? *Int. Med. J.*, 38, 149.

Beran RG (1998) Confidentiality and the Management of Patients who Fail to Comply with Doctor's Advice Not To Drive: A Survey of Medico-Legal opinion in Australia, *Seizure* 6; 1-10.

Beran RG (2003) Informed Consent, A Legal Requirement in the Management of Patients with Epilepsy. *Med. Law* 22;155-84.

Beran RG (2004) Epilepsy and the Defence Forces. *ADF Health* 5; 85-88.

Beran RG (2005) An Analysis and Overview of the Guidelines for Assessing Fitness to Drive for Commercial and Private Vehicle Drivers, *Internal Medical Journal,* 35: 364-8.

Beran RG (2006) The Ethics of Excluding Women who become Pregnant While Participating in Clinical Trials of Anti-epileptic Medications. *Seizure* 15; 563-70.

Beran RG (2008) Epilepsy and Law. *Epilepsy and Behaviour* 12; 644 – 651.

Beran RG, Ainley LAE, Beran ME (2007) Opinions, Attitudes and Practices of Australian Neurologists with regards to Epilepsy and Driving. *Int Med J* 37; 251-7.

Beran RG, Devereux JA (2007) Road not taken: Lessons to be Learned from Queen v Gillett *Internal Medical Journal,* 37; 336 – 9.

Beran RG, Devereux JA, McLin W, Lehman C, Falk-Petersen J, de Boer HM, Finucane A (2008) *Legal concerns and effective advocacy strategies in Epilepsy-A Comprehensive Text Book* Vo 3 Engel J, Pedley TA (Eds) Lippincott-Raven, Philadelphia at 2277-2282.

Beran RG, Weber S, Sungaran R, Venn N, Hung A (2004) Review of the Legal Obligations of the Doctor to Discuss Sudden Unexplained Death in Epilepsy (SUDEP) – A Cohort Controlled Comparative Cross-Matched Study in an Outpatient Epilepsy Clinic. *Seizure* 13; 523-28.

Black AB (2003) Confidentiality – Confidentiality and Driver Licensing Authorities, *Med Law* 22; 333-44.

Bolam v Friern Hospital Management Committee [1957] 1 WLR 582.

Carran MA, Kohler CG, O'Connor MJ (1999) Marital Status After epilepsy Surgery. *Epilepsia* 40; 1755-60.

CASA (2003) *Civil Aviation Safety Regulations 1998 (CASR) 1st Ed* Office of Legal Council, ACT, Australia Part 67 at 21-33.

Chaplin VE, Western A Tomson T (1998) Factors Associated with Employment Problems of People with Established Epilepsy. *Seizure* 7; 299-303.

Civil Aviation Safety Authority (CASA) (2003) *Designated Aviation Medical Examiner's Handbook*, CASA, Phillip ACT.

Collins JA (1990) Psychological Well-being and Epilepsy: An Empirical Study *Epilepsia* 31; 418-26.

Confederation of Australian Motor Sports (CAMS) (1989) *Medical Standards,* CAMS, Sydney at 4.

Dansky LV, Andermann E, Anndermann F (1980) Marriage and Fertility in Epileptic Patients. *Epilepsia* 21; 261- 71.

Devereux JA (2002) Epilepsy and Driving Licences *Med Law* 21: 121-32.

Disability Discrimination Act 1992 (Cth) Australia.

Finucane AK (1999) Legal Aspects of Epilepsy. *Neurology Clinics* 17; 235-43.

Fisher RS, Parsonage M, Beaussart M, Bladin P, Masland R, Sonnen AE, Remillard G (1994) Epilepsy and Driving: An International Perspective, Joint Commission on Drivers' Licensing of the International Bureau for Epilepsy and the International League Against Epilepsy, *Epilepsia* 35; 675-84.

Freckleton I., Petersen K. (2006) Disputes and dilemmas in health law: An overview - in *Disputes and Dilemmas in Health Law* Federation Press, Sydney at 3 Gillett v Regina [2006] NSWCCA 370.

Halverson and Ors v Dobler; Halverson by his tutor v Dobler [2006] NSWSC Hurley D (2007) When Epileptic Patients Crash: Legal Airbags Protect Most Neurologists but Buckle your Seat Belt Just the Same. *Neurology Today*, 7, 18-19.

Ipp DA (2002) Review of the Law of Negligence, Cth of Australia, Canberra.

Jang RW, Man-Son-Hing M, Molnar FJ, Hogan DB, Marchall SC, Auger J. Graham ID, Korner-Bitensky N, Tomlinson G, Kowgier ME, Naglie G (2007) Family Physicians' Attitudes and Practices Regarding Assessments of Medical Fitness to Drive in Older Persons. *J Gen Intern Med* 22; 531-43.

Johnston JC (2004) Liability of Neurologists –in *Legal Medicine 6th edition* Sanbar S, Firestone MH (Eds) ACLM Mosby, USA at 474-481.

Krauss GL, Ampaw L, Krunholz A (2001) Individual State Driving Restrictions for People with Epilepsy in the US. *Neurology* 57; 1780-85.

Krumholz A, Fisher RS, Lesser RP, Hauser WA (1991) Driving and Epilepsy: A Review and Reappraisal. *JAMA* 265; 622-26.

Lowns v Woods [1996] *Aust torts Reports* 81-376 at 63, 165-63,166.

Mani KS (1997) Legal Discrimination from Negative to Positive *Med Law* 16; 367-74.

Masia SL, Devinski O, (2000) Epilepsy and Behaviour: A Brief History *Epilepsy and Behaviour* 1; 27-36.

McLachlan RS, Starrevels E, Lee MA (2007) Impact of Mandatory reporting on Accident Risk in Epilepsy, *Epilepsia* 48;1500-5.

Meek M (1999) *The Australian Legal System 3rd Ed* LBC Information Services at 117-126.

Ooi WW, Gutrecht JA (2000) International Regulations for automobile driving and Epilepsy, *Journal of Travel Medicine,* 7;1-4.

Rogers v Whitaker (1992) 175 CLR 479. See Harden v Dalrymple, 883 F. Supp. 963 (D.Del.1995). *Cf. Praesel v Johnson*, 41 Tex. Super Ct. J. 630 (1998).

Shanahan EM, Sladek RM, Phillips P (2007) Medical Aspects of Fitness to Drive. What do Public Hospital Doctors Know and Think? *Int. Med. J.* 37; 372-76.

Shostak S, Ottman R (2006) Ethical, Legal and Social Dimensions of Epilepsy Genetics *Epilepsia* 47; 1595 -1602.

Somerville E, Granot R, Black A, Beran RG, Harvey A (2008) A proposed algorithm to determine fitness to drive in patients with epilepsy" *Australian and New Zealand Association of Neurologists (ANZAN) – Annual Scientific Meeting,* Brisbane, Australia.

Sutton C, Beran RG (1983) The Role of the Health System in Reducing the Stigma Attached to Epilepsy. *Aust. J. Soc. Issues* 18;203-208.

Tarasoff v Regents of the Univ. of Cal., 551 P. 2d 334 (Cal.1976). *See Osborne v USA*, No 30115 (W. Va. July 3, 2002).

Taylor DC, Falconer MA (1968) Clinical, Socio-economic and Psychological Changes After Epilepsy Surgery. *Br. J. Psychiatry* 114; 1247-61.

Van Hoorebeek, Gale C (2008) Sharia Law and the Qur'an: Providing Islamic Jurisprudential Modules *Education, Business and Society: Contemporary Middle Eastern Issues* 1; 138-144.

Wacks R (2008) Law's roots – in *Law – A Very Short Introduction* Oxford, Oxford University Press, Oxford at 1-35.

West MD, Dye AN, McMahon BT (2006) Epilepsy and Workforce Discrimination: Population Characteristics and Trends. *Epilepsy and Behaviour* 9; 101 -5.

Wilks J (2000) Scuba Diving and Snorkelling Safely on Australia's Great Barrier Reef. *J Travel Med* 7; 283-89.

Woods v Lowns (1995) 36 NSWLR 344.

In: Social Epileptology
Editors: J. Pinikahana and C. Walker
ISBN 978-1-60876-228-6

Chapter 8

EPILEPSY, CULTURE, IDENTITY AND WELLBEING: A STUDY OF THE SOCIAL, CULTURAL AND ENVIRONMENTAL CONTEXT OF EPILEPSY IN CAMEROON

Pascale Allotey **[*]** ***and Daniel Reidpath***
School of Health Sciences and Social Care,
Centre for Public Health Research
Brunel University, Uxbridge Middlesex, United Kingdom

ABSTRACT

Epilepsy presents an identity of exclusion which at multiple levels hinders the ability to engage with one's community. This paper describes an exploratory, mixed methods study (n=42) of the relationship between the social, cultural and environmental context and the experience of living with epilepsy in Cameroon. Participants were identified as "epileptics;" consequently restrictions placed on them reduced their ability to perform other traditional roles, affected their social value and excluded them from their communities. Participants detail the effects of their reduced "social value" and the challenges they face in attempts to be reintegrated as productive and functioning members of society.

Keywords: stigma; subjective well being; social value; exclusion.

[*] Correspondence: Professor Pascale Allotey, Chair of Race and Diversity, School of Health Sciences and Social Care and Centre for Public Health Research. Brunel University, Uxbridge Middlesex UB8 3PH. United Kingdom. Email: pascale.allotey@brunel.ac.uk

INTRODUCTION

In functioning societies, an individual's ability to contribute to the society is critical to the social and economic investment of the society in the individual (Komter, 1996; Trivers, 1971). We have extended this argument to suggest that where resources are particularly limited, the markers of individuals' ability to engage in this reciprocal exchange are based on social constructs and include *inter alia* gender, ethnicity, life stage (age), health states (see Reidpath, Chen, Gifford, and Allotey, 2005). Some of these are fluid and labile such as being a child or a patient with a short term acute illness; others more rigid such as gender, race or chronic disease status. As identities, they may be revealed to or hidden from others according to need and capacity. Individuals embody a multiplicity of these identities, the characteristics of which are implicitly used to determine their social value. Furthermore, the environment is critical to enabling or restricting the capacity of individuals to raise or lower their perceived social value. Thus individuals perceived as incapable of contributing to the society are of low social value, and their access to social (and economic) goods and services are curtailed resulting in exclusion, marginalisation, stigmatisation and discrimination (Reidpath, Chen, Gifford, and Allotey, 2005).

To illustrate, in sub-Saharan Africa, congenital deafness often results in profound developmental retardation and disability because of the lack of access to screening for early detection and management. Unable to interact 'normally' with their social and physical environment, individuals become socially isolated and are socially stigmatised (Kiyaga and Moores, 2003; Olusanya, Luxon, and Wirz, 2005). The discrimination suffered by the disabled, evidenced by restricted access to goods and services and other societal engagement is well documented (Groce and Scheer, 1990; Scheer and Groce, 1988). Based on the argument above, for reasons relating to both lack of structure and capacity, the deaf are considered non-contributing members of the community. They are perceived to be of low social value and 'unworthy' of investment (Reidpath, Chen, Gifford, and Allotey, 2005). By contrast, in a study in Martha's Vineyard in the US, the deaf were included in all aspects of the community's life. The community recorded a high prevalence of congenital deafness (1 in 155) and as a result both the hearing and deaf could communicate in sign language. In the absence of the communication disorder, the deaf were 'normal' contributing members of the population (Groce, 1985) and there was therefore no justification for deafness to be a marker of lower social value.

The experience, severity and outcome of diseases are therefore determined not only by the clinical and pathological processes but also by the patient's capacity to engage with their physical, social and cultural environment during the disease state. This conceptual framework offers a useful approach to the exploration of the experience, impact and context of chronic illness in resource poor settings. Chronic illness is, by definition, inveterate, may require long term expenditure of resources depending on the level of severity. The condition often becomes the primary identity by which the patient defines themselves (Faircloth, 1998; Jacoby, Snape, and Baker, 2005). The research described in this paper is a study designed to explore the continuing engagement of people with a chronic illness - epilepsy - with their communities. The study describes the effects of structure and context on the experience and severity of epilepsy. Epilepsy was selected because it is relatively common, and while it is considered of to be of low to moderate severity clinically (Murray and Lopez, 1996:p413) there is a growing body of research, particularly in the applied health social sciences that highlights its strong social impact (Baker, 2002; Baskind and Birbeck, 2005; Jacoby, Snape, and Baker, 2005; Nubukpo et al., 2004). The objective was to develop detailed descriptions of the experience of epilepsy as it relates to other identities with socially constructed social values such as gender (Allotey and Gyapong, 2005) and to socio-economic status and across rural and urban environments.

EPILEPSY

Epilepsy describes a group of disorders of cerebral function characterised by a pattern of repeated, sudden brief attacks of altered consciousness, motor activity or sensory phenomena known as seizures. The seizures are a symptom of the underlying neurological dysfunction, which in some cases is due to brain tumours, scar tissue from trauma to the brain, or a progressive neurological disease (Schachter, 2003). In most cases however, epilepsy is idiopathic with no apparent pathological basis for the seizures. Seizures can be unpredictable, putting the person and those around them into potentially dangerous situations (World Health Organization, International Bureau for Epilepsy, and International League Against Epilepsy, 1997). With treatment, seizures can be controlled in approximately 70% of cases. Where the cause is identified and treatable, the prognosis for the total remission of seizures is very good (Global Campaign against Epilepsy, 2003; Kwan and Sander, 2004) giving people with epilepsy (PWE) a close-to-average level of functioning within society.

Historically and almost universally however, epilepsy has been associated with the mystical; with demonic possession, witchcraft or spiritual delinquency (Carod and Vazquez-Cabrera, 1998; Temkin, 1971). Contemporary lay interpretations remain negative and the condition is highly stigmatized. Recent reviews of available data compiled from across developed and developing countries (including Cameroon, the site of the present study) on the role of stigma in epilepsy demonstrate a persistent and widely held perception of PWE as violent, antisocial and "retarded" (Jacoby, 2002).

In recognition of its hidden status, the World Health Organization launched the *Global Campaign against Epilepsy* (Global Campaign against Epilepsy, 2003). One of the major concerns of the campaign was for PWE in resource poor settings, where the burden of the condition is not well recognized. In Sub-Saharan Africa, for instance, the prevalence of epilepsy is estimated to be much higher than Europe or North America, ranging between 14.5/1000 in Zambia (Birbeck and Kalichi, 2004) and 35/1000 in Benin (Debrock et al., 2000); compared to the North American/European average of 5-8/1000 (Laporte et al., 2006).

It is estimated that less than 15% of cases in resource poor countries are appropriately diagnosed (Meinardi, Scott, Reis, and Sander, 2001). Between 65-95% remain untreated and most of these are in rural areas (Baskind and Birbeck, 2005). Research into the reasons for under-reporting has focused largely on the public perceptions of PWE, internalized stigma associated with seizures and the discrimination against PWE (Carod and Vazquez-Cabrera, 1998; Dalrymple and Appleby, 2000; Doughty, Baker, Jacoby, and Lavaud, 2003; Jacoby, 2002; Tekle-Haimanot et al., 1991). While stigma is well established as a major challenge in the management of epilepsy, there is a limited understanding of the broader context in which the condition is experienced in resource poor settings and consequently how different contexts and identities of PWE affect the severity of the condition. How does the condition affect the daily lives of PWE and how do external, contextual factors interact and mitigate the lived experience? Are there gender differences in experiences; are the social networks and supports available in rural communities sufficient to overcome the psychosocial aspects of the condition? This paper describes an exploratory study of the social, cultural and environmental context of epilepsy experienced by a sample of PWE in Cameroon and the effects of the condition on their subjective wellbeing (SWB). The findings of the study provide potentially new ways of conceptualising the experience of epilepsy and alternative models for intervention to address the social forces that affect epilepsy management.

METHODS

The study was a cross-sectional, descriptive study, using both qualitative and quantitative methods to develop detailed descriptions of epilepsy in a developing country context.

Setting

The setting of the study was Cameroon, a central African country on the coast with a population of about 15.5 million people. Cameroon is typical of many developing countries, particularly in Africa, with approximately 30% unemployment and 40% of its population estimated to be living below the poverty line (the nominal USD$1 per day)(Central Intelligence Agency, 2000). It has a GDP per capita (purchasing power parity) of USD$2000 (Central Intelligence Agency, 2000) ranking it among the poorest countries in the world. English and French are the official languages, but there are approximately 24 local languages and dialects spoken throughout the country. The prevalence of epilepsy in Cameroon is estimated to exceed 30 per 1,000 and communities have identified the condition as being a major health concern (Kamgno, Pion, and Boussinesq, 2003).

Tertiary health facilities are provided in provincial and district hospitals, primary care is provided through integrated health centres. Health resources are limited with approximately one physician for every 8,000 persons (Preux et al., 2000). For most, particularly in rural communities, traditional healers still present the primary health care contact (Kamagno, Pion and Boussinesq, 2003).

Sample

There are often clear differences in the health indicators for rural and urban populations that relate to infrastructure, access to care, social support networks and geographical contexts (Reidpath, Allotey, Kouame, and Cummins, 2001). Rurality was therefore one of the variables identified for the research. Urban and rural samples were drawn from two independent sources. The urban sample was identified through a Catholic Health Centre in Yaoundé (Centre de Santé Mental Benoit). Most of the rural sample was drawn from villages along the Sanaga River north of Yaoundé – an area recorded as having a high prevalence of epilepsy; the reasons remain unclear (Kamgno, Pion, and Boussinesq, 2003; Nchoji Nkwi and Tioko Ndonko, 1989; Preux et al., 2000). The rural participants were identified by traditional healers and local health workers. Potential participants were contacted directly by the research team and asked if they would be willing to participate.

Criteria guiding inclusion were established for participation:

- Age 25-35 to cover peak years of productivity.
- Epilepsy (with patent seizures[1]) for at least five years.
- Living in the community.
- Seizure frequency: less than 1 seizure per day and more than 1 every 2 months[2]

Twenty of the participants came from urban Yaoundé and 22 were from its rural hinterland. Twenty-three (23) males (mean age =24.5, sd=4.9) and 19 females (mean age 24.2, sd=3.4) participated in the study (Table 1). All participants had a minimum of 3 years of primary education and there were 2 urban participants, both male, with tertiary education. Socio-economic status was also of potential interest. However as a result of the sampling strategy it was difficult to make that a specific inclusion criterion. Some data on socioeconomic status was collected based on estimated household income, which indicated that most of the participants were in a low income category (see Table 1). Two men were in paid employment and the rest of the sample either considered themselves invalids and unable to work (n=9), were studying (4 men and 5 women, all from the urban sample), were not and never had sought employment outside the home (8 women) or had been unable to obtain employment despite a desire to be employed (n=14).

Procedures

Participants were visited on two separate occasions. On the first visit, consent for participation was obtained, and where participants met the inclusion criteria, a first (structured) interview was conducted. The structured interview comprised a series of adapted scales, principally the SF12-(Ware, Kosinski, and Keller, 1998) to measure health related quality of life (HRQoL) and the Comprehensive Quality of Life Scale (ComQoL) to measure subjective wellbeing (SWB)(Cummins, 1997). Although it has been slightly modified since its use in this study (Cummins, 2005) the ComQoL was selected because it is a simply administered, highly researched and cross-culturally validated instrument for measuring SWB (Cummins, 1997). It is based on a 7-item scale in which each question is related to one of seven domains, of wellbeing, which have been proposed on both theoretical and empirical grounds (Cummins, 1997). Specifically, the scale measures satisfaction with material possessions, health, and achievement in life, relationships, safety, community, and happiness. When linearly transformed to a 100 point scale, it can be referenced to an international "gold standard" for SWB (Cummins, 1998).

[1] The criterion of patent seizures meant that witnesses could externally verify the occurrence of a seizure. This was particularly important for the inclusion because some of the participants reported that they had not seen a doctor.

[2] This criterion was introduced to assist in the identification of PWE in the absence of a clinical diagnosis.

Table 1. Characteristics of the Cameroon participants with epilepsy

	Urban	*Rural*	Total
Male - Income (monthly)			
<20,000 CFA(≈ US$38) - below the poverty line	1	6	7
20,000 – 50,000 CFA	4	5	9
50,000 – 100,000 CFA (≈ US$96) lower income	5	0	5
>100,000 CFA (≈ US$192) - middle income	2	0	2
Male Total	12	11	23
Female- Income (monthly)			
<20,000 CFA(≈ US$38) - below the poverty line	0	6	6
20,000 – 50,000 CFA	4	5	9
50,000 – 100,000 CFA (≈ US$96) lower income	2	0	2
>100,000 CFA (≈ US$192) - middle income	2	0	2
Female Total	8	11	19
Total	20	22	42

In the first interview, demographic information, and a brief clinical history were also recorded. At the end of the first interview participants were invited to engage in a longer in-depth interview. Thirty of the 42 participants agreed.

Photo Voice (Wang and Burris, 1997) was used to collect rich contextual, qualitative data for the second interview. Photo Voice is a participatory research technique that enables a compilation of visual images generated by the participant that provide insight into the factors that create their reality. Each of the 30 participants was provided with a disposable camera and instructed in its use. Participants were asked to take photographs depicting aspects of their daily lives, particularly focusing on how their health condition affected their functioning within their community. The disposable cameras were collected, and the films developed by the research team prior to the second interview. At the in-depth interviews, participants were asked to select six of the developed photographs based on the ones they perceived as most important to their lives. These were then used as prompts for the interviews. In addition, open ended questions were posed to explore the effects of gender and rurality on the experience of the condition.

Ethics

The research was approved by the Human Research Ethics Committee at The University of Melbourne, Australia and by the Research Ethics Committee at the Institut de Formation et de Reserches Demographiques (IFORD), the collaborating institution in Cameroon. All participants involved gave individual consent following a full description of the purpose of the study and the nature of their involvement. Separate consent was obtained for the use of Photo Voice. There were no adverse outcomes anticipated from the study and none were recorded.

Data Analysis

The SWB scores from the ComQoL were linearly transformed to lie on a 100 point scale. Exploratory and descriptive techniques were used in the analysis of the data, with a focus on relationships between the quality of life measures (SF12 and ComQoL), and gender and rurality. The analyses were also used to inform the analysis of the interview data, and vice-versa. The quantitative data were analysed using STATA, a statistical software package for quantitative data analysis, management and graphics (StataCorp, 2006).

Data from the in-depth interviews, supported by the photo voice data were analysed using a grounded theory approach (Schreiber, 2001), guided principally by the underlying assumption that gender and rurality would influence the experience of the condition. Coding was done by the lead field researcher in Cameroon and as well as one of the principal investigators (PA) who also verified consistencies in themes. Initial coding was done around the broad thematic areas of the seven domains of wellbeing in the ComQoL and inter-relationships between these areas and the broader gender and rurality categories were explored.

RESULTS

In the process of setting up the research, discussions with officials of the Cameroon Public Health Department highlighted the challenges they faced with the rise in chronic and non-communicable diseases including epilepsy. The lack of resources and the need to prioritise issues such as poverty alleviation meant that non-communicable disease were not included in the four top health priorities for 1998-2008 (Reidpath, Allotey, Kouame, and Cummins, 2001) and this was reflected in the availability and quality of health care for PWE, particularly for those in rural communities.

Quantitative Findings: Health and Wellbeing

There were no major differences between the rural and urban samples, including in socio-economic status. It is likely that those in a higher socio-economic group with epilepsy would not access services through the networks used to sample for this study and this is a clear limitation of the sampling strategy. All but six of the 42 participants were on anti-epileptic medication at the time of the interviews; four of the un-medicated participants came from the urban sample and two from the rural sample. The high treatment rate (85%) is not surprising again given the sampling strategy through health facilities and healers. As a result of poor diagnosis, national treatment figures are non-existent. However in a 10 year cohort study in a district within the same region of our study, 42% of identified PWE had been on medication at some stage during the follow up period although treatment had not been constant (Kamgno, Pion, and Boussinesq, 2003).

Reported compliance depended on affordability and availability at any particular point in time. Forty participants reported that although they took their medications as often as they could, it was not always possible to maintain a regular supply[3]. Rural participants had a long way to travel to the nearest available health centre and transportation was expensive. There were also occasions when the prescribed medication was not available at the health centre dispensary or at a private chemist's, or were not affordable. The problems with poor compliance are therefore predictable. Two of the rural participants were on traditional treatments and reported that for the cost of the pharmaceuticals, they were not sufficiently convinced of their efficacy to warrant the expense.

The time reported by participants since their last seizure is one, albeit imperfect, proxy measure of the severity of the epilepsy. Figure 1 shows a Kaplan-Meier style graph of the time since participant's experienced their last seizure. Fifty percent of participants had experienced a seizure within the 30 days prior to the first interview. A log-rank test for differences between survival curves shows no significant difference between the time since the last seizure for those on medication and those who were not (Chi-squared=2.67, df=1, p=.10) (Collett, 2003).

The average SWB (mean = 54.2, 95%CI: 49.2 - 59.3) was significantly lower than the "set point" of 60 to 70 anticipated by the work of Cummins (1998). Disaggregating the measure of SWB into its component dimensions allows one to examine the type of impact that epilepsy has on wellbeing. On might, for instance, imagine that the impact of epilepsy would lie exclusively in the domain of health rather than in other domains such as material goods, safety, or happiness.

Because the SWB scale is based on an equally weighted sum of the seven individual dimensions, all other things being equal one would expect that, on average, each of the dimensions would contribute equally to a person's overall sense of SWB. If this was the case then each dimension should contribute 14.3% (i.e., 100%/7) of the overall SWB score (or .143 as a proportion). Figure 2 shows a plot of the mean proportion (and 95% confidence intervals) of the SWB scores contributed by each of the individual dimensions – a reference line has been added at .143. It is known that in the sample, the mean level of SWB is significantly below the anticipated set-point. If the mean proportion was around .143 on all dimensions of wellbeing, it would indicate that wellbeing was uniformly affected by epilepsy. It is clear, however, that the impact of epilepsy is not evenly distributed across the dimensions. The two dimensions of Health and Relationships are outliers (see Figure 2). Health contributes significantly less to the overall SWB score and Relationships contribute significantly more, supporting the importance of exploring those social contextual factors in chronic disease. Explanations for the distribution are offered in the qualitative analysis and descriptions provided below.

The 12 items from the SF12 scale were not uniformly well completed and due to inconsistencies most of the data were excluded from the analysis. The reasons given by the research assistants included the lack of relevance to people's lives and difficulties in understanding the question. However, the first question of the SF12 which is the standard five-point scale of self-rated health, from "poor" through to "excellent", was completed by all participants. Sixty-two percent of participants (n=26) rated their health as "poor" and 90% (n=38) rated it as "poor" or "fair". The reasons for the low self-rated health are discussed later with reference to the qualitative data.

[3] The project team raised money to obtain medications for some of the respondents.

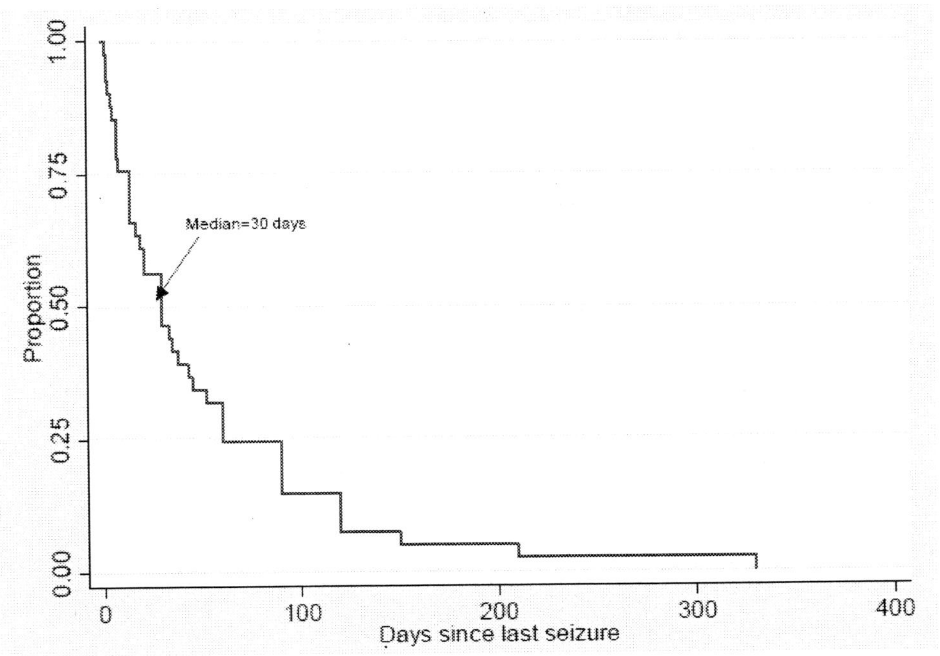

Figure 1. Time since last seizure.

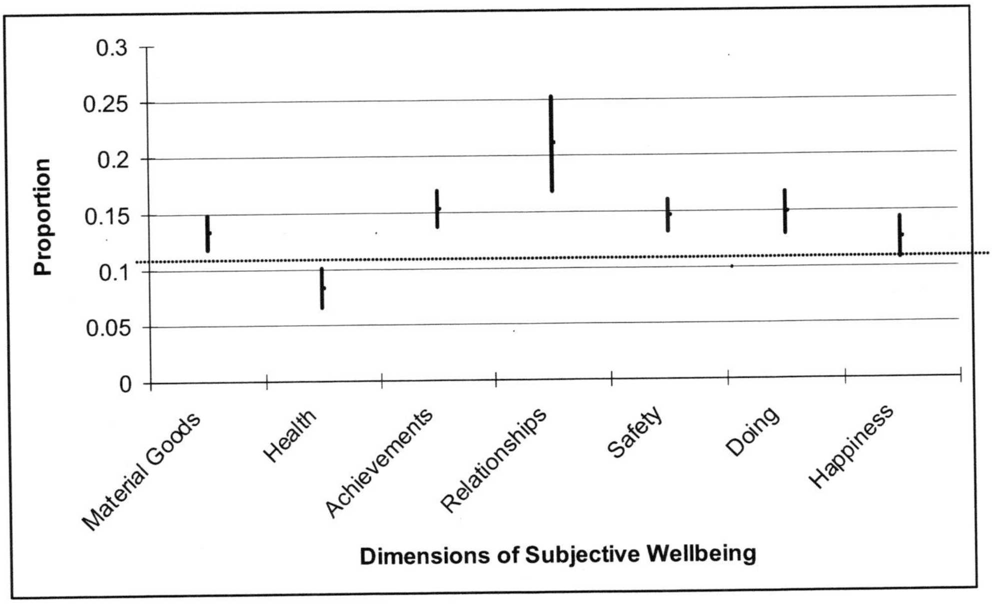

Figure 2. Reported subjective wellbeing across the 7 ComQoL domains.

There were no statistically significant differences between the mean SWB nor the self rated health of participants based on gender, socio-economic status or rurality.

QUALITATIVE FINDINGS: LIVING WITH EPILEPSY

1. Understanding Epilepsy – The Epileptic Identity

None of the participants was able to identify any specific pathology related to the cause of their seizures. Consistent with explanations in other studies in Sub-Saharan Africa most attributed their condition to supernatural forces including bad luck, jealousy, witchcraft, and divine punishment (Nchoji Nkwi and Tioko Ndonko, 1989; Tekle-Haimanot et al., 1991).

In their description of epilepsy, they talked specifically about the seizures. While they did not often recall details, the seizures were the central focus of what they understood the condition to be. There were also descriptions of heightened vulnerability to spirits, curses and other forms of evil during a seizure, in addition to physical injuries. All participants spoke of intense feelings of humiliation about the incontinence that occurred during seizures. For most, seizures were unpredictable but occurred about twice a month. However, in the descriptions of themselves as people living with epilepsy, the condition took on a greater role than just the seizures. Most identified themselves as "disabled," "chronically ill," and "always unwell".

I hardly go out, and when I do I can only go as far as the cock crows [the distance over which a cock's crow can be heard]. (female, 28 years, rural sample)

I have to be constantly bedridden because of this disease. (male 22 years old, urban sample)

Some described their non-seizure symptoms of epilepsy to include generalised itching and rash, sleepiness and dizziness. It would appear from the literature, however, that these symptoms are well-documented side effects of the anti-epileptic medication (Aiken and Brown, 2000; Diop, de Boer, Mandlhate, Prilipko, and Meinardi, 2003). The perception of the chronic nature of epilepsy was reinforced through the health care system. Participants reported that they were advised by medical and nursing staff to "take things easy." The formal advice also included the need to avoid exposure to the sun and all forms of strenuous exercise, including sexual intercourse. A range of dietary treatments and restrictions were also recommended, often by both health care workers and traditional healers suggesting that regardless of medical knowledge, traditional beliefs about the condition permeated both forms of care. Dietary treatments included substantial amounts of locally available herbs such as mistletoe and various tree barks mixed with palm oil. Administration was also in the form of smoke inhalations, baths and topical administration following abdominal scarification. There has been some toxicity reported from herbal preparations (Preux et al., 2000). Restrictions included high protein foods such as red meat, fish and eggs, and sweet foods such as sugarcane and sweet potatoes.

The identity assumed by the sick role heavily restricted the ability of the PWE to engage in productive activity. This was reinforced both by internalizing of the sick role, the constant tiredness and the supporting advice from health practitioners that they not engage in activities. For carers and other members of the community, therefore, a person diagnosed with epilepsy became a person to be supported; a consumer of resources who made limited or no contribution. Food restrictions and other dietary requirements increased the workload of carers again consuming extra social and economic resources.

2. Impact of Epilepsy on Daily Activities

While there were clear differences in the quality of experiences, being a PWE pervaded all aspects of the lives of the participants regardless of gender. This was evident in the descriptions of their roles and powerfully depicted by the images captured through PhotoVoice. For instance, they were culturally prohibited from approaching or crossing over large bodies of water. Explanations for this taboo range from a belief that looking into water may cause their "heads to turn and cause a fit," their presence could offend the spirits in and around the river, or more simply, they may drown if they had a seizure while in the water. Drowning has been identified as one of the top three causes of death in PWE. In a cohort study of 158 PWE, almost 20% of the 37 reported deaths were from drowning during a seizure (Kamgno, Pion, and Boussinesq, 2003). Sixteen participants in the sample in our study were from fishing families along the Sanaga River and eight had been fishermen prior to their first seizure. Their livelihoods were therefore removed (and diets restricted) once the diagnosis of epilepsy was established. In addition, those who lived in communities that required commuting over water became isolated from family and other supports.

Other situations that PWE were advised to avoid included exposure to direct sunlight and heights. Whereas heights may expose PWE to greater risk of injury from falls, there is no evidence that sunlight poses a risk. Quite the contrary, anti-epileptic medication is known to increase the metabolism of vitamin D, and lack of exposure to sunlight may increase these effects (Fitzpatrick, 2004).

Whether the restriction on activity is well-founded (heights) or based on local beliefs (sunlight), employment options for PWE is greatly reduced, particularly in manual jobs outdoors, including common casual occupations that involved tree climbing such as fruit picking and palm wine tapping. One participant had been in a white-collar job (with the presidential guard), but reported having problems with his memory. He eventually was relieved of his duties because of frequent time-off work and apparent vagueness.

The people I worked with said I am becoming more and more disturbed so they sent me away. For the moment they only call me when there is a serious thing that needs my attention. When I get there I only look and tell them what to do and then I come back. I have no opportunity to advance in the job because of this thing [epilepsy].

The inability to work made supporting families very difficult.

This illness has greatly paralyzed me, since I am doing nothing. I was driving but now I can't do it anymore because I am sick and I have fits [seizures] frequently, which hinders me from doing my work. My wife is no longer with me. You should know that with women, when one does not have money she cannot stay with you. (Male urban respondent – 29 years)

None of the women were in paid employment. However, even within the domestic environment, living with epilepsy presented restrictions in gendered role expectations. Women living with their families, particularly in the urban sample, were not allowed to go to the market unless accompanied by someone else - to ensure that they were safe, but also to avoid if possible, the disclosure of their condition to the wider community. The women were also concerned about the risk of burns because of the use of open fires for cooking during the day and for lighting at nights. The risk meant that cooking, an important domestic role was often not possible. Burns are a common co-morbidity of PWE, with injuries occurring particularly during seizures (Carod and Vazquez-Cabrera, 1998). Interestingly, with this sample, burns were almost equally reported in men (n=4) and women (n=3), although the men did not spontaneously raise burns as a concern associated with the condition. Research from other parts of Africa suggests that the presence of burn scars in PWE establishes a definitive mark that indicates that the condition is incurable and that both the physical and spiritual prognosis for the individual is poor (Baskind and Birbeck, 2005; Preux et al, 2000). The advice to avoid open fires is therefore taken very seriously.

3. Impact of Epilepsy on Relationships with Others

With the large focus on stigma in the epilepsy literature, we had anticipated poor performance on the relationships domain of the quality of life measure. In broad terms however, the participants in this study reported satisfaction with the relationships with people around them. This was expressed largely as gratitude for being looked after in spite of the disease (and an implied perception of unworthiness of the care). However, beyond the discussion about gratitude, details on relationships and social support varied considerably. There were no consistent differences between the rural and urban samples. The urban sample, in general felt more anonymous and unless they had had a public seizure, they were content not to be known as an 'epileptic.' However, they did report that they lacked strong close personal social supports. The participants in the rural communities generally lived with extended families in larger households. However there were also reports of family crises and rifts, with accusations of jealousy. Two participants reported that family members had used witchcraft to afflict them with epilepsy because of their potential for success or their successful achievement and relationships with those family members were no longer maintained.

A further concern, expressed more consistently by the male participants, was the effect that the restriction on sexual intercourse placed on development of relationships. Nineteen participants reported that they had to abstain from sexual intercourse on advice from their doctors. Fourteen of these were male and they expressed concern about what this abstinence also did to their self-esteem.

Because of this illness, I cannot get work and I have to stay home all the time. Now the doctors also say that I cannot bed a woman. What is my purpose in this life with only relatives to look after me all the time?

The medical doctors who are treating this condition forbid us from having sexual intercourse or sexual partners. Even the doctors know that you cannot have sex with this disease.

Concerns about close personal relationships for women participants were mostly related to marriage and children. There were eight single parents amongst the participants, all of whom were women and all of whom lived with their parents. The relationships ended for two main reasons: the partner found out late about the epilepsy; or had known about the condition but did not want to make the long term commitment that would be required following the birth of a child. Seizures remain a major reason for rejection of potential marital unions by families across Africa and this finding was consistent in this study (Kamgno, Pion, and Boussinesq, 2003).

As expected, stigmatization was raised as a major issue for the participants in both urban and rural areas and across genders. Most participants reported high levels of discrimination, with one of the urban participants reporting that "money does not stop the stigma of this disease". In other words, epilepsy is so stigmatising that wealth is not protective from the social opprobrium. Several participants also reported having been expelled from school because their seizures were considered disruptive to others in the classroom. Findings from other research support this experience (Kamgno, Pion, and Boussinesq, 2003). Thirty out of the 42 participants had their education interrupted as a result of seizures. They reported that they had been openly mocked and ridiculed even within their own homes, where they were occasionally not allowed to eat with the rest of the family. One of the participants reported:

The neighbours treated me like a mad person. They would not let me talk to their children because they were afraid I would contaminate them or something. And when I was in the street the children would point at me and say there is the mad man and shout at me to go away like a stray dog.

Participants in the urban areas generally reported that they thought stigma would be less in rural areas although this was not evident in the study. In spite of the reduced health care infrastructure in rural areas, five urban participants were keen to move there. They thought rural areas would also be safer given the lower levels of road traffic. There are no data however on seizure related car crashes so it is unclear how important this concern was.

Another woman from Yaoundé reported that moving to a rural area carried a greater risk of exposure to witchcraft during seizures. This statement supports a belief expressed by this participant that seizures were inflicted on people for the purpose of reducing their vulnerability to curses and witchcraft. Since witches were largely located in rural villages, this made living in Yaoundé a safer option for this participant. We were unable to ascertain in our study how widespread this belief was.

Discussion

The findings reported represent a cursory glimpse into the lives of 42 individuals with epilepsy in Cameroon. The findings do not address the complexities of the range of seizures, socio-economic backgrounds or pre-morbid social status of PWE. Limited resources also precluded a design that would enable the involvement of the broader social networks of PWE in the study. Nonetheless, the findings provide us some insights into the lives of those who identify and are identified as PWE.

Participants in the study took on an identity of a PWE; an identity that was largely defined by the restrictions imposed on them by traditional and clinical health systems and cultural beliefs and social attitudes to epilepsy. The internalization of chronically ill patient was evident in their self reported health status, in the subjective well being scores and in the qualitative data. Clinically however, the chronic sick role adopted within this identity appears to be unjustified. As previously described, with treatment, and in the absence of seizures, most PWE can engage in normal activities while avoiding situations which would harm them and others in case of a seizure (World Health Organization, International Bureau for Epilepsy, and International League Against Epilepsy, 1997).

However, the persistent structural barriers to treatment were evident. Poor access to anti-epileptic drugs made compliance with treatment difficult and for some, restrictions on movement also contributed to poor compliance. The time since last seizure graph provides a good illustration of the poor control of seizures in spite of treatment, with supporting qualitative data of the inability to maintain consistent treatment. Ensuring consistent access and compliance has been identified as one of the greatest challenges of epilepsy management (Preux et al., 2000) and is likely to be a problem in sub-Saharan Africa across a number of diseases that require long-term treatment.

For the participants in this study, their conformity to the culturally and structurally imposed restrictions, paradoxically also reduced their ability to perform their traditional roles, impacted on their social value and excluded them from engaging with the community. Societies function on the ability of individuals to undertake various roles and responsibilities within the community and the ability of individuals to undertake their roles is critical to being a worthy member (Reidpath, Chen, Gifford, and Allotey, 2005; Walzer, 1981). Identities such as gender, through which roles are undertaken, interact with other identities to mitigate one's social value. This was demonstrated for instance by the descriptions of inability neither to perform sexually nor to provide for the family.

The combined experiences described within the framework of social valuation and functioning status are useful for exploring the dynamics of stigmatization, particularly for conditions like epilepsy. Interventions to address stigmatization have traditionally focused on education campaigns to overcome ignorance, dispel myths about the condition and foster more positive attitudes towards PWE (Baskind and Birbeck, 2005; Diop, de Boer, Mandlhate, Prilipko, and Meinardi, 2003; Jilek-Aall, Jilek, Kaaya, Mkombachepa, and Hillary, 1997; Millogo and Siranyan, 2004). The advantage of this framework is that it offers the potential for interventions that could increase one's social value through identifying strategies that overcome obstacles to contributing to the community. It provides information on points at which structural barriers to effective functioning can be addressed. For instance, alternatives to open fires for cooking could be explored, as well as low technology devices for farming and protection to ensure continuing livelihoods. The argument for providing livelihoods is not necessarily new. However, there is a tendency in occupational therapy, particularly with those labeled as chronically ill or disabled, for alternative skills to be of low social value. In a study conducted at the same time with people with paraplegia in Cameroon, participants spoke about the tendency for rehabilitation to focus on providing them with skills that were not important (Reidpath, Allotey, Kouame, and Cummins, 2001). In describing their poor quality of life, for instance the men in the paraplegia study spoke about being taught tasks that were traditionally women's work. Others described performing skills at an equivalent level of children, having to make toys and mend shoes. Restoring function and capability to enable an increase in social value and choices for health are therefore critical.

Conclusion

The management and control of disease in resource poor settings in general and in Sub-Saharan Africa in particular is undoubtedly a major challenge. With a new focus on chronic diseases, there is a clear need for approaches that take into account the longer term demand not only on economic but also social resources. Addressing the resource problems will clearly go a long way to improving the availability and quality of care and the living conditions and contexts in which people live. However in the short term, there are strategies that can be adapted to begin to alleviate some of the suffering.

Current priorities in epilepsy management are to address the treatment gap (Coleman, Loppy, and Walraven, 2002; Diop, de Boer, Mandlhate, Prilipko, and Meinardi, 2003; Meinardi, Scott, Reis, and Sander, 2001), overcoming the stigma associated with the condition in order to increase diagnosis and treatment. However the focus needs to extend to the ongoing experiences of PWE. Epilepsy presents an identity of exclusion, which at multiple levels takes away the freedom to participate. Increasing the ability to participate in one's community at some level is an important feature of general wellbeing and quality of life.

ACKNOWLEDGMENTS

The research was funded by a grant from the Global Forum for Health Research. The authors would like to acknowledge Dr Aka Kouamé and Professor Robert Cummins who collaborated in the larger research project from which this paper draws and the research teams in Yaoundé and Melbourne who assisted in data collection. The research was conducted when PA was at the University of Melbourne and DDR was at Deakin University in Australia.

REFERENCES

Aiken, P. S., and Brown, W. M. (2000). Tretament of epilepsy: existing therapies and future developments. *Frontiers in Bioscience, 5*, e124-152.

Allotey, P., and Gyapong, M. (2005). The gender agenda in the control of tropical diseases: a review of current evidence. *The Special Topics in Social, Economic and Behavioural (SEB) Research, TDR/STR/SEB/ST/05.1*(4).

Baker, G. A. (2002). The psychosocial burden of epilepsy. *Epilepsia, 43*, 26-30.

Baskind, R., and Birbeck, G. (2005). Epilepsy care in Zambia: A study of traditional healers. *Epilepsia, 46*(7), 1121-1126.

Baskind, R., and Birbeck, G. L. (2005). Epilepsy-associated stigma in sub-Saharan Africa: The social landscape of a disease. *Epilepsy and Behavior, 7*(1), 68-73.

Birbeck, G. L., and Kalichi, E. M. N. (2004). Epilepsy prevalence in rural Zambia: a door-to-door survey. *Tropical Medicine and International Health, 9*(1), 92-95.

Carod, F. J., and Vazquez-Cabrera, C. (1998). Witchcraft and epilepsy in traditional indigenous medicine. *Revista De Neurologia, 26*(154), 1064-1068.

Central Intelligence Agency. (2000). CIA Worldbook of Facts. Retrieved 26.Jan.2001, 2001, from http://www.odci.gov/cia/publications/factbook/geos/cm.html

Coleman, R., Loppy, L., and Walraven, G. (2002). The treatment gap and primary health care for people with epilepsy in rural Gambia. *Bulletin of the World Health Organization, 80*(5), 378-383.

Collett, D. (2003). *Modelling Survival Data in Medical Research* (2nd Edition ed.). Boca Raton, FL: Chapman and Hall.

Cummins, R. A. (1997). Assessing quality of life for people with disabilities. In R. I. Brown (Ed.), *Quality of Life for Handicapped People* (pp. 116-150). Cheltenham, UK: Stanley Thomas.

Cummins, R. A. (1998). The second approximation to an international standard of life satisfaction. *Social Indicators Research, 43*, 307-334.

Cummins, R. A. (2005). Moving from the quality of life concept to a theory. *Journal of Intellectual Disability Research, 49*(10), 699-706.

Dalrymple, J., and Appleby, J. (2000). Cross sectional study of reporting of epileptic seizures to general practitioners. *BMJ, 320*(7227), 94-97.

Debrock, C., Preux, P. M., Houinato, D., Druet-Cabanac, M., Kassa, F., Adjien, C., et al. (2000). Estimation of the prevalence of epilepsy in the Benin region of Zinvie using the capture-recapture method. *International Journal of Epidemiology, 29*(2), 330-335.

Diop, A. G., de Boer, H. M., Mandlhate, C., Prilipko, L., and Meinardi, H. (2003). The global campaign against epilepsy in Africa. *Acta Tropica, 87*(1), 149-159.

Doughty, J., Baker, G. A., Jacoby, T., and Lavaud, V. (2003). Cross-cultural differences in levels of knowledge about epilepsy. *Epilepsia, 44*(1), 115-123.

Faircloth, C. A. (1998). Epilepsies, identities, and difference: Horizons of meaning for individuals with an epilepsy. *Qualitative Health Research, 8*(5), 602-617.

Fitzpatrick, L. A. (2004). Pathophysiology of bone loss in patients receiving anticonvulsant therapy. *Epilespy and Behavior, 5*(Suppl 2), S3-15.

Global Campaign against Epilepsy. (2003). *Epilepsy. Out of the Shadows*. Heemstede, The Netherlands: International League Against Epilepsy / World Health Organization / International Bureau for Epilepsy.

Groce, N., and Scheer, J. (1990). Cross-Cultural Perspectives on Disability - Introduction. *Social Science and Medicine, 30*(8), R5-R6.

Groce, N. E. (1985). *Everyone here spoke sign language: Hereditary deafness on Martha's Vineyard*. Boston: Harvard University Press.

Jacoby, A. (2002). Stigma, epilepsy, and quality of life. *Epilepsy and Behavior, 3*(6), S10-S20.

Jacoby, A., Snape, D., and Baker, G. A. (2005). Epilepsy and social identity: the stigma of a chronic neurological disorder. *Lancet Neurology, 4*(3), 171-178.

Jilek-Aall, L., Jilek, M., Kaaya, J., Mkombachepa, L., and Hillary, K. (1997). Psychosocial study of epilepsy in Africa. *Social Science and Medicine, 45*(5), 783-795.

Kamgno, J., Pion, S. D. S., and Boussinesq, M. (2003). Demographic impact of epilepsy in Africa: Results of a 10-year Cohort study in a rural area of Cameroon. *Epilepsia, 44*(7), 956-963.

Kiyaga, N. B., and Moores, D. F. (2003). Deafness in sub-Saharan Africa. *American Annals of the Deaf, 148*(1), 18-24.

Komter, A. E. (1996). Reciprocity as a Principle of Exclusion: Gift Giving in the Netherlands. *Sociology, 30*(2), 299-316.

Kwan, P., and Sander, J. W. (2004). The natural history of epilepsy: an epidemiological view. *J Neurol Neurosurg Psychiatry, 75*(10), 1376-1381.

Laporte, A., Rouvel-Tallec, A., Grosdidier, E., Carpentier, S., Benoit, C., Gerard, D., et al. (2006). Epilepsy among the homeless: prevalence and characteristics. *Eur J Public Health*, ckl011.

Meinardi, H., Scott, R. A., Reis, R., and Sander, J. (2001). The treatment gap in epilepsy: The current situation and ways forward. *Epilepsia, 42*(1), 136-149.

Millogo, A., and Siranyan, A. S. (2004). Knowledge of epilepsy and attitudes towards the condition among schoolteachers in Bobo-Dioulasso (Burkina Faso). *Epileptic Disorders, 6*(1), 21-26.

Murray, C. J. L., and Lopez, A. D. (Eds.). (1996). *The Global Burden of Disease* (Vol. 1). Cambridge, MA: Harvard School of Public Health.

Nchoji Nkwi, P., and Tioko Ndonko, F. (1989). The epileptic among the Bamileke of Maham in the NDE Division, West Province of Cameroon. *Culture, Medicine and Psychiatry, 13*(4), 437-448.

Nubukpo, P., Clement, J. P., Houinato, D., Radji, A., Grunitzky, E. K., Avode, G., et al. (2004). Psychosocial issues in people with epilepsy in Togo and Benin (West Africa) - II: Quality of life measured using the QOLIE-31 scale. *Epilepsy and Behavior, 5*(5), 728-734.

Olusanya, B., Luxon, L., and Wirz, S. (2005). Screening for early childhood hearing loss in Nigeria. *J Med Screen, 12*(3), 115-118.

Preux, P. M., Tiemagni, F., Fodzo, L., Kandem, P., Ngouafong, P., Ndonko, F., et al. (2000). Antiepileptic therapies in the Mifi Province in Cameroon. *Epilepsia, 41*(4), 432-439.

Reidpath, D., Chen, K., Gifford, S., and Allotey, P. (2005). He hath the french pox: stigma, social value and social exclusion. *Sociology of Health and Illness, 27*(4), 468-489.

Reidpath, D. D., Allotey, P. A., Kouame, A., and Cummins, R. A. (2001). *Social, Cultural and Environmental Contexts and the Measurement of the Burden of Disease: An Exploratory Study in the Developed and Developing World.* Melbourne: Key Centre for Women's Health in Scoiety, The University of Melbourne.

Schachter, S. (2003). Overview of epilepsy and seizures. In S. Schachter and L. Anderman (Eds.), *The brain storms village: epilepsy in our world* (pp. 1-4). Philadelphia Lippincott, Williams and Wilkins.

Scheer, J., and Groce, N. (1988). Impairment as a Human Constant - Cross-Cultural and Historical Perspectives on Variation. *Journal of Social Issues, 44*(1), 23-37.

Schreiber, R. (2001). The 'how to' of grounded theory: Avoiding the pitfalls. In R. Schreiber and P. Noerager Stern (Eds.), *Using Grounded Theory in Nursing* (pp. 55–84). New York: Springer Publishing.

StataCorp (2006). Stata SE 9.2 College Station, TX: StataCorp.

Tekle-Haimanot, R., Abebe, M., Forsgren, L., Gebre-Mariam, A., Heijbel, J., Holmgren, G., et al. (1991). Attitudes of rural people in central Ethiopia toward epilepsy. *Social Science and Medicine, 32*(2), 203-209.

Temkin, O. (1971). *The falling sickness*. Baltimore: Johns Hopkins Press.

Trivers, R. L. (1971). The evolution of reciprocal altruism. *Quarterly Review of Biology, 46*, 35-57.

Walzer, M. (1981). The distribution of membership. In P. G. Brown and H. Shue (Eds.), *Boundaries: National Autonomy and its Limits* (pp. 1-35). Totowa, NJ: Rowman and Littlefield.

Wang, C., and Burris, M. A. (1997). Photovoice: concept, methodology, and use for participatory needs assessment. *Health Educ. Behav., 24*(3), 369-387.

Ware, J. E., Kosinski, M., and Keller, S. D. (1998). *SF-12: How to Score the SF-12 Physical and Mental Health Summary Scales*. Boston, MA: Health Assessment Lab., New England Medical Centre.

World Health Organization, International Bureau for Epilepsy, and International League Against Epilepsy. (1997). *Global Campaign Against Epilepsy: Out of the shadows.* Geneva: WHO, IBE, ILAE.

This paper has been published in the Journal of Health Psychology, 12(3), 431-443, 2007 http://online.sagepub.com

In: Social Epileptology
Editors: J. Pinikahana and C. Walker
ISBN 978-1-60876-228-6

Chapter 9

KNOWLEDGE, ATTITUDES AND EPILEPSY

John O. Elliott*[*,1], Sheri Hart[1] and Christine Charyton[2]
[1]The Ohio State University, Department of Neurology
395 West 12th Avenue, 7th Floor
Columbus, Ohio, United States, 43210
[2]The Ohio State University, Department of Psychology
1827 Neil Avenue, 130 Lazenby Hall
Columbus, Ohio, United States, 43210

ABSTRACT

In 2002, a global campaign organized by the International League Against Epilepsy (ILAE) was called to bring epilepsy "out of the shadows". An extensive amount of international literature has been published regarding knowledge and attitudes towards epilepsy over the past 50 years. Of specific interest are studies of the general population and educational settings (teachers/student peers). While knowledge and attitudes vary widely in different regions of the world, common themes in the population research emerge. In general, the populations in developing countries have less knowledge and more negative attitudes towards epilepsy. Prospective studies in the U.S., Germany, Hungary and Korea have found improvements in knowledge over time, but more modest changes in negative attitudes. More enlightened attitudes in the U.S. are thought to be related to an overall improvement in public attitudes towards diseases; improved control of seizures by medication, educational efforts by professional and lay societies regarding epilepsy; employment by a number of major industries of persons with epilepsy and more reasonable legal regulations concerning immigration, marriage and motor vehicle licenses. Knowledge and attitudes are mediated by socio-cultural factors as well as by personal experience. Educational settings are thought to be ideal for interventions to improve knowledge and attitudes towards epilepsy in the general population. The international literature suggests teachers also have limited knowledge and attitudes that promote stigma. Most teachers indicate an interest in learning more about epilepsy. The reduction of health related stigma in school settings would go a long way to improving acceptance and dispelling centuries old myths. Education about epilepsy in the school

* Telephone: 614-293-6219; Fax: 614-293-4688; Email: john.elliott@osumc.edu

setting would also go a long way to improve educational outcomes for PWE. To improve public knowledge of epilepsy and to overcome negative attitudes, social marketing approaches have been suggested. These include protesting inaccurate depictions of people with epilepsy (PWE) in the media, education of PWE and key social groups as well as increasing the public's contact with PWE. Education and social marketing programs alone are not cost effective or sustainable without substantial funding and high levels of political will. Continued advocacy by PWE, health professionals and epilepsy support organizations is vital for improving knowledge and beliefs in the general public.

INTRODUCTION

The history of epilepsy has been summarized by one writer as "4,000 years of ignorance, superstition and stigma followed by 100 years of knowledge, superstition and stigma" (Kale, 1997). Persons with epilepsy (PWE) not only have to cope with the complex demand of a chronic illness, but also have to deal with health-related stigma and prejudice in employment and education. Health–related stigma has been defined by Weiss and Ramakrishna (2006) as "a social process or related personal experience characterized by exclusion, rejection, blame or devaluation that result from experience or reasonable anticipation of an adverse social judgment about a person or group identified with a particular health problem." (p. 536). Of the 40 million PWE worldwide, 80% live in developing countries (Institute of Medicine, 2001). With proper medical treatment, seizures can be controlled in approximately 70% of cases (Allotey and Reidpath, 2007). PWE in developed countries have significantly better access to treatment, however in developing countries, the World Health Organization has estimated that 80% to 90% of PWE receive inadequate or no treatment (Scott, Lhatoo, and Sander, 2001; Shorvon and Farmer, 1988).

A global campaign organized by the International League Against Epilepsy (ILAE) in 2002 was called to bring epilepsy "out of the shadows". Keys objectives were stated as: 1) to increase awareness among health professionals and the general public of epilepsy as a universal and treatable brain disorder, 2) to raise epilepsy to a new plane of acceptability in the public domain, 3) to improve education about epilepsy, 4) to identify the needs of people with epilepsy and 5) to encourage governments to address the needs of people with epilepsy. If negative population attitudes towards epilepsy could be eradicated through public education it would act as primary prevention of many psychiatric and social consequences of epilepsy just as the reduction of birth trauma, brain infections and accidents would prevent many cases of epilepsy from developing at all (Bagley, 1972).

An extensive amount of international literature has been published regarding knowledge and attitudes towards epilepsy over the past 50 years. A literature review was completed using electronic searches through PubMed (http://www.ncbi.nlm.nih.gov) of "epilepsy" combined with "knowledge", "beliefs" and "attitudes". These searches resulted in 1,895 hits for knowledge, 1,054 for attitudes and 1,274 for attitudes. These were separated into five themes: population research, patients, health professionals, schools (teachers and students) and educational programs targeted towards epilepsy. This chapter will focus on two areas: population research and school settings (teachers and students). For interested readers a previously published review by the authors covered health professionals, caregivers and patients (Elliott and Shneker, 2008).

While knowledge and attitudes vary widely in different regions of the world, common themes in the population research emerge. These focus on 1) whether people are familiar with epilepsy, 2) if they know anyone with epilepsy, 3) if they seen anyone have a seizure, 4) whether they object to their children playing with someone who has epilepsy, 5) if they consider persons with epilepsy be employed in the same jobs as those without epilepsy, 6) epilepsy as a mental illness and 7) what they regard as the causes of epilepsy.

A discussion of interventions for the general population as well as where future efforts should be targeted would be beneficial to the epilepsy community. Thus we hope the literature review presented in this chapter will benefit health professionals (neurologists, epileptologists, psychiatrists, general practitioners, psychologists, social workers) and staff in epilepsy associations, epilepsy foundations and epilepsy societies around the world who are working with people with epilepsy.

GENERAL POPULATION RESEARCH

Surveys of public attitudes help identify misconceptions and misperceptions. Such information also helps in suggesting what efforts may alleviate the problems that come from misinformation. Epilepsy continues to be shrouded in misinformation (McLin and de Boer, 1995). Throughout history persons with epilepsy have been stigmatized by misperceptions such as being possessed by evil spirits. In developing countries epilepsy is often thought to be infectious (Andermann, 1995). Stigma in epilepsy is thought to be the result of information management (what to disclose about their condition and to whom). The process of concealing epilepsy is not always voluntary. This leads to planning in order to avoid high-risk situations that could lead to disclosure. These factors contribute to feelings of stigma (Jacoby, Baker, Steen, Potts, and Chadwick, 1996). However for stigmatization to continue to affect the individual with epilepsy they must accept society's devaluation (McLin and de Boer, 1995). Persons with epilepsy will be less able to overcome such stereotypes while society's collective beliefs, which vary dramatically around the world, are accepted. Stereotypes and discriminatory behaviors in epilepsy result not from the individual's abilities but those ascribed to the group. Attitudes towards people with epilepsy are thought to be influenced by the degree of knowledge people have about the condition.

A study of perceptions about stigma, education and public awareness from the perspective of PWE found 89% did not believe the general public was well-informed about epilepsy (Paschal et al., 2007). When asked what the most common misperceptions were; 63% ranked "People do not know how to react to seizures" followed by "All epilepsy patients experience severe seizures" 51%, "Epilepsy is a mental illness" 37%, "Epilepsy is passed from parent to child" 22%, "Epilepsy is contagious" 20% and "Persons with epilepsy should be avoided" 19%. When asked what methods would be the most effective for educating the general public, 52% ranked television advertisements, 47% information in doctor's offices, 42% workplace programs, 38% educational pamphlets, 24% radio advertisements, 23% billboards and 18% extension services (Paschal et al., 2007).

United States

In the United States, Caveness and Gallup conducted a series of seven surveys of persons > age 21, every five years, over a thirty year period from 1949 to 1979 (Caveness, 1949; Caveness, 1954; Caveness, 1960; Caveness, Merritt, Gallup, and Ruby, 1965; Caveness, Merritt, and Gallup, 1969; Caveness, Merritt, and Gallup, 1974; Caveness and Gallup, 1980). The surveys were conducted with assistance from George Gallup and the American Institute of Public Opinion who were well known for conducting public election polls. A set of questions were developed that focus on 1) whether people are familiar with epilepsy, 2) do they know anyone with epilepsy, 3) have they seen anyone have a seizure, 4) would they object to their children playing with someone who has epilepsy, 5) should persons with epilepsy be employed in the same jobs as those without epilepsy, 6) is epilepsy a mental illness and 7) what are the causes of epilepsy. A summary of the U.S. results are displayed in Table 1.

Knowledge and attitudes towards epilepsy improved dramatically over the 30 years. The percentage of people who reported they had heard or read about epilepsy remained high > 90%. Over time, more people indicated they knew someone with epilepsy (57% in 1949 vs. 63% in 1979). The percentage who reported they had seen a seizure stayed in the 56 to 61% range. The percentage of people reporting they would object to their children associating with child with epilepsy decreased from 24% to 6%. Although, 18% reported they objected to their son or daughter marrying a person with epilepsy, this question was only asked in 1979. The percentage of people who reported they objected to employment for persons with epilepsy decreased from 35% to 9%. The perception that epilepsy was a mental illness also dropped from 13% to 3%. Caveness and Gallup were also interested in tackling if people knew the causes of epilepsy. In general, more people reported knowing appropriate causes of epilepsy over the course of the surveys (43% vs. 61%).

To follow up on the work of Caveness, a Gallup survey was conducted in 1987 by LaMartina in conjunction with the Epilepsy Foundation of America (LaMartina, 1989). Results were similar in terms of the percentage of people who reported they had heard or read about epilepsy (92%), however 16% indicated they believed that epilepsy was a form of mental illness. LaMartina asked more detailed questions about attitudes towards specific career choices for persons with epilepsy. Between 9 and 13% of respondents believed PWE should not be employed in jobs such as a supervisor, jobs that involved handling food, teaching school and acting as an elected official. A much larger percentage believed PWE should not be employed in the armed forces (41%) or in a job that involved driving a bus or a truck (66%). When asked about treatment, 82% knew that prescription medications were one way of controlling epilepsy, but 68% said they would place something hard between the teeth and 52% said they would restrain or hold a person down during a seizure.

Recent U.S. studies have assessed knowledge, attitudes and beliefs through other methods. The Centers for Disease Control (CDC) HealthStyles Survey assessed epilepsy knowledge in the general population through a mail-based survey targeted to a representative sample (Kobau and Price, 2003). Twenty-five percent of the 4,397 respondents considered themselves knowledgeable about epilepsy. Thirty percent indicated they knew someone with epilepsy. Half indicated they had witnessed a seizure first hand and 57% said they had seen a seizure on television. However, only one-third indicated they knew what to do if someone had a seizure. Respondents indicated they had primarily heard about epilepsy through friends or family or through television.

In response, the CDC has funded other projects to develop other measures for use in population research such as the "Attitudes and Beliefs about Living with Epilepsy" instrument (DiIorio et al., 2004; Kobau, DiIorio, Anderson, and Price, 2006). Participants with less education had more negative attitudes. Attitudes towards treatment were favorable; 75% believed with treatment most people can go a year or more without a seizure; 76% felt that for most people doctors can prevent seizures with drugs and 82% felt for most people with epilepsy, seizures are well controlled with drug treatment. As for symptoms of epilepsy, 33% thought every time a person has a seizure they have convulsions, only 12% thought all people have the same type of seizure, 33% thought all people with epilepsy lose consciousness, 85% recognized that some seizures may last only a few seconds, 67% recognized that a person can have a warning before a seizure and 75% recognized that stress may cause some seizures. Misperceptions were also found; 16% of 651 respondents felt epilepsy was a type of mental illness, 73% thought there is a high likelihood of death every time someone has a seizure and 66% thought you should put something in a person's mouth during a seizure (DiIorio et al., 2004). Television programs have a big influence on knowledge and attitudes towards epilepsy in the United States. Unfortunately, much of this influence has been tainted with inaccuracies.

A follow up validation study of 4,345 participants in a stratified random sample from the ConsumerStyles mail survey found 83% moderately or strongly disagreed with the statement "I believe people with epilepsy are not as smart as other people who do not have epilepsy" (Kobau, DiIorio, Anderson, and Price, 2006). Roughly 4% of respondents moderately or strongly agreed that people with epilepsy should not marry. Four percent moderately or strongly agreed with the statement "I believe people with epilepsy are mentally ill." Participants had more mixed views of risk and safety concerns related to driving, operating heavy machinery or babysitting a child for PWE.

In a recent assessment of the U.S. population, significantly less Hispanics were knowledgeable about epilepsy compared to the non-Hispanic population (Sirven, Lopez, Vazquez, and Van Haverbeke, 2005). However, in comparison to the previous U.S. studies significantly higher percentages of both populations believed epilepsy was hereditary. The Hispanic population was also more likely to perceive epilepsy to be caused by eating undercooked meat, lack of spiritual faith, lack of intelligence, evil spirits or from being in close proximity to someone with epilepsy. U.S. Hispanics were also more likely to overprotect someone with epilepsy (68% vs. 11%). Culturally, some of these differences may be the result of Hispanic Americans being more likely to seek help for somatic complaints than for psychological concerns (Koss, 1990).

A small study of misperceptions of persons at a shopping mall (n = 202) which is not shown in Table 1 found 49% believed people with epilepsy have more personality problems than people in general (Gouvier, Brown, Prestholdt, and Hayes, 1995). Low rates of misconceptions were found in everyday activities such as persons with epilepsy cannot marry and have children (3%) or need to restrict themselves to sedentary sports (9%). Sixty-four percent believed forcing something hard between the teeth was appropriate first aid and many endorsed restraining a person during a seizure. Forty-six percent believed that seizure medicines were dangerously addictive.

Table 1. Public knowledge and attitudes towards epilepsy - United States

Question		1949 (n=2,696)	1 954 (n=1,511)	1 959 (n= 1,520)	1 964 (n=1,600)	1 969 (n=1,551)	1 974 (n=2,682)	1 979 (n=1,539)	1 987 (n=1,002)	2 002 (n=4,397)	2 004 (n=651)	2 004 (n=760) H ispanic	2 004 (n=272) non-Hispanic	2 006 (n=4,345)
		Percentage answering "yes"												
1.	Ever heard/read about epilepsy	92	90	93	95	94	94	95	92	-	-	79	93	-
2.	Knows someone with epilepsy	57	-	-	61	65	62	63	56	34	-	49	47	-
3.	Has seen a seizure	56	-	-	59	59	61	59	-	52	-	-	-	-
4.	Objects to children associating	24	22	18	9	9	5	6	-	-	-	-	-	-
5.	Objects to marriage	-	-	-	-	-	-	18	-	-	-	-	-	4
6.	Objects to employment	35	22	11	9	12	8	9	-	-	-	-	-	-
7.	Epilepsy is a mental illness	13	7	4	4	4	2	3	16	-	16	-	-	4
8.	Epilepsy is contagious	-	-	-	-	-	-	-	-	-	-	6	1	-
9.	What do you think is the cause of epilepsy													
	Don't know	57	-	58	39	40	41	39	49	-	-	55	64	-
	Nervous system disease	18	-	16	17	14	16	16	12	-	-	-	-	-
	Brain disease, disorder	4	-	11	21	16	10	20	19	-	78	63	47	-
	Hereditary or birth defect	12	-	13	10	19	15	15	11	-	-	61	56	-
	Other diseases, injury	3	-	4	11	7	7	7	4	-	-	58	53	-
	Mental or emotional	1	-	-	4	4	3	2	-	-	-	-	-	-
	Blood disorders	2	-	1	3	3	2	1	-	-	-	-	-	-
	Miscellaneous	7	-	4	2	2	4	2	5	-	-	-	-	-

Table 2. Public knowledge and attitudes towards epilepsy - Europe

	Percentage answering "yes"																		
	Poland	Finland	Italy	Denmark	New Zealand	Hungary	Hungary	Austria	Greece	Czech Republic	Czech Republic	Switzerland	England	England	Bosnia Herzegovina				
	1970	1 980	1 985	1 992	1 997	1 994	2 000	2 000	2 006	1 981	2 002	2 003	1 969	2 004	2 008				
Question	(n=1,370)	(n=2,272)	(n=1,043)	(n=1,038)	(n=400)	(n=1,000)	(n=1,000)	(n=2,128)	(n=750)	(n=372)	(n=235)	(n=2,053)	(n=NR)	(n=1,694)	(n=1,000)				
10. Ever heard/read about epilepsy	95	95	73	97	95	92	94	89	94	78	94	92	-	99	91				
11. Knows someone with epilepsy	57	49	61	60	73	56	52	40	39	-	-	68	-	-	41				
12. Has seen a seizure	77	45	52	50	67	58	55	36	51	-	-	60	-	-	33				
13. Object to children associating	15	19	11	7	2	19	17	11	14	29	13	2	15	5	15				
14. Object to marriage	51	-	-	-	5	53	41	15	66	-	-	5	-	6	-				
15. Object to employment	36	-	15	11	55	38	41	9	58	26	26	23	7		-				
16. Epilepsy is a mental illness	40	-	8	-	1	15	17	11	15	50	29	4	-	19	6				
17. Epilepsy a type of MR	-	-	-	-	-	-	-	-	19	-	-	-	-	-	-				
18. Supernatural phenomena	-	-	-	-	-	-	-	-	5	-	-	-	-	-	-				
19. Never or rarely cured	-	-	31	-	-	-	-	-	-	78	-	-	-	-	-				
20. High risk of passing it on	-	-	-	-	-	-	-	-	58	-	-	-	-	-	-				
21. Children attend normal school	-	-	-	-	-	-	-	-	-	-	-	9	0	-	-	-			
22. What do you think is the cause																			
Don't know	20	36	16	27	32	20	45	29	14	-	-	6	-	-	56				
Nervous system disease	49	-	2	8	-	8	-	-	4	1	67	-	-	6	0	-	5	0	2
Brain disease, disorder	39	-	10	33	39	42	12	25	92	-	-	46	-	57	1				
Hereditary	-	-	11	37	7	12	2	22	43	-	-	35	-	-	17				
Birth defect	-	-	10	27	2	1	10	6	32	-	-	20	-	-	-				
Accidents	36	-	-	22	-	-	-	-	-	-	-	-	-	44	-				
Other diseases, injury	-	-	1	-	-	3	-	-	-	-	-	-	-	-	-				
Mental or emotional	11	-	-	6	-	20	25	11	32	-	-	26	-	13	2				
Blood disorders	-	-	-	2	-	1	-	2	4	-	-	3	-	-	-				
Miscellaneous	7	-	-	6	-	4	-	-	17	-	-	2	-	-	-				

Notes: MR = mental retardation. While New Zealand is in the South Pacific, we chose to group it with Europe since it is Western country based on similar language and customs. NR = sample size not reported.

College graduates and people with postgraduate education had fewer misperceptions compared to those with less than a high school education. The most cited sources of information about epilepsy were friends (36%), weekly magazines (31%), documentaries (22%) and movies or drama (20%).

As a whole the consecutive U.S. surveys suggest as knowledge of the causes of epilepsy increases it results in more positive attitudes. In many studies a more detailed breakdown of the questions by demographics found less knowledge and poorer attitudes in those with less education, older age, manual workers and those who live in the Southern region of the United States. Residents of metropolitan areas also have more favorable attitudes (Baumann, Wilson, and Wiese, 1995).

Europe

Based on the research conducted by Caveness and Gallup, many surveys have been conducted in Europe using the similar questions (Bagic, Bagic, and Zivkovic, 2009; Canger and Cornaggia, 1985; Diamantopoulos, Kaleyias, Tzoufi, and Kotsalis, 2006; Hills and MacKenzie, 2002; Iivanainen, Uutela, and Vilkkumaa, 1980; Jacoby, Gorry, Gamble, and Baker, 2004; Jensen and Dam, 1992; Krämer, 2003; Mirnics, Czikora, Zavecz, and Halasz, 2001; Novotna and Rektor, 2002; Office of Health Economics, 1971; Spatt et al., 2005; Zielinski, 1974). The results of the European surveys are displayed in Table 2.

The percentage of people who reported they had heard or read about epilepsy ranged from 73% in Italy (1985) to 99% in England (2004). Overall the percentage of Europeans (excluding Germany) who had heard or read about epilepsy was 91%. The percentage of people who reported they knew someone with epilepsy ranged from 39% in Greece (2006) to 73% in New Zealand (1997). Overall the percentage of people in European countries (we have included New Zealand based on language and customs) who report knowing someone with epilepsy was 54%. The percentage of people who reported witnessing a seizure ranged from 36% in Austria (2000) to 77% in Poland (1974) with an average of 53% across countries. The percentage of respondents reporting that they would object to their child associating with a child who has epilepsy ranged from 2% in New Zealand (1997) and Switzerland (2003) to 29% in the Czech Republic (1981), with an average of 13% overall. Objections to marriage ranged dramatically in Europe from 5% in Switzerland and New Zealand to 66% in Greece. Negative attitudes towards employment ranged dramatically from 7% in England (2004) to 58% in Czech Republic. The belief that epilepsy is a form of mental illness ranged dramatically from 1% in New Zealand to 50% in the Czech Republic (1981). The percentage of people who indicated they didn't know the cause of epilepsy ranged from 6% in Switzerland to 56% in Boznia/Herzegovina (2009).

Several countries conducted follow up surveys. In England between 1969 and 2004 there was a significant drop in negative attitudes towards employment of PWE and children associating with another child with epilepsy (Jacoby et al., 2004; Office of Health Economics, 1971). Hungary conducted two public surveys 6 years apart and found a significant drop in negative attitudes towards employment and marriage of PWE, but no change in attitudes towards children associating with another child with epilepsy (Mirnics et al., 2001). The Czech Republic conducted a survey of public attitudes in 1981 and 1997-1998 (Novotna and

Rektor, 2002) of persons attending a secondary dentistry clinic at a university medical school. While the location of the study was the same it was not population based.

Germany

West Germany conducted random probability sample research of public attitudes using the same methodology as the U.S. studies by Caveness; see Table 3 (Diehl, 1975; Diehl and Hauck, 1975; Thorbecke, 1987; Finke, 1981; Hauck, 1968). There was little change in the percentage of people who reported they had ever heard or read about epilepsy with an average of 86%. The percentage of people reporting they would object to their children associating with another child with epilepsy dropped from 37% in 1967 to 15% in 1996. The percentage of people objecting to employment also dropped from 31% in 1976 to 11% in 1996, while the percentage who reported they believed epilepsy was a mental illness has not dropped much between 1967 and 1996 (27% to 20%).

Table 3. Public knowledge and attitudes towards epilepsy - Germany

	Percentage answering "yes"				
	West Germany 1967	West Germany 1973	West Germany 1978	West Germany 1984	West Germany 1996
Question	(n=NR)	(n=1,998)	(n=2,007)	(n=2,023)	(n=NR)
23. Ever heard/read about epilepsy	84	88	90	83	86
24. Knows someone with epilepsy	-	-	-	33	41
25. Has seen a seizure	-	-	-	32	38
26. Object to children associating	37	27	23	23	15
27. Object to marriage	-	-	-	30	21
28. Object to employment	31	21	20	18	11
29. Epilepsy is a mental illness	27	31	23	25	20
30. What do you think is the cause					
Don't know	-	-	-	30	21
Nervous system disease	-	-	-	33	33
Brain disease, disorder	-	-	-	29	29
Hereditary	-	-	-	-	25
Birth defect	-	-	-	12	-
Accidents	-	-	-	-	-
Other diseases, injury	-	-	-	-	12
Mental or emotional	-	-	-	-	9
Blood disorders	-	-	-	-	4
Miscellaneous	-	-	-	-	-

Notes: NR = sample size not reported.

The summary provided in Table 2 indicates a much wider range of attitudes and beliefs in the Europe towards epilepsy in comparison to the United States. Such differences may be explained by many factors. The largest differences are likely due to educational level and cultural attitudes. In addition, the variability of the attitudes may also be in part to due to the type of survey design used. Studies conducted in England (1969), Poland (1974), Italy (1985), Denmark (1992) and Austria (2005) used the same questions and random probability sample methodology as the U.S. (Bagic et al., 2009; Jensen and Dam, 1992; Spatt et al., 2005). Studies from Finland (1980) and England (2004) used a postal method (Iivanainen et al., 1980; Jacoby et al., 2004), while others were conducted in healthcare settings (Diamantopoulos et al., 2006; Novotna and Rektor, 2002). Some observed differences may be related to difficulties in the translation of questions into the variety of languages spoken throughout Europe.

Africa

Ten studies of public knowledge and attitudes towards epilepsy have been conducted in Africa over the past 35 years (Andriantseheno and Rakotoarivony, 2000; Atadzhanov, Chomba, Haworth, Mbewe, and Birbeck, 2006; Kabir, Abubakar, Kabir, and Farinyaro, 2005; Mbewe, Haworth, Atadzhanov, Chomba, and Birbeck, 2007; Moross, 1974; Ndoye et al., 2005; Njamnshi, Angwafor, Tabah, Jallon, and Muna, 2008; Nyame and Biritwum, 1997; Rwiza et al., 1993; Tekle-Haimanot et al., 1991), see Table 4. The percentage of people who reported they had heard or read about epilepsy ranged from 89% in Ethiopia (1991) to 100% in Nigeria (2005). The percentage of people who reported they knew someone with epilepsy ranged from 49% in South Africa (1974) to 98% in Zambia (2006). The percentage of people who reported witnessing a seizure ranged from 27% in Nigeria (2005) to 95% in Zambia (2006). The percentage of respondents reporting that they would object to their child associating with a child who has epilepsy ranged from 16% in Zambia (2007) to 65% in Ethiopia (1991). Objections to marriage ranged dramatically from 16% in Ghana (1997) to 76% in Cameroon (2008). Negative attitudes towards employment range of 13% in Ghana (1997) to 75% in Ethiopia (1991). The belief that epilepsy is a form of mental illness ranged dramatically from 1% in Zambia (2007) to 35% in Cameroon (2008). Around 45% of respondents in Africa had the belief that epilepsy is contagious, except for Ghana (11%) and Nigeria (18%). The percentage of people who indicated they didn't know the cause of epilepsy ranged from 25% in Senegal and Nigeria to 68% in Tanzania (1993).

All studies from Africa involved face-to-face interviews conducted in the native language of that country or region. Studies from Ethiopia (Tekle-Haimanot et al., 1991), Madagascar (Andriantseheno and Rakotoarivony, 2000), Senegal (Ndoye et al., 2005) and Tanzania (Rwiza et al., 1993) were population based using either random sampling methodology or widespread door-to-door surveying of a specific area. Studies from Cameroon (Njamnshi et al., 2008), Ghana (Nyame and Biritwum, 1997) and Zambia (Atadzhanov et al., 2006; Mbewe et al., 2007) involved convenience based samples. The two studies from Zambia focused on clerics and police officers, while the study from Cameroon interviewed people in a hospital setting. The study from Ghana interviewed government workers and the general public.

Table 4. Public knowledge and attitudes towards epilepsy in Africa

Question	S. Africa 1974 (n=NR) Afrikaans	S. Africa 1974 (n=NR) English	Tanzania 1993 (n=3,256)	Madagascar 1997 (1,392)	Zambia 2006 (n=225)	Zambia 2007 (n=175)	Senegal 2005 (n=2,263)	Nigeria 2005 (n=200)	Ghana 1997 (n=380)	Ethiopia 1991 (n=1,546)	Cameroon 2008 (n=302)
	Percentage answering "yes"										
31. Ever heard/read about epilepsy	-	-	-	90	97	98	-	100	99	89	99
32. Knows someone with epilepsy	63	49	-	-	98	92	-	-	-	-	90
33. Has seen a seizure	62	51	35	-	95	85	66	27	-	86	88
34. Object to children associating	- -	-	-	-	17	16	42	-	-	65	43
35. Object to marriage	-	-	-	26	57	43	68	-	16	74	76
36. Object to employment	25	16	-	34	-	-	-	-	13	75	35
37. Epilepsy is a mental illness	- -	-	-	-	8	1	-	-	8	2	35
38. Epilepsy is contagious	-	-	41	47	43	-	35	18	11	45	46
39. Never or rarely cured/controlled	-	-	17	16	-	-	-	-	-	-	-
40. What do you think is the cause											
Don't know	-	-	68	33	-	-	25	25	45	52	30
Nervous system disease	42	7	-	-	-	-	-	-	-	-	38
Brain disease, disorder	30	14	3	-	76	77	76	19	-	-	28
Hereditary	-	-	18	37	-	36	-	20	32	5	16
Birth defect, mental retardation	7 2	-	-	31	30	64	-	-	-	-	-
Accidents, injury	-	-	2	-	62	21	72	7	7	1	-
Mental, emotional, excessive worry	-	-	-	-	13	7	35	-	-	-	16
Blood disorders	-	-	-	-	25	31	-	-	-	-	39
Divine punishment, evil spirits, witchcraft	-	-	-	-	7	4	51	16	28	30	34
High fever, infection	-	-	-	-	-	-	58	12	4	-	-
Alcohol and drug abuse	-	-	-	-	-	-	-	-	6	-	-
Miscellaneous	-	-	-	-	-	-	-	-	15	1	-

Notes: NR = sample size not reported/

Table 5. Public knowledge and attitudes towards epilepsy - Middle East and India

		Percentage answering "yes"								
		Jordan	UAE	Turkey	Kuwait	Pakistan	Pakistan	North India	South India	Sri Lanka
		2007	1998	2006	2008	2007	2007	1995	2000	1984
	Question	(n=16,044)	(n=892)	(n=582)	(n=784)	(n=487)	(n=57)	(n=1,000)	(n=487)	(n=1,784)
41.	Ever heard/read about epilepsy	88	75	81	98	88	90	92	99	-
42.	Knows someone with epilepsy -	-	56	47	52	65	28	77	-	77
43.	Has seen a seizure	52	34	54	56	-	-	55	-	67
44.	Object to children associating	52	7	28	28	-	-	43	11	-
45.	Object to marriage	88	68	62	72	18	53	66	29	-
46.	Object to employment	56	10	46	55	-	-	-	46	-
47.	Epilepsy is a mental illness	9	-	12	50	-	-	15	27	-
48.	Epilepsy is contagious -	-	1	-	4	33	19	-	-	-
49.	Never or rarely cured/controlled	-	-	-	-	-	-	-	-	-
50.	What do you think is the cause	-								
	Don't know	28	9	36	-	-	-	20	-	-
	Nervous system disease	85	12	-	-	-	-	-	-	55
	Brain disease, disorder	78	17	42	-	-	-	-	-	66
	Hereditary	44	16	7	46	-	31	-	31	42
	Birth defect, mental retardation	-	5	1	-	-	-	-	-	-
	Accidents, injury -	-	16	4	-	-	-	-	-	52
	Mental, emotional, excessive worry -	-	16	16	-	52	-	-	-	-
	Blood disorders -	-	-	1	-	-	-	-	-	-
	Divine punishment, evil spirits, witchcraft	15	13	-	25	39	-	-	15	18
	High fever, infection -		-	-	-	-	-	-	-	-
	Alcohol and drug abuse -		-	-	-	-	-	-	-	-
	Miscellaneous 31		-	4	-	-	-	-	-	23

Notes: UAE = United Arab Emirates.

Table 6. Public knowledge and attitudes towards epilepsy - Asia

Question	China 1990 (n=1,278)	Taiwan 1995 (n=2,610)	Hong Kong 1999 (n=233)	Hong Kong 2002 (n=1,128)	Malaysia 1998 (n=379)	Malaysia 2000 (n=839)	Indonesia 2004 (n=1,000)	Myanmar 2002 (n=296)	Vietnam 2003 (n=1,000)	Vietnam 2006 (n=2,005)	Laos 2007 (n=332)
	Percentage answering "yes"										
51. Ever heard/read about epilepsy	93	87	96	58	99	91	97	82	55	67	-
52. Knows someone with epilepsy	77	70	27	19	38	56	-	25	46	52	-
53. Has seen a seizure	72	56	57	55	62	33	84	78	49	49	-
54. Object to children associating	57	18	11	11	9	20	-	44	19	36	-
55. Object to marriage	87	72	44	32	43	48	8	71	56	82	39
56. Object to employment	53	49	10	-	13	58	21	86	58	66	-
57. Epilepsy is a mental illness	16	7	10	10	9	23	-	25	24	10	34
58. Epilepsy a type of mental retardation	-	-	-	-	-	-	-	-	-	-	-
59. Epilepsy is contagious	-	-	-	3	-	-	12	-	-	-	49
60. Supernatural phenomena	-	-	-	-	-	-	-	-	-	-	34
61. Never or rarely cured	-	-	-	51	-	-	-	-	-	-	43
62. What do you think is the cause											
Don't know	40	34	15	-	26	17	-	27	7	31	-
Nervous system disease	-	-	-	-	-	-	-	-	-	-	-
Brain disease, disorder	25	20	48	-	12	30	-	33	77	50	66
Hereditary	17	28	50	-	25	69	49	23	19	27	42
Birth defect	12	14	29	-	24	13	-	42	7		7
Accidents, injury	-	-	-	-	-	-	-	-	-	-	47
Other diseases	-	-	-	-	-	-	-	-	-	-	-
Mental or emotional	17	8	-	-	8	24	-	36	21	-	
Blood disorders	2	2	-	-	2	6	-	13	9	-	
Malnutrition	-	-	-	-	-	-	-	-	-	-	-
Divine punishment	-	-	-	-	-	-	-	-	-	-	26
Miscellaneous	4	3	-	-	8	2	-	-			

The Middle East and India

Six studies of public knowledge and attitudes towards epilepsy have been conducted in the Middle East (Awad and Sarkhoo, 2008; Bener, al-Marzooqi, and Sztriha, 1998; Daoud, Al-Safi, Otoom, Wahba, and Alkofahi, 2007; Demirci, Dönmez, Gündoğar, and Baydar, 2007; Naeem et al., 2007; Shafiq et al., 2007) and three in India (Gambhir, Kumar, Singhi, and Goel, 1995; Radhakrishnan et al., 2000; Seneviratne, Rajapakse, Pathirana, and Seetha, 2002), see Table 5. People from the Middle East and India appear to have more negative attitudes towards epilepsy compared to the United States, especially in their attitudes towards marriage and employment. This is likely due to a strong belief that epilepsy is primarily inherited. A wide range of negative attitudes related to children was found by region. In South India, 11% reported objecting to their children associating with a child who has epilepsy. In North India, 43% objected to the same issue.

The belief that epilepsy is contagious varies widely throughout the Middle East and India. Areas of Pakistan lack resources and access to Western medicines. Populations of India and Pakistan also have the expectation that physicians address diet and lifestyle issues. This may result in people seeking care for epilepsy from a traditional healer first (Shafiq et al., 2007). However, those who had learned about epilepsy from a health care provider or the media were more likely to know that epilepsy is treatable. Knowledge of improper first aid (putting an object in a person's mouth during a seizure or pulling their tongue) was also high, 88% in Kuwait (Awad and Sarkhoo, 2008; Otoom, Al-Safi, Sequeira, and Alkofahi, 2006). In Turkey, most respondents recommended harmful first aid measures such as placing a person on their back, inserting a knife or a fork in their mouth, compressing on the person and pouring water on them (Demirci et al., 2007). In the Kuwait, 77% of respondents indicated their major sources of knowledge about epilepsy included: friends/relatives (49%), mass media (34%), school or university (14%) and other sources such as seminars about public health education (3%). Participants were also asked if they were willing to obtain more information about epilepsy (Awad and Sarkhoo, 2008). The preferred sources of information to learn more about epilepsy included the internet (39%), library (24%), physicians (37%), pharmacists (4%) and other sources (13%) which included brochures, mass media and seminars about public health education. The preference for electronic information over a physician speaks to the importance of technology and the need for accurate information about epilepsy to be available on the World Wide Web.

Studies from Jordan (Daoud et al., 2007), United Arab Emirates (Bener et al., 1998), Kuwait (Awad and Sarkhoo, 2008), North India (Gambhir et al., 1995) and South India (Radhakrishnan et al., 2000) were population based using either random sampling methodology or widespread door-to-door surveying of a specific area. The United Arab Emirates study used a postal method. Studies from Turkey (Demirci et al., 2007), Pakistan (Shafiq et al., 2007; Shafiq et al., 2008) and Sri Lanka (Senanayake and Abeykoon, 1984) did not use random sampling methods. Due to the significant number of resources required, population surveys are not practical in many parts of the world. Telephone and postal access is also a major limitation in many developing countries.

Asia

Eleven studies of public knowledge and attitudes towards epilepsy have been conducted in Asia (excluding South Korea) (Chung, Chang, Lai, and Lai, 1995; Fong and Hung, 2002; Gunadharma, 2004; Lai et al., 1990; Le, Dinh, and Jallon, 2006; Lim, Tan, Lim, and Tan, 1999; Ramasundrum, Mohd Hussin, and Tan, 2000; Tran et al., 2007; Tuan, Cuong, Allebeck, Chuc, and Tomson, 2007; Win and Soe, 2002; Wong, Chung, and Wong, 2004), see Table 6. The percentage of people who reported they had heard or read about epilepsy in Asia ranged from 55% in Vietnam (2003) to 99% in Malaysia (1998) with an average of 83%, see Table 6. The percentage of people who reported they knew someone with epilepsy ranged from 19% in Hong Kong (2002) to 77% in China (1990). The percentage of people who reported witnessing a seizure ranged from 33% in Malaysia (2003) to 84% in Indonesia (2004) with an average of 55% across countries. The percentage of respondents reporting that they would object to their child associating with a child who has epilepsy ranged from 9% in Malaysia (1998) to 57% in China (1990). Objections to marriage ranged dramatically in Asia from 8% in Indonesia to 87% in China, with an average of 53%. Negative attitudes towards employment were high with a range from 10% in Hong Kong (1999) to 86% in Myanmar (2002), with an average 46%. The belief that epilepsy is a form of mental illness ranged dramatically from 7% in Taiwan (1995) to 34% in Laos (2007), with an average of 17%. The percentage of people who indicated they didn't know the cause of epilepsy ranged from 7% in Vietnam (2003) to 40% in China (1990). In Asia a lack of accurate medical and psychological education is evident in comparison the United States.

All studies from Asia involved face-to-face native language interviews. Studies from Vietnam (Le et al., 2006; Tuan et al., 2007) and China (Fong and Hung, 2002), used random sampling procedures like the U.S. studies. Others used convenience samples conducted in various settings (streets, parks, markets, shopping areas, temples, schools and hospitals) (Chung et al., 1995; Lai et al., 1990). The study from Laos focused on PWE, one of their family members and a random sample of local villagers (Tran et al., 2007). In general, the Asian countries have particularly negative attitudes towards children associating with another child with epilepsy, marriage, employment and the belief that epilepsy is a mental illness. Higher education is linked with better understanding of epilepsy, its management and a reduction of prejudice however it did not change attitudes towards marriage and employment much. It is believed some negative beliefs in the Asian countries may also derive from traditional Chinese medicine which considers epilepsy a genetic disease (Choi-Kwon et al., 2004).

South Korea

Seven studies of public knowledge and attitudes towards epilepsy have been conducted in South Korea (Choi-Kwon et al., 2004; M. K. Kim, Cho, Shin, and Kim, 1994; M. K. Kim et al., 2003; Y. Lee, Kim, Lim, Yi, and Park, 1997; Park et al., 1996), see Table 7. Studies from South Korea found an average of 93% of respondents had heard or read about epilepsy, see Table 7 (Choi-Kwon et al., 2004; M. K. Kim et al., 1994; M. K. Kim et al., 2003; Y. Lee et al., 1997; Park et al., 1996). Objections to children associating with someone who has epilepsy were as high as 50%, but the most recent study in 2004 only 18% reported such objections.

Table 7. Public knowledge and attitudes towards epilepsy - South Korea

		Percentage answering "yes"						
		South Korea	South Korea	South Korea	South Korea	South Korea	South Korea	South Korea
		1971	1992	1996	1997	1995	1999	2004
		(n=NR)	(n=587)	(n=802)	(n=1,722)	(n=820)	(n=715)	(n=918)
	Question	pre				post		
63.	Ever heard/read about epilepsy	94	90	-	-	93	98	92
64.	Knows someone with epilepsy	-	42	-	-	-	-	-
65.	Has seen a seizure	-	-	-	-	55		64
66.	Object to children associating	-	-	47	-	50	40	18
67.	Object to marriage	-	-	91	-	94	89	62
68.	Object to employment	-	-	58	-	52	51	63
69.	Epilepsy is a mental illness	-	45	-	-	34	22	5
70.	Epilepsy is contagious	-	14	11	-	13	12	2
71.	Supernatural phenomena	-	-	-	-	-	-	3
72.	Never or rarely cured	-	-	-	-	-	-	25
73.	High risk of passing it to child	-	-	-	-	-	-	47
74.	What do you think is the cause							
	Don't know	-	9	11	-	-	-	-
	Nervous system disease	-	24	34	-	-	-	-
	Brain disease, disorder	-	21	-	48	34	30	30
	Hereditary	36	42	30	24	29	24	-
	Birth defect	-	3	-	-	-	-	-
	Accidents, injury	-	8	28	-	27	17	-
	Other diseases	-	-	-	-	-	-	-
	Mental or emotional	-	13	35	22	34	22	-
	Blood disorders/infection	-	4	-	5	9	6	-
	Malnutrition	-	-	31	-	31	23	-
	Divine punishment	-	-	63	-	62	52	-
	Miscellaneous	-	5	-	-	-	-	-

Notes: NR = sample size not reported.

Negative attitudes towards employment were also high with a range from 51 to 63%. Objections to marriage were the highest of any area around the globe (89 to 94% in three studies). Fortunately, in the most recent study the percentage of respondents objecting to marriage has dropped some to 62%. Belief that epilepsy is a mental illness was reported in the range of 22 to 45%, with a large drop in the most recent study to 5%. In the earlier studies 11 to 14% thought epilepsy is contagious. The most recent study found this belief dropped to 2%. Two Korean studies were conducted in the same village in 1995 and 1999. Some improvements were found, however the belief that epilepsy is a form of divine punishment remained strong (M. K. Kim et al., 2003). Koreans indicated their main sources of knowledge were neighborhood/relatives (78%), mass media (15%) and school (6%) (Choi-Kwon et al., 2004). Some of the Korean studies used other standardized methods such as interviewing every 10th house in a geographic area or picking names in a consistent way from a phone book (Choi-Kwon et al., 2004; Kim et al., 1994). Attitudes and beliefs were sampled in various settings (streets, parks, markets, shopping areas, temples, schools and hospitals) (Kim et al., 2003). The use of non-random sampling techniques may be related to customary procedures for research in these areas and/or a lack of resources to conduct random sampling techniques.

The trends of improvement outside the U.S. in knowledge and beliefs towards epilepsy may be explained by educational level, by easier access to information and possibly by sociopolitical changes that have taken place over the past few decades as well as through specific interventions and campaigns about epilepsy (Diamantopoulos et al., 2006). It is believed that face to face interviews may also elicit more social desirable responses (Spatt et al., 2005) however, in many countries, respondents were not apprehensive about voicing very negative attitudes towards epilepsy. Cultural definitions of epilepsy are likely to affect comparisons across regions. It is also possible that in the process of translation the meaning and implication of questions may be obscured. This highlights the importance of using the terminology or vernacular used by that population to describe epilepsy and seizures within a survey.

Education Setting Population Research

Teacher Attitudes and Beliefs towards Students with Epilepsy

Children with epilepsy are an educationally vulnerable group and educational staff need to be aware of the additional support the students may need (Tidman, Saravanan, and Gibbs, 2003). Children with chronic neurological conditions are more likely to experience problems academically compared to those with non-neurological health problems (Howe, Feinstein, Reiss, Molock, and Berger, 1993). Previous research has also found that children with epilepsy to have difficulty with academic achievement that would be predicted by their intellectual ability (Seidenberg and Berent, 1992; Sturniolo and Galletti, 1994).

Teachers in primary and secondary schools are in a position to have an important impact on ongoing education of the child with epilepsy and thereby subsequent employment and self-reliance. As with the general population, ignorance of causes, treatment options and acute seizure management facilitates the propagation of prejudices and consequent unjust attitudes and harmful behaviors. The perception of persons with epilepsy being contagious, supernaturally afflicted or mentally ill is prevalent in many developing countries and to some extent in the developed world. These ill-informed perceptions about the causes of epilepsy likely contribute to negative attitudes regarding proper socialization, intelligence, and employability of persons with epilepsy. Furthermore, ignorance about acute seizure management can lead to injurious behaviors by the very individuals appointed to protect the child with epilepsy should a seizure occur in the educational setting. Again mirroring the general population, familiarity with epilepsy and higher levels of education ameliorate prejudicial attitudes and behaviors. Moreover, negative attitudes have been demonstrated to be remediable with focused educational interventions. Worldwide, the literature suggests that in order to address gaps in knowledge and beliefs towards epilepsy there is a need for targeted educational interventions for educators.

United States and Canada

Only a handful of surveys have been completed on the experiences and attitudes relating to epilepsy of teachers in the United States and Canada, see Table 8 (Bishop and Slevin, 2004; Bishop and Boag, 2006; Katzenstein, Fastenau, Dunn, and Austin, 2007; Price, Murphy, and Cureton, 2004; Young et al., 2002). These few surveys indicate some degree of negative attitude towards children with epilepsy, and acknowledgement of lack of formal education in dealing with this population. Price et al. (2004) sampled 28 special needs educators regarding confidence in managing a seizure emergency (Price et al., 2004). Prior to focused education, 50% expressed a lack of confidence in their knowledge regarding what actions to take in the event of a first-time seizure and in working with the families of children with epilepsy.

Bishop and Slevin (2004) surveyed 135 elementary and middle school teachers in Kentucky, U.S. documenting a poor familiarity of the respondents with children with epilepsy (Bishop and Slevin, 2004). Only 58% knew someone with epilepsy and 44% had ever had a student with epilepsy. However, 89% felt that they had had inadequate training about epilepsy. Overall this population endorsed a minimally positive attitude toward children with epilepsy, with 30% scoring in the negative range and greater than 10% endorsing negative attitudes more than one standard deviation below the mean. These attitude scores were significantly correlated with years of teaching experienced, with the more experienced teachers showing more positive attitudes toward children with epilepsy. This work was expanded upon with a survey conducted in 512 elementary and middle school educators across the United States (Bishop and Boag, 2006). Regarding knowledge of epilepsy, 49% felt knowledgeable about epilepsy, 65% felt prepared to handle a seizure in their classroom, 56% felt they had sufficient training in first aid for seizures and 14% endorsed having adequate training in epilepsy during their teaching education. Regarding attitudes toward children with epilepsy, the study documented the range of negative to positive attitudes on a Likert scale from negative three to three. In general the surveyed population had positive attitudes toward children with epilepsy endorsing equal rights (2.73), ability to marry (2.40) and have children (2.41), having normal intelligence (2.87), and not being contagious (2.96). Further, only 1.2% viewed epilepsy as a mental illness. Some negative residua were documented including a perception of a higher propensity to develop criminal tendencies (-2.28), less of a chance of equal employment (-2.01) and decreased life expectancy (-1.73) with expectation of a deteriorating condition (-1.49). Beyond simple attitude, it has been demonstrated by Katzenstein et al (2007) that teacher rating of the academic performance of students with epilepsy was significantly lower in those for whom the teacher was aware of the condition versus those for whom the teacher was not, despite equal measures of performance on objective testing between the two groups (Katzenstein et al., 2007).

Table 8. School teacher knowledge and attitudes towards epilepsy – USA, Europe and South America

Question	U	SA 2004 (n= 135)	USA 2 006 (n=512)	England 1 992 (n=142)	Holland 1 996 (n=169)	Spain 1 990 (n=1,283)	Greece 2 005 (n=300)	Croatia 2 003 (n=216)	Brazil 2 001 (n=300)	Brazil 2 007 (n=100)
		P ercentage answering "yes"								
75.	Ever heard of or read about epilepsy	-	-	-	-	-	-	-	99	-
76.	Knows someone with epilepsy	58	-	-	-	-	-	-	87	-
77.	Has a friend or family member with epilepsy/seizures	-	-	-	24	29	-	-	-	-
78.	Has had a student with epilepsy	44	-	57	65	28	24	-	-	50
79.	Has seen a seizure	-	-	69	78	-	-	-	85	79
80.	Has seen a seizure at school	-	-	-	-	-	9	-	-	-
81.	Object to children associating	-	-	-	-	-	-	-	-	-
82.	Object to marriage of their child	-	10	-	-	-	-	-	-	-
83.	Object to employment	-	3	-	-	-	-	-	-	-
84.	Epilepsy is a mental illness	-	1	-	-	-	1	-	-	-
85.	Epilepsy is a brain disorder or malfunction	-	-	77	-	-	85	-	-	-
86.	Epilepsy is inherited	-	15	66	68	-	-	-	-	-
87.	Epilepsy is contagious	-	2	-	-	-	-	-	2	1
88.	Epilepsy a type of mental retardation	-	2	-	-	-	1	-	-	51
89.	Caused by supernatural phenomena or spirits	-	-	-	-	-	-	-	-	-
90.	Never or rarely cured	-	-	-	-	-	17	-	-	-
91.	AEDs affect mood, memory, learning, drowsiness	-	72	60	86	-	-	-	-	-

Table 8. (Continued)

92. Have below average intelligence	-	-	0				-	23			-	-	2			6
93. More likely to have learning problems	-		-		15	18	-			15		53	-			-
94. More likely to have behavioral problems	-	-	-	77					-	10		54		-	-	
95. Prefer placement in special classrooms or schools	-		2		4		5		25	6		-		-		-
96. Would help a student with epilepsy	-	-	-	-	-	-	-	-	-							
97. Afraid to have a student with epilepsy	-		-		64		-		-	2		36		4		-
98. Is there discrimination against PWE	-	-	-	-	-	-	-	89								-
99. Improper first aid knowledge	-	56			-	36			-	. 77		-	-	26		
100. Believes social activities should be limited	-	-	-	-	-	-	-	-	-							
101. Believes sports or strenuous activities should be limited	-	3			-	-	-	-	-	-	-					
102. Had inadequate information/training about epilepsy	89	86		77	8				89	-		-		56	-	
103. Desired more training on epilepsy	-		95	92		63	-			-		91	-			89

Table 9. School teacher knowledge and attitudes towards epilepsy – Asia, India and the Middle East

	Percentage answering "yes"											
	Thailand	Thailand	Taiwan	Japan	Indonesia	Pakistan	India	India	Pakistan	Turkey	Turkey	Turkey
	1999	2005	2001	2008	2001	2007	1997	2008	2007	2004	2004	2007
	(n=100)	(n=102)	(n=216)	(n=16)	(n=84)	(n=535)	(n=116)	(n=568)	(n=535)	(n=346)	(n=346)	(n=275)
Question										pre	post	
104. Ever heard of or read about epilepsy	58	-	-	-	100	-	-	97	-	69	90	-
105. Knows someone with epilepsy	-	-	-	-	-	34	32	-	34	59	61	-
106. Has a friend or family member with epilepsy/seizures	-	22	-	-	-	-	-	8	-	-	-	30
107. Has had a student with epilepsy	34	-	-	-	-	-	27	12	-	-	-	-
108. Has seen a seizure	-	-	-	-	-	-	57	-	-	72	71	79
109. Has seen a seizure at school	-	-	-	-	-	-	-	-	-	-	-	-
110. Object to children associating	3	-	-	-	25	-	-	38	-	6	2	-
111. Object to marriage of their child	36	-	-	-	56	74	-	87	74	74	76	-
112. Object to employment	-	-	-	-	-	-	-	-	-	14	2	-
113. Epilepsy is a mental illness	30	-	-	-	57	-	-	14	-	18	7	24
114. Epilepsy is a brain disorder or malfunction	10	78	-	50	-	-	-	44	-	-	-	-
115. Epilepsy is inherited	-	75	-	-	35	22	50	16	22	-	-	-
116. Epilepsy is contagious	3	-	-	-	20	10	-	5	10	2	4	-
117. Epilepsy a type of mental retardation	-	-	-	-	-	-	-	-	-	-	-	-
118. Caused by supernatural phenomena or spirits	-	1	-	-	4	1	-	6	1	-	-	-
119. Never or rarely cured (or untreatable)	47	16	-	33	-	23	-	21	23	-	-	-
120. AEDs affect mood, memory, learning, drowsiness	-	-	-	-	-	-	73	-	-	-	-	-
121. Have below average intelligence	38	-	-	-	-	-	-	32	-	-	-	-
122. More likely to have learning problems	-	-	-	-	49	-	67	-	-	-	-	-
123. More likely to have behavioral problems	-	-	-	-	-	-	-	-	-	-	-	-

Table 9. (Continued)

124. Prefer placement in special classrooms or schools	15	-	30	-	-	11	11	21	11	6	1	30
125. Would help a student with epilepsy	-	-	-	-	-	-	-	-	-	-	-	-
126. Afraid to have a student with epilepsy	10	64	-	-	-	-	-	32	-	-	-	-
127. Is there discrimination against PWE	-	-	-	-	-	-	-	-	-	-	-	-
128. Improper first aid knowledge	86	-	-	-	-	50	65	57	50	59	2	56
129. Believes social activities should be limited	-	-	-	-	-	-	-	-	-	91	94	-
130. Believes sports or strenuous activities should be limited	-	-	-	0	-	-	58	-	-	7	6	-
131. Had inadequate information/training about epilepsy	-	-	-	-	85	-	68	-	-	-	-	35
132. Desired more training on epilepsy	-	-	-	-	-	-	-	-	-	-	-	-

Table 10. School teacher knowledge and attitudes towards epilepsy - Africa

	Percentage answering "yes"						
	Nigeria 2002	Nigeria 2005	Nigeria 2005	Senegal 2004	Zambia 2006	Zimbabwe 1997	Bobo Diolaaso 2004
Question	(n=125)	(n=118)	(n=460)	(n=373)	(n=159)	(n=165)	(n=260)
133. Ever heard of or read about epilepsy	-	-	92	-	96	89	98
134. Knows someone with epilepsy	-	-	-	-	79	-	77
135. Has a friend or family member with epilepsy	-	-	-	-	40	15	-
136. Has had a student with epilepsy	23	17	-	-	-	-	-
137. Has seen a seizure	70	-	78	-	84	71	91
138. Has seen a seizure at school	-	55	-	-	-	-	-
139. Object to children associating	-	-	-	-	3	18	-
140. Object to marriage of their child	-	-	95	-	56	24	-
141. Object to employment	-	-	-	-	-	44	-
142. Epilepsy is a mental illness	-	-	10	-	0	12	31
143. Epilepsy is a brain disorder or malfunction	71	-	28	69	81	4	43
144. Epilepsy is inherited	46	56	16	-	-	35	8
145. Epilepsy is contagious	29	32	31	24	28	23	12
146. Epilepsy a type of mental retardation	-	-	-	-	-	-	-
147. Caused by supernatural phenomena or spirits	22	61	28	-	20	1	-
148. Never or rarely cured	-	-	-	27	-	-	14
149. AEDs affect mood, memory, learning, drowsiness	-	-	-	-	-	-	-
150. Have below average intelligence	-	28	19	-	24	-	19
151. More likely to have learning problems	27	-	-	-	-	-	-
152. More likely to have behavioral problems	52	-	-	-	-	-	-
153. Prefer placement in special classrooms or schools	50	70	33	63	7	17	15
154. Would help a student with epilepsy	-	-	85	66	-	-	-
155. Afraid to have a student with epilepsy	63	-	-	-	-	10	-
156. Is there discrimination against PWE	-	-	-	-	-	-	-
157. Improper first aid knowledge	-	45	-	53	-	4	-
158. Believes social activities should be limited	-	-	-	-	-	-	-
159. Believes sports or strenuous activities should be limited	70	-	-	-	-	-	-
160. Never received information or training about epilepsy	99	-	-	-	-	-	-
161. Desired more training on epilepsy	-	-	-	99	-	-	-

Table 11. Student knowledge and attitudes towards epilepsy

	Percentage answering "yes"													
	USA	Canada	Poland	Poland	Italy	Malaysia	Brazil	Brazil	Brazil	Brazil	South India	Tanzania	South India	Cameroon
	2002	2002	2005	2006	2007	2005	1998	2007	2007	2007	2006	1994	2001	2008
	(n=19,441)	(n=191)	(n=181)	(n=315)	(n=344)	(n=289)	(n=355)	(n=248)	(n=258)	(n=116)	(n=1,213)	(n=426)	(n=253)	(n=910)
						pre						post		
	High		Secondary	High school	Gen pop	Middle					High	Secondary		Secondary
Question	School	Univ	School	1st yr Med	Univ	Univ	Univ	Univ	Univ	Univ	School	School	Univ	School
162. Ever heard/read about epilepsy	52	100	98	96	91	87	96	-	93	-	98	-	71	95
163. Knows someone with epilepsy	21	-	46	-	-	-	68	-	-	-	43	-	55	73
164. Has a friend or family member with epilepsy	-	-	-	-	24	6	-	-	18	-	-	-	-	-
165. Has seen a seizure	-	-	-	26	57	56	67	-	42	-	-	83	30	76
166. Has seen a seizure at school	-	-	-	-	-	-	-	-	-	-	-	-	-	-
167. Object to sit and play with child who has epilepsy	4	5	-	-	-	-	4	-	-	-	13	46	-	-
168. Object to dating or marrying someone with epilepsy	11	4	-	-	-	-	20	21	13	2	-	81	31	64
169. Object to employment	8	14	-	48	-	-	45	8	6	0	71	-	27	43
170. Epilepsy is a mental illness	19	9	12	-	-	40	2	6	11	0	59	3	-	38
171. Epilepsy is contagious	4	-	9	-	16	5	-	-	-	-	14	61	13	50
172. Never or rarely cured	-	8	-	-	13	1	4	-	-	97	99	53	54	-
173. Knows how to perform first-aid seizure management	-	-	2	-	-	20	-	28	-	-	-	-	-	-
174. Improper first aid knowledge	-	-	71	70	-	-	-	-	14	1	37	14	-	-
175. AEDs cause side effects	-	-	-	-	-	-	-	-	-	-	55	-	-	-
176. Believes activities should be limited	-	-	-	-	-	12	-	-	53	98	-	-	-	-
177. Children with epilepsy should not be allowed to attend school	9	-	-	-	-	-	-	-	-	-	-	59	13	-

178. Believes someone with epilepsy has low intelligence	-	-	-	-	-	-	-	4	-	-	-	93	-	-
179. Believes epilepsy is shameful illness or isolated	-	-	8	-	-	64	-	-	-	-	-	-	10	-
180. What do you think is the cause of epilepsy														
Don't know	-	35	77	-	33	69	23	-	-	-	-	54	39	25
Nervous system disease	-	-	5	-	71	-	49	95	-	-	-	-	-	-
Brain disease, disorder, infection	-	-	-	76	-	-	-	-	-	-	50	8	71	26
Hereditary	-	45	3	42	28	67	6	-	33	17	34	19	57	26
Birth defect, mental retardation	-	33	-	-	15	-	-	-	30	5	-	20	63	-
Accidents, head injury	-	25	4	74	19	-	3	87	-	-	-	15	-	-
Mental, emotional, excessive worry	-	-	7	-	26	40	7	3	-	-	-	-	63	16
Blood disorders	-	-	-	-	-	-	-	-	-	-	-	-	-	14
Divine punishment or evil spirits	-	-	-	-	-	5	-	-	-	-	11	4	26	26
High fever or infection	-	-	-	-	2	-	3	29	-	-	-	-	31	-
Stroke	-	26	-	-	-	-	-	-	-	-	-	-	-	-
Miscellaneous/Other -	-	-	-	4	-	11	-	-	-	-	-	56		

Europe

Studies in European countries have included the United Kingdom, Denmark, Greece, Spain and Croatia, see Table 8 (Bannon, Wildig, and Jones, 1992; Herranz Fernandez et al., 1990; Kaleyias, Tzoufi, Kotsalis, Papavasiliou, and Diamantopoulos, 2005; Madsen, 1996; Prpic et al., 2003). A wide range of familiarity with epilepsy was demonstrated in the reviewed studies. Rates of having taught a student with epilepsy were 24% in the study conducted in Greece, 28% in Spain, 57% in England and 65% in Denmark. Teachers endorsed having a friend or family member with epilepsy at a rate of 24% in Denmark and 29% in England. There were clear perceptions of a need for further education with 36% of those surveyed in Croatia and 82% of those from stating that they did not know enough about epilepsy and 63% of the Danish and 91% Croatian teachers endorsing a need for further education regarding epilepsy. Of concern is the lack of information about providing first aid during a seizure. Of teachers surveyed in Greece 77% did not feel able to render first aid in this situation. Sixty-four percent of English teachers surveyed did not feel confident supervising children with epilepsy. This lack of education amongst teachers was also demonstrated to lead to the endorsement of harmful behaviors such as placing a handkerchief in the mouth (Denmark 35%; England 11 and 15%) and restraining the child's limbs (Denmark 19% England 5 and 18%).

Attitudes and beliefs studied in the European teaching community touched upon the axes of the perception of behavioral problems and subnormal intelligence in students with epilepsy as well as the opinion as to the type of setting in which the student was to be best educated. Some teachers perceived the students with epilepsy having greater difficulty mastering school work (England 15%, Croatia 53%), with a minority perceiving these students as frankly less intelligent (England 0 and 5%, Greece 2%, Denmark 18%, Spain 23%) and only a minor fraction regarding epilepsy as a form of mental retardation (Greece 1%).

Prognosis for treatment of epilepsy was generally positive with only 9% of teachers in the Greek study believing that epilepsy was almost never controlled and 84% in the English study believing the outlook was mostly good. There was a definite perception of behavioral problems in students with epilepsy. Fifty-four percent of teachers surveyed in Croatia believed that there were behavioral pattern differences in students with epilepsy. A minority of teachers surveyed in Greece (10%) believed that epilepsy was usually associated with behavioral problems while a large majority or teachers surveyed in Denmark (77%) believed that students with epilepsy were maladjusted and aggressive. A minor fraction of teachers in the Greek study (1%) believed that epilepsy itself was a psychological problem. Negative perceptions of intelligence and behavioral issues can translate into an unwillingness to work with students with epilepsy. In the Greek cohort 2% felt awkward or completely negative about working with a student with epilepsy. Fifty-two percent of this same population endorsed that having a student with epilepsy in class creates problems, 50% stating that anxiety for the teacher was a major contributing factor. Positively, teachers in England (92%, 97%) and Denmark (94%) overwhelming thought that students with epilepsy should all or mostly be educated in mainstream schools and in the Greek study only 6% would desire a student with epilepsy be transferred to another school. However, 25% of teachers in the Spanish study thought that students with epilepsy needed to attend special schools or needed complementary help.

South America

There were only two studies identified for the region of South America – both in Brazil, see Table 8. Dantas et al. (2001) surveyed 300 teachers (Dantas, Cariri, Cariri, and Ribeiro-Filho, 2001). In this group, familiarity with epilepsy was somewhat more than the counterparts surveyed in the United States. Eighty-seven percent knew someone with epilepsy and 85% had witnessed an epileptic seizure. However, only 43% felt knowledgeable in rendering first aid during a seizure. This included specific endorsement of harmful behaviors such as pulling on the tongue (17%) and oral insertion of an object (4%). In general, endorsement of negative attitudes was quite low with minimal endorsement for believing epilepsy to be contagious (2%), children with epilepsy to be of subnormal intelligence (2%) and objecting to have a child with epilepsy in the class (4%). As with studies of the general population, the higher the level of training the teacher had completed the more positive their attitude toward the students with epilepsy.

Fernandes et al. (2007) surveyed knowledge and attitudes toward epilepsy in 100 elementary school teachers (Fernandes et al., 2007). Again, most teachers had seen a seizure (79%) but 50% stated they had never taught a student with epilepsy and 89% desired to learn more about epilepsy. Not knowing how to proceed during a seizure (26%) and harmful behaviors such as pulling on the tongue (24%) were endorsed by respondents. In regards to attitudes, there were significant majorities endorsing epilepsy as a treatable condition, allowing their own children to play with a child with epilepsy, women with epilepsy being able to bear children, persons with epilepsy being able to marry, and epilepsy not being associated with a failure in life.

Asia

Studies in Taiwan, Japan, Thailand and Indonesia somewhat less positive attitudes toward students with epilepsy in the teaching population in areas of general attitude towards persons with epilepsy and the intellectual ability of a student with epilepsy (Hsieh and Chiou, 2001; Kankirawatana, 1999; Okumura and Watanabe, 2008; Rambe and Sjahrir, 2002; Tiamkao et al., 2005). In one Thai study 34% of teachers recalled having had a student with epilepsy in class and 28% endorsed having someone with epilepsy in their family. Knowledge about epilepsy was poor. In the Indonesian study 85% did not feel well informed about epilepsy and 86% of the teachers in a survey from Thailand did not know proper first aid measures for seizures. This misinformation included endorsement of potentially dangerous behaviors such as placing a spoon/gag in the student's mouth (Thailand 64%, 73%) and restraining the student (Thailand 27%, 30%). A large minority (38%) of teachers in a Thai study believed that children with epilepsy are of lower intelligence and 15% felt special classes were required for students with epilepsy. Teachers in the Taiwan study were significantly more concerned about aggression from students with epilepsy compared to those with asthma. Thirty percent preferred to not have a student with epilepsy in their class while 10% of a sample in Thailand 10% endorsed being afraid to have a child with epilepsy in their class. Attitudes toward epilepsy in general were mixed. Many teachers thought that epilepsy was untreatable (Thailand 16%, 47%; Japan 33%). Endorsed etiologies for epilepsy also demonstrated levels of stigmatism. Epilepsy was felt to be caused by an infectious agent in

15% of teachers in a Thailand sample and to be considered to be contagious by a minority of others (Thailand 3%, Indonesia 2%). Eleven percent in a sample of Thai teachers believed epilepsy was caused by eating pork. Epilepsy was significantly associated with mental illness. In the Taiwan study children with epilepsy were significantly more associated with insanity than children with asthma while 30% of a Thai sample believed children with epilepsy have a higher incidence of insanity. Many teachers endorsed epilepsy as a frank form of mental disease (Thailand 18%; Indonesia 57%). A very small minority endorsed superstitious beliefs involving the etiology of epilepsy including an ancestor's sin (Indonesia 4%), divine punishment (Thailand 1%), and demonic possession (Thailand 1%). The prejudicial views of persons with epilepsy were somewhat translated into views about appropriate social interactions. A significant minority (43%) of the Indonesia sample believed that persons with epilepsy can not work like other people. Most of the teachers would allow their children to play with a child with epilepsy (Thailand 95%, Indonesia 75%) and endorse the right to marry (Thailand 98%; Indonesia 79%) and have children (Thailand 90%). However, only a minority of teachers would allow their child to marry a person with epilepsy (Thailand 41%; Indonesia 44%).

The Middle East and India

Studies in Turkey, India and Pakistan documented similar familiarity with and attitudes about epilepsy as those found in the Asian studies (Akhtar et al., 2007; Aydin and Yildiz, 2007; Bekiroglu, Ozkan, Gurses, Arpaci, and Dervent, 2004; Pala and Vankar, 1997; Thacker, Verma, Ji, Thacker, and Mishra, 2008). Level of familiarity with epilepsy was similar to that found in Western nations. Fifty-nine percent of teachers surveyed in a Turkish and 27% in the Pakistani study knew someone with epilepsy. There were varying degrees of admitting to having a friend or relative with epilepsy with 30% in a Turkish population and 32% and 7% in separate Indian studies. Only one Indian study queried the number of teachers having taught a child with epilepsy with a result of 27%.

Self-perceived ability to handle seizures was poor in two Turkish (24%, 41%) educational communities and in one Indian (16%) educational community. There were very frequent endorsements of dangerous behaviors in response to seizures. Restraining limbs from jerking was endorsed in 29% of a Turkish population and 85% in an Indian population while insertion of various objects into the mouth was also felt to be appropriate (India 40%, 85%; Pakistan 21%). Fifty percent of an Indian teaching population desired more information regarding epilepsy. Indian educational communities endorsed a view of students with epilepsy being educationally challenged with 67% believing that students with epilepsy were more likely to have learning problems; 56% stating that students with epilepsy were educationally subnormal and 32% believing that students with epilepsy had below average intelligence. Despite this, only 11% and 21% of separate Indian teaching populations favored special schools for students with epilepsy, although in one community 32% of teachers would prefer not to have a student with epilepsy in their class. The Pakistani teaching population had similar attitudes with only 75% stating that a student with epilepsy could be successful in a normal class. In comparison, one Turkish study documented that 93% of teachers believed mainstream schooling was appropriate. Success in life was viewed as possible by 82% of Turkish teachers, but only 19% of Indian teachers felt the outlook was mostly good for students with epilepsy. Such mixed attitudes towards students with epilepsy suggest that through education and additional training we may be able to overcome misperceptions and improve acceptance in the educational settings around the world.

Epilepsy was felt by the majority to be a treatable condition in Turkey (87%), in India (62%, and in Pakistan (62%). Etiologies of epilepsy were felt to be transmissible, psychological or supernatural by a minority of teachers. Ninety-eight percent of Turkish teachers knew epilepsy was not contagious and a small minority of those surveyed in Pakistan (10%) and India (3%, 5%) believed the condition was transmissible. In Turkey 18% of teachers felt that epilepsy was a psychological disease; 14% of Indian teachers felt persons with epilepsy had a higher incidence of insanity with 1.1% of Indian teachers marking epilepsy as caused by insanity. A minimal number of respondents endorsed supernatural causes of epilepsy such as possession or magic (India 6%, Pakistan 1%). Attitudes regarding persons with epilepsy in society varied widely. Ninety-nine percent of Turkish teachers would accept a colleague with epilepsy and 86% would offer a person with epilepsy a job. The ability to marry was endorsed by the majority of teachers in Turkey (90%) and Pakistan (74%). However, only 59% of Turkish teachers would themselves marry a person with epilepsy and fewer still would allow their child to marry a person with epilepsy (Turkey 26%, India 11%). Having children was deemed appropriate for PWE by a majority of teachers (Pakistan 70%, Turkey 83%) but in India 38% would not allow their child to play with a child with epilepsy. In the Middle East and India, attitudes and beliefs toward epilepsy are most favorable in Turkey. This may partly be explained by Turkish society being more westernized in comparison to other nations in this region.

Africa

Attitudes in educators regarding epilepsy were significantly more negative and fraught with ignorance and superstition in the African samples gathered from Burkina Faso, Nigeria, Senegal, Zambia and Zimbabwe (Alikor and Essien, 2005; G. L. Birbeck, Chomba, Atadzhanov, Mbewe, and Haworth, 2006; Mielke, Adamolekun, Ball, and Mundanda, 1997; Millogo and Siranyan, 2004; Ndour et al., 2004; Ojinnaka, 2002; Sanya, Salami, Goodman, Buhari, and Araoye, 2005). There was a wide range of variability in endorsed familiarity in either knowing someone with epilepsy (Zimbabwe 15%, Nigeria 18%, Burkina Faso 77%, Zambia 79%) or having a family member with epilepsy (Zambia 40%). Despite familiarity perceived and actual knowledge base was poor. In Senegal, 84% of teachers surveyed felt their knowledge not adequate and 99% desired more training. This suggests it would very helpful to capitalize on this recognized need by providing an epilepsy specific educational intervention.

The lack of training was evident in responses recorded to questions regarding first aid during a seizure. In a Zimbabwe sample of educators, 72% were unsure what to do in response to a seizure and many (4% Zimbabwe, 53% Senegal) would perform potentially dangerous interventions. Of the multiple harmful interventions endorsed, placing an object in the patient mouth and or pulling their tongue was among the more prevalent (Burkina Faso 5%, 28%, Nigeria 89%) followed by restraining the child (Nigeria 41%), feeding the child cow's urine (Nigeria 25%) and putting the child's feet in hot water or fire (Nigeria 18%). Teachers' estimate of the intelligence of a student with epilepsy were negative in a minority who believed that children with epilepsy were always of lower intelligence (Nigeria 28%, 19%, Burkina Faso 19%) and would never be able to attain the highest educational level possible (Nigeria 16%). However, a majority of teachers (57%) in Burkina Faso thought that idiocy was a consequence of epilepsy. There was significant reluctance expressed in willingness to teach a student with epilepsy. Although the majority of teachers would be willing to teach a child with epilepsy in a normal classroom (Zambia 61%, 45%, Zimbabwe 83%, Senegal 84%, Nigeria 86%) there was a distinct preference that students with epilepsy be taught in special schools (Senegal 63%, Zambia 50%, Nigeria 73%, 33%, 25%). Further concerning, teachers expressed not wanting to be involved in teaching a student with epilepsy (Nigeria 63%, Zimbabwe 17%), frankly objecting to a student with epilepsy being in their class (Burkina Faso 15%) and suggesting that a child with epilepsy be withdrawn from school entirely (Nigeria 48%).

The negative views of students with epilepsy are likely to be a reflection of negative stereotypes regarding epilepsy in general. There was a low expectation by teachers that epilepsy was a treatable condition (Senegal 73%, Nigeria 47%) and endorsements that it was specifically always refractory (Zimbabwe 40%). There were significant concerns that epilepsy was infectious, especially any saliva from the mouth of a victim during a seizure (Burkina Faso 12%; Zimbabwe 23%; Senegal 24%; Zambia 28%; Nigeria 29%; 31%, 32%; Zambia 51%). Mental illness was frequently but not universally felt to be a cause or consequence of epilepsy (Zambia 0%, Nigeria 10%, Zimbabwe 12% and Burkina Faso 31%). Moreover, superstitious beliefs were prevalent with 29% of teachers in Senegal stating that epilepsy was a supernatural affliction and other teachers endorsing more specific etiologic beliefs such as possession (Zambia 20%; Nigeria 22%, 28%, 61%), witchcraft (Nigeria 6%; Zambia 17%) and curses from God (Zambia 2%).

Social association was affected by the generally negative outlook toward persons with epilepsy, especially associations involving marriage. In general most teachers would allow their child to play with a child with epilepsy (Zambia 97%, Zimbabwe 83%). Only 80% of teachers surveyed in Zimbabwe would agree to work with a person with epilepsy and just over half (56%) would agree to employ one. Seventy-six percent of teachers in the Zimbabwe sample would consider marrying a person with epilepsy but only 44% of the respondents in Zambia would allow their child to marry and 95% of Nigerian teachers surveyed would adopt a negative stance toward their child marrying a person with epilepsy.

Peers of Students with Epilepsy

Students in primary and secondary schools function as the peer group for persons with epilepsy in the educational setting. Surveys of this population reflect the findings of research in general and teaching populations. In general, level of knowledge and the culture setting have significant impact on the attitudes of students toward persons with epilepsy. In one survey of teenagers and young adults with epilepsy spanning 16 countries 36% kept their condition a secret for fear of being treated differently (Baker et al., 2008).

Primary School

Little research has been done to document the attitudes of primary school children. One Brazilian study demonstrated a lack of knowledge in a small sample (n = 24) of children aged 9 to 11 years old (Fernandes, Cabral, Araujo, Noronha, and Li, 2005). Twenty percent of these students did not know what epilepsy was, while 16% believed that epilepsy was a contagious disease. A similar study by a group in Ontario, Canada demonstrated significant improvement in positive attitudes towards PWE with educational programs, but baseline attitudes were not reported (Martiniuk, Speechley, Secco, Campbell, and Donner, 2007).

Secondary School

Surveys in secondary schools demonstrate patterns of belief similar to those found in the teaching population. Low but significant levels of misinformation were uncovered in the more western populations surveyed with more fear and superstition being documented in the India and Africa (Matuja and Rwiza, 1994; Njamnshi et al., 2008; Pandian, Santosh, Kumar, Sarma, and Radhakrishnan, 2006). Universally these prejudices were documented to be less in populations having higher education (graduate school versus high school populations) and, where studied, amendable to educational intervention. Much of the prejudice surrounding epilepsy likely comes from misperceptions of what the disease is and how it is caused. Seven percent of high school student surveyed in one study viewed PWE as dangerous. Four percent of these same students believed that epilepsy was contagious (Martiniuk et al., 2007).

Similar numbers documenting fears of "catching" epilepsy can be found in other surveys in western countries (Poland 9%, Italy 16%) (Mecarelli et al., 2007; Zielinska, Klos, and Talarska, 2005). Likewise, only 14% of a group of Indian high school students endorsed this belief. However, this misconception was much more prevalent in populations surveyed in Africa with 50% endorsement by students in Cameroon (Njamnshi et al., 2008) and 61% endorsement by students in Tanzania (Matuja and Rwiza, 1994). Aside from the view of epilepsy as contagious, there is also a harmful perception of epilepsy as a mental disorder. Nineteen percent of high school students surveyed in the United States believed this to be true while 12% of students in Poland also endorsed this idea. Eight percent of Brazilian students thought that an appropriate treatment for epilepsy was psychological or psychiatric (Reno, Fernandes, Bell, Sander, and Li, 2007). Surprisingly 56% of an Italian population classified epilepsy as a psychiatric disease (Mecarelli et al., 2007). Similar numbers were found in Cameroon (38%) and India (59%). Superstition was evident in Indian and African samples with 11% of Indian students surveyed believing epilepsy was caused by ancestor sin, 22% of the same student would treat epilepsy with exorcism, and 4% of students surveyed in Tanzania believing in an etiology of evil spirits.

These fears generated by the perceived etiologies of epilepsy are compounded by the beliefs in the adverse effects and permanence of the disease. Nine percent of students surveyed in the United States believe that CWE do not usually attend regular schools (Austin, Shafer, and Deering, 2002), while 93% of secondary students in Tanzania believe all PWE are mentally subnormal. Thirteen percent of Italian students endorsed the belief that PWE can never recover while 53% of Indian students and 54% of Tanzanian students believed that epilepsy can not be cured.

Prejudices toward PWE are translated into low expectations and social isolation. Again, this is less prevalent but still present in more western cultures. There is a widespread belief that PWE can or should not be employed amongst those who were surveyed: (U.S. 8%, Cameroon 41%, India 71%), marry and/or have children (U.S. 8%, Italy 12%, India 41%, Cameroon 64%, Tanzania 81%). In Poland 92% of students surveyed would accept a PWE as a friend, but in the United States sample 11% would refuse to date a PWE. In India and Africa the prejudice endorsed was more extreme. Many students would object to associating with, sitting in the same class as or playing with a PWE (India 13%, Cameroon 25%). In Tanzania, 54% would not allow a sibling to sit in the same class with a PWE and 59% would not allow a PWE to attend school at all.

Post-Secondary School

University students in general endorsed lower levels of misconceptions regarding epilepsy than less educated individuals, but did still reflect cultural biases in their region. Epilepsy was considered to be contagious by 14% of students in a Malaysian university student population (Ab Rahman, 2005) and 13% in a similar population in South Africa (Peltzer, 2001). Yet despite this improvement in knowledge, there is still lingering fears surrounding PWE with 30% of the Malaysian student population studied endorsing that PWE are dangerous.

The perception of epilepsy associated with mental illness was still apparent in this more educated group. Some of this misperception may be due to comorbid depression and anxiety which is common in PWE (Tellez-Zenteno, Patten, Jette, Williams, and Wiebe, 2007). Although a very low percentage of Brazilian university and 1st and 6th year medical students endorsed mental illness as the actual etiology for epilepsy (0%, 13%, 3%) there were still minor perceptions that epilepsy predisposed one to developing serious psychiatric illness (11%, 9%, 3%) (Caixeta, Fernandes, Bell, Sander, and Li, 2007). Similar low grade misinformation was documented in a sample of Canadian college students, 9% of whom endorsed insanity as a cause for epilepsy (Young et al., 2002). Much higher levels of this belief were documented in Malaysia (40%) and South Africa (63%) with residual superstitions also apparent in the answer choice of evil spirits as causative to epilepsy (Malaysia 5%, South Africa 26%) (Ab Rahman, 2005; Peltzer, 2001). Poor cognition resultant from epilepsy was a documented belief at low levels in 1st and 6th year Brazilian medical students (3%, 8% respectively) and poor perceived prognosis was indicated by 53% of Brazilian and 14% of Malaysian university students.

Imposition of social isolation on PWE was less prevalent in the university samples compared to secondary schools. In the Brazilian medical student population 82% of 1st year students and 89% of 6th year students would marry a PWE. In South Africa 78% of students surveyed stated a PWE could marry while 69% would marry a PWE themselves. Conversely, there were small percentages of university students who would object to themselves or a relative marrying a PWE (Canada 4%, Brazil 16%, and South Africa 20%). In the Canadian university population 11% believed that PWE should not have children. Employment opportunities for PWE were positively regarded with 92% and 89% of 1st and 6th year Brazilian medical students willing to employ a PWE and 73% of South African university students affirming that PWE are employable. Low numbers of university students in Canada

(14%) and Brazil (6%, 7%) did not deem PWE employable. Minimal actual isolation was endorsed in this sample with only 13% of South African university students desiring PWE being physically separate from other students. Four percent of Brazilian and five percent of Canadian university students would object to their child associating with a child with epilepsy.

CULTURE

Perceptions of Epilepsy in Non-Western Societies

Southeast Asians (consisting of Muslims, Sikhs and Hindus) and Africans tend to have the belief that epilepsy is caused by mystical or spiritual reasons such as possession or delinquency (Allotey and Reidpath, 2007; Ismail, Wright, Rhodes, Small, and Jacoby, 2005). This belief that epilepsy is caused by spiritual possession (called jinn) is also widespread in Muslims in the UK and India. Sikhs and Hindus believe that epilepsy is the result of sins from a past life. In native tribes from Central and South America, just the pronunciation of the word 'epilepsy" is taboo (Carod-Artal and Vazquez-Cabrera, 2007). In China the moral blame for an individual's epilepsy encompasses his or her whole family (Andermann, 1995).

Many of the African studies found a large percentage of people believe that epilepsy is contagious and this belief was not influenced by age, gender or education level (Rwiza et al., 1993). Many also believe in supernatural causes and this belief was also not reduced by higher educational attainment (Ndoye et al., 2005; Nyame and Biritwum, 1997; Tekle-Haimanot et al., 1991). A third of Christian Zambian clerics also endorsed spiritual causes. A majority (89%) recommended a doctor while 34% recommended a traditional healer (Atadzhanov et al., 2006). In Ethiopia 89% did not know what to do for someone having a seizure (Tekle-Haimanot et al., 1991). In rural areas of Africa close family ties, communal living arrangements and traditional belief systems are thought to be a big determinant of stigmatization (Baskind and Birbeck, 2005). In Africa one's place in the community and family unit is also a major determinant of self-perception (Baskind and Birbeck, 2005).

Most importantly, PWE from these cultures do not share these beliefs themselves. Some PWE do discuss their conditions of epilepsy in fatal terms such as "the will of Allah." However, in most cases spiritual beliefs did not prevent people from searching for the cause of their epilepsy or from taking steps to seek treatment or a cure (Ismail, Wright, Rhodes, and Small, 2005). In Nepal, traditional healers (called Jhankri) make house calls and use methods such as fainting attacks, water over the forehead, casting anti-spell on water for PWE to drink, herbal medicine and offering their spiritual being an offering (Rajbhandari, 2004). Supernatural explanations include bad luck, jealousy, witchcraft and divine punishment (Allotey and Reidpath, 2007). In one study 100% of Nigerians laypersons believed that epilepsy was contagious (Awaritefe, 1989). Many users of alternative medicine in non-Western cultures have secondary education with a higher percentage being illiterate (Danesi and Adetunji, 1994).

Cultural beliefs about epilepsy and attribution to spiritual possession underpin health seeking behavior (Snape, Wang, Wu, Jacoby, and Baker, 2009). In a small ethnographic study from China respondents only rarely acknowledged spiritual causes, many however described epilepsy as "a fate not as good as death" (Snape et al., 2009). Participants also expressed great economic suffering as a consequence of long term treatment. Almost half of PWE from Lagos used spiritual healing. Common forms included prayers, fasting and holy water or oil. PWE drank or bathed in herbal preparations. An alternate explanation would suggest that people may not seek treatment for epilepsy with AEDs if epilepsy is not viewed as a condition that can be treated by Western medicine (Scott et al., 2001) or from a preference for traditional medicine (Andermann, 1995).

Obstacles for PWE in Non-Western Societies

Obstacles for PWE in developing countries include a treatment gap, a poor understanding of epilepsy and a lack of sufficient resources (Rajbhandari, 2004; Scott et al., 2001). PWE from these countries lack information with proper medical health information may have language barriers, literacy barriers and may express dissatisfaction with general practitioners (Danesi and Adetunji, 1994; Ismail, Wright, Rhodes, Small, and Jacoby, 2005). Developing countries do not have organized health care systems, record keeping is poor and research is minimal (Krishnamoorthy, Satishchandra, and Sander, 2003).

In sub-Sahara Africa, 67% to 75% of rural populations have no access to health care facilities (Slikkerveer, 1982). A large percentage of people in Africa reported they had witnessed a seizure compared to studies from the U.S., Europe and Asia and reported epilepsy prevalence rates are as high as 6% in some African countries (Njamnshi et al., 2008; Rwiza et al., 1993). The wide treatment gap in Africa may explain these results. In Senegal 23% of persons with epilepsy never received treatment (Ndoye et al., 2005). These gaps have prompted calls for improved health care delivery and guarantees of an adequate supply of inexpensive AEDs within basic health services (Tekle-Haimanot et al., 1991). Use of indigenous medicine practices is also common in Africa (Rwiza et al., 1993). Utilization studies in the Phillipines, Pakistan and Equador suggested that 80% to 90% of PWE were not receiving antiepileptic medication (Danesi and Adetunji, 1994; Ellison, Guvener, Feksi, Placentia, and Shorvon, 1989). Many PWE from developing nations use alternative medicines since they do not have access to allopathic medicine (Danesi and Adetunji, 1994).

In developing countries, specialists are primarily concentrated in the urban centers while much of the population lives in villages (Krishnamoorthy et al., 2003). The ideal neurologist to population ratio is 1 per 100,000 however the ratio is 1 to 8 million (Africa) and 1 per 2.4 million in India (Murthy, 2003). Access to specialists is minimal in some countries, for example, there are only 500 neurologists for the entire population of 1 billion in India (Krishnamoorthy et al., 2003). Cultural attitudes, a lack of prioritization, poor health system infrastructure and inadequate supplies of most AEDs are all serious barriers to care. These barriers are compounded when cultural beliefs do not recognize Western treatment methods as valid for epilepsy. To help overcome such barriers epilepsy must be described in culturally relevant terms. In Malawi seizures were explained to result from a scar on the brain and this resulted in a high rate of AED take up and compliance (Watts, 1989). It will be difficult to close the treatment gap until poverty and inequalities of health are also dealt with at the local, national and global levels (Scott et al., 2001).

Mistaken views need to be educated and negative attitudes need to be replaced with positive attitudes (Awaritefe, 1989). There is an evident need for accessible, high quality mental health, educational and medical services regardless of socioeconomic status and ethnicity (Wu et al., 2008). Racial and ethnic minority groups continue to be underserved in developed countries like the U.S. (Sue, 1988) and they are more likely to avoid mental health services due to the notion of a double stigma of ethnicity and mental health (Wu et al., 2008). The minimization of cultural problems does not imply that treatment should match cultural expectations (Sue and Zane, 1987). Furthermore, all ethnic minority groups have significantly higher dropout rates from mental health treatment than Caucasians (Sue and Zane, 1987). In developing countries the treatment gap will only be closed by addressing poverty and inequalities in income (Scott et al., 2001). All health personnel should be familiar with local beliefs regarding health and illness (Andermann, 1995) especially when it comes to epilepsy.

Employment and Improved Legal Regulations

Caveness suggested more enlightened attitudes in the U.S. were likely due to an overall improvement in public attitudes towards diseases such as tuberculosis, syphilis and cancer; improved control of seizures by medication, educational efforts by professional and lay societies regarding epilepsy; employment by a number of major industries of persons with epilepsy and more reasonable legal regulations concerning immigration, marriage and motor vehicle licenses (Caveness et al., 1969; Caveness and Gallup, 1980). Worldwide, persons with epilepsy are known to have significant difficulties obtaining and maintaining employment (Bautista and Wludyka, 2007; Chaplin, 2005; de Boer, 2005; S. A. Lee, 2005; Smeets, van Lierop, Vanhoutvin, Aldenkamp, and Nijhuis, 2007; Varma, Sylaja, George, Sankara Sarma, and Radhakrishnan, 2007). It has long been recognized that employment is a necessary step in the rehabilitation process. However a large scale, one year, community-based educational program using local broadcasting, newspapers, flyers and movies had little effect on changing employers' attitudes about hiring someone with epilepsy in the short term (Sands and Zalkind, 1972). A more recent prospective U.S. study found employer attitudes maintained a positive change over 30 years (Hicks and Hicks, 1991).

In the U.S., the Americans with Disabilities Act of 1990 provided more sweeping legislation against discrimination in employment settings (Troxell, 1997). Outside the U.S. employers still report significant concerns over hiring someone with epilepsy (Jacoby, Gorry, and Baker, 2005). However, company size and previous experience employing PWE positively impacted attitudes in the United Kingdom. In addition, many employers were willing to make accommodations for PWE. Helping PWE overcome these barriers is critical as one survey found many PWE feel the experience of being refused a job or having been unemployed regarded this as a declaration of incompetence (Ekermo, 1975).

Laws enforcing sterilization of persons with epilepsy as well as bans on marriage have been repealed in the last 50 years in many areas of the world (McLin and de Boer, 1995). However, social policies are still in their infancy in other countries. In India a marriage can be annulled for recurrent attacks of insanity or epilepsy. In China the moral blame for an individual's epilepsy encompasses his or her whole family (Andermann, 1995). In the developing world overcoming such views is vital to improving knowledge and beliefs about epilepsy.

Recommendations for Addressing Public Education about Epilepsy

Studies also found older age, type of employment, unfamiliarity with epilepsy and the belief that epilepsy was a form of mental illness were associated with more negative attitudes towards epilepsy (Diamantopoulos et al., 2006; Spatt et al., 2005). These groups may be the best to target educational campaigns. Logistic regression analyses found knowledge of epilepsy was an independent predictor, even more so than general education. This is important in that public awareness campaigns can influence epilepsy specific knowledge as where increasing general educational level in society is a much bigger issue (Spatt et al., 2005).

Educational programs have shown improvement in knowledge and attitudes regardless of the method used (Gutteling, Seydel, and Wiegman, 1986). Educational campaigns in community settings, work sites, schools, churches and stores have been suggested as a method to improve general population knowledge (Kobau and Price, 2003). Social marketing approaches include protesting inaccurate depictions of PWE in the media, education of PWE and key social groups and increasing the public's contact with PWE (Birbeck, 2006; Rusch, Angermeyer, and Corrigan, 2005). Such methods must balance the message that PWE are "no different than you and me" with "they are different and deserve special treatment" (Birbeck, 2006).

Protesting Inaccurate Depictions in the Media

Due to rapid expansion and accessibility of the media and the internet, people now have greater access to information and resources. However, 31% of print media stories about epilepsy contained gross errors, scientific inaccuracies, exaggerated claims and overestimates of the risks of dying during a seizure (Krauss, Gondek, Krumholz, Paul, and Shen, 2000). Television programs and movies continue to portray epilepsy in a negative light (Baxendale and O'toole, 2007). These include drama based medical programs that have medical consultants who could guard against promoting improper information and dangerous first aid procedures. This would suggest that negative attitudes, stereotypes and incorrect information portrayed in the media continue to influence the consciousness of the general population. This has prompted the Epilepsy Foundation in the U.S. to respond very strongly to such egregious representations of epilepsy (Coelho, 2006). Unfortunately, little is known about the effectiveness of such "protest" efforts against prejudices (Rusch et al., 2005). Such approaches demand a lot of resources which may distract people from learning new information that disconfirms the stigmatizing stereotypes.

Patient Education

Education of PWE through programs and social support groups may help reduce the health burden of epilepsy, improve access and quality of care, decrease the emotional impact of epilepsy and improve social policy making and advocacy (Birbeck, 2006). Patient education has been shown to be effective for improving health outcomes such as reduced medication needs, reduced duration of treatment and hospitals stays, improvements in risk reducing behavior and reduction of risk factors (Keulers, Welters, Spauwen, and Houpt, 2007).

Educational interventions for persons with epilepsy have been developed around the world. The modular service package for epilepsy (MOSES) program, that uses a total of fourteen, 1-hour sessions over 2 days, showed improvement in patient knowledge, coping, seizure outcome and treatment therapy satisfaction six months after the intervention (May and Pfafflin, 2002) for those in the intervention group. While successful, the MOSES program is however limited in its ability to be replicated as it was developed in German and presently no manuals or materials are available in other languages. In addition, due to the length of the program it may only be suitable for patients who are highly motivated and have only slight cognitive and learning deficits.

A shorter 6 hour program was developed in Norway (Helde, Brodtkorb, Brathen, and Bovim, 2003). The two main aims were: 1) to provide general information about epilepsy focusing on individual problems of the patient and 2) to allow the participants to share their own experiences of coming to terms with the diagnosis/living with epilepsy. This nurse-led intervention followed by two years of extended nurse follow up and counseling was studied in a randomized, controlled trial (Helde et al., 2003). The program was shown to improve quality of life (based on the QOLIE-89) in areas specific to health discouragement, medication effects and physical role limitations for the intervention group but not the control group. No outcomes related to knowledge were evaluated or reported.

A two day psycho-educational program from Nigeria found a significant decrease in depression level psychoneurotic traits based on the Crown-Crisp experiential index as well as a significant increase in knowledge (Olley, Osinowo, and Brieger, 2001). The program focused on three modules: background, diagnosis/management and living with epilepsy. This is the only educational program to document an influence on psychopathology. This program also has limited ability to be replicated as it was developed in a specific culture and presently no manuals are available in other languages.

In the U.S. only one educational program has documented improvements in patients. The Sepulveda Epilepsy Education program, now known as the Seizures and Epilepsy Education (SEE) program demonstrated increases in knowledge, a significant decrease in fear of seizures and a significant decrease in hazardous medical self-management practices in the treatment group compared to those on a wait-list control group (Helgeson, Mittan, Tan, and Chayasirisobhon, 1990). The SEE program is a two-day weekend program designed to provide medical education and psychosocial therapy. No changes in outcome measures related to seizure frequency, mood, anxiety, and self-efficacy or on subscales of the Washington Psychosocial Seizure Inventory were seen.

Education for Key Social Groups

Focused programs tailored for key social groups are thought to play an important role in either promoting or alleviating stigma (Birbeck, 2006). Such programs are thought to be more cost effective than mass social marketing campaigns. Key social groups who are known to have a great influence on knowledge and attitudes about epilepsy include health professionals and educators. Research from Australia in the 1980's revealed general practitioners' negative attitudes and a bias towards a psychological instability for those with controlled uncomplicated epilepsy and mixed opinions towards personal relationships. On the positive side they had positive attitudes towards education, intelligence and employment (Beran and Read, 1983). A follow up study by the same investigators found some improvement in attitudes with exception of attitudes towards emotional and behavioral problems (Frith, Harris, and Beran, 1994). Similar patterns of negative and positive attitudes have been found for physicians in Oman (Al-Adawi et al., 2001).

A lack of effective teaching about epilepsy in medical schools was identified over 30 years ago (Stores, 1975) and this effect seems to have persisted (Gomes, 2000). Epilepsy seminars designed for medical students have improved knowledge but not attitudes (Mason, Fenton, and Jamieson, 1990). It has been recommended that medical education address student's beliefs and attitudes as well as for providing adequate knowledge and skills in managing epilepsy (Mason et al., 1990).

A didactic epilepsy workshop for community professionals (school teachers, mental health staff and public health nurses) that utilized presenters with epilepsy helped improved both knowledge and comfort (Appolone, Romeis, Gibson, McLean, and Howard, 1979). A recent study confirms targeted education for medical students improves knowledge and confidence while decreasing stigma in the primary setting. A one year follow up found this improvement was maintained (Noronha et al., 2007). A similar program for health professionals focused on the bio-psycho-social aspects of epilepsy was able to improve knowledge, attitudes and perceptions (Fernandes, Noronha, Sander, Bell, and Li, 2007) however knowledge was still below 50%, stressing the need for ongoing educational programs.

Lack of public awareness, availability of social services and the cost of antiepileptic drugs were identified as the three greatest health system barriers to positive outcomes identified by health professionals in epilepsy (Hayes, Melin, Dupuis, Murray, and Labiner, 2007). Eighty-one percent of neurologists in another study believed that the public was not adequately informed about epilepsy and frequent misperceptions still focus on epilepsy being primarily hereditary or a mental illness. A television campaign was most often suggested as the best method for public education by practitioners (Hawley et al., 2007). To make mass media campaigns more effective it has been suggested that language of different segments of society be used to take out labels and improve social acceptance (Li et al., 2007).

Fear is thought to be one of the key factors in prejudice (Bagley, 1972). Therefore it is generally believed that measures to improve knowledge will ameliorate prejudices (Spatt, Langbauer, and Mamoli, 1998). While education level is negatively correlated with the perception of stigma (Fernandes et al., 2007) ending the stigma of epilepsy may reside in reaching the young while they are still forming their values and societal attitudes (Coelho, 2006). Population studies from the United States show persons with a history of epilepsy report lower educational attainment, lower household income and poorer health status compared to those without epilepsy (Elliott, Moore, and Lu, 2008; Kobau et al., 2007; Kobau et al., 2008). Educational attainment improves health both directly and indirectly through work and economic conditions, psychosocial resources and a healthy lifestyle (Ross and Wu, 1995).

Contact with PWE

Health education is often written for the large public who has no direct experience with the topic. Contact with PWE is thought to enhance educational efforts to reduce stigma (Rusch et al., 2005). However, one study found that persons with direct behavioral experiences with epilepsy showed less change of attitude and knowledge after participating in a health education intervention (Gutteling et al., 1986). This suggests that people with direct personal experiences can be expected to be less effected than those with indirect experiences.

While direct experience with someone who has epilepsy may not be feasible on a large scale contact to PWE can also be achieved through educational films. A 1955 study of college students and community adults examined the effects of a Veteran's Administration film called "Seizure" (Rose, Peace, and McBride, 1955). The film was designed to create a more favorable view towards epilepsy and explain the needless injury to PWE caused by negative society views. In a ranking of the fifteen most feared socio-physical handicaps, epilepsy ranked as one of the three most feared among participants. The movie was then used as an educational intervention. The most improvement in attitudes was found in those of middle socio-economic level, who were not in health professions, in pre and post scores analyses of expressed attitudes towards epilepsy. In a three month follow up there was only a slight decrease in improved attitudes towards epilepsy.

RECOMMENDATIONS

While positive changes in knowledge and beliefs towards serious health problems, including epilepsy, have occurred in many areas of the world there is still much that needs to be done (Weiss and Ramakrishna, 2006). The most important step in overcoming negative attitudes and beliefs towards epilepsy involves education of the general public. Educational interventions to improve attitudes and beliefs towards epilepsy must take into account the cultural aspect of diverse societies. The reduction of health related stigma in school settings would go a long way to improving acceptance and dispelling centuries old myths that continue to pervade society. Education about epilepsy in the school setting would also go a long way to improve educational outcomes for PWE.

Studies have documented the burden of stigma in epilepsy, but few have compared epilepsy to other chronic health problems. Little is known about the effects of stigma on the delay of appropriate help-seeking as well as treatment drop out and effectiveness. Further research is needed to evaluate the effects of social change and stigma reducing interventions in the general population. Community understanding and social policies need to be developed through scientific understanding to avoid laws and health policies that are influenced by stereotypes and prejudices. We also need to develop simple, clear and unambiguous messages about epilepsy for the general public. Such messages need to take into account ethnic and cultural differences (i.e., acknowledge cultural differences and practice respect concerning accepted roles of men and women, value of traditional medicine versus Western medicine, favorite or forbidden foods, manner of dress and body language) when appropriate (U.S. Department of Health and Human Services, 2005). We must also collaborate and learn from stigma research and policies that have been studied in other areas. Mental health research is one area that is directly relevant to our efforts (Rusch et al., 2005) especially when many PWE suffer disproportionately from comorbid mental illnesses (Tellez-Zenteno et al., 2007).

CONCLUSIONS

While knowledge and attitudes vary widely in different regions of the world, common themes in the population research emerge. In general, populations of non-industrialized countries have more negative attitudes towards epilepsy. Knowledge and attitudes are mediated by socio-cultural factors as well as by personal experience. Educational settings are thought to be ideal for interventions to improve knowledge and attitudes towards epilepsy in the general population. Students with chronic illnesses, such as epilepsy, can encounter negative attitudes towards their learning abilities as well as fear and misunderstanding among their fellow students and teachers. The current literature suggests teachers have knowledge and attitudes similar to the general population. They also indicate an interest in learning more about epilepsy. Educational settings are a perfect place to dispel myths and misperceptions. Such as strategy will help decrease stigma while improving public attitudes over the long term. The developing world (Asia, India and Africa) are all place where efforts to improve public education should be focused. Education and social marketing programs alone are not cost effective or sustainable without substantial funding and high levels of political will. Continued advocacy by epilepsy support organizations is vital for improving knowledge and beliefs in the general public. Advocacy organizations are also crucial for building and maintaining a strong sense of confidence in personal abilities and the persistence that individuals with epilepsy need to make the most of their lives in the broader society.

REFERENCES

Ab Rahman, A. F. (2005). Awareness and knowledge of epilepsy among students in a Malaysian university. *Seizure, 14*, 593-596.

Akhtar, S. W., Ali, S.:. A.,S.M., Sonija, A. L., Husainuddin, Mogal, Z., Iqbal, Z., et al. (2007). Survey of knowledge, attitude and practice of epilepsy among 535 schoolteachers in five cities of Pakistan. *Neurology Asia 2007, 12 Suppl 1*, 99-100.

Al-Adawi, S., Al-Ismaily, S., Martin, R., Al-Naamani, A., Al-Riyamy, K., Al-Maskari, M., et al. (2001). Psychosocial aspects of epilepsy in Oman: Attitude of health personnel. *Epilepsia, 42*, 1476-1481.

Alikor, E. A., and Essien, A. A. (2005). Childhood epilepsy: Knowledge and attitude of primary school teachers in Port Harcourt, Nigeria. *Nigerian Journal of Medicine, 14*, 299-303.

Allotey, P., and Reidpath, D. (2007). Epilepsy, culture, identity and well-being: A study of the social, cultural and environmental context of epilepsy in Cameroon. *Journal of Health Psychology, 12*, 431-443.

Andermann, L. F. (1995). Epilepsy in developing countries. *Transcultural Psychiatry, 32*, 351-384.

Andriantseheno, L. M., and Rakotoarivony, M. C. (2000). Sociocultural aspects of epilepsy in Madagascar. K.A.P. survey carried out in Antananarivo. *Bulletin De La Societe De Pathologie Exotique, 93*, 247-250.

Appolone, C., Romeis, J., Gibson, P., McLean, W., and Howard, G. (1979). An epilepsy workshop for professionals. *Epilepsia, 20*, 127-132.

Atadzhanov, M., Chomba, E., Haworth, A., Mbewe, E., and Birbeck, G. L. (2006). Knowledge, attitudes, behaviors, and practices regarding epilepsy among Zambian clerics. *Epilepsy and Behavior, 9*, 83-88.

Austin, J. K., Shafer, P. O., and Deering, J. B. (2002). Epilepsy familiarity, knowledge, and perceptions of stigma: Report from a survey of adolescents in the general population. *Epilepsy and Behavior, 3*, 368-375.

Awad, A., and Sarkhoo, F. (2008). Public knowledge and attitudes toward epilepsy in Kuwait. *Epilepsia, 49*, 564-572.

Awaritefe, A. (1989). Epilepsy: The myth of a contagious disease. *Culture, Medicine and Psychiatry, 13*, 449-456.

Aydin, K., and Yildiz, H. (2007). Teachers' perceptions in central turkey concerning epilepsy and asthma and the short-term effect of a brief education on the perception of epilepsy. *Epilepsy and Behavior, 10*, 286-290.

Bagic, A., Bagic, D., and Zivkovic, I. (2009). First population study of the general public awareness and perception of epilepsy in Bosnia and Herzegovina. *Epilepsy and Behavior, 14*, 154-61.

Baker, G. A., Hargis, E., Hsih, M. M., Mounfield, H., Arzimanoglou, A., Glauser, T., et al. (2008). Perceived impact of epilepsy in teenagers and young adults: An international survey. *Epilepsy and Behavior, 12*, 395-401.

Bannon, M. J., Wildig, C., and Jones, P. W. (1992). Teachers' perceptions of epilepsy. *Archives of Disease in Childhood, 67*, 1467-1471.

Baskind, R., and Birbeck, G. L. (2005). Epilepsy-associated stigma in sub-Saharan Africa: The social landscape of a disease. *Epilepsy and Behavior, 7*, 68-73.

Baumann, R. J., Wilson, J. F., and Wiese, H. J. (1995). Kentuckians' attitudes toward children with epilepsy. *Epilepsia, 36*, 1003-1008.

Bautista, R. E., and Wludyka, P. (2007). Factors associated with employment in epilepsy patients. *Epilepsy and Behavior, 10*, 89-95.

Baxendale, S., and O'toole, A. (2007). Epilepsy myths: Alive and foaming in the 21st century. *Epilepsy and Behavior, 11*, 192-196.

Bekiroglu, N., Ozkan, R., Gurses, C., Arpaci, B., and Dervent, A. (2004). A study on awareness and attitude of teachers on epilepsy in Istanbul. *Seizure, 13*, 517-522.

Bener, A., al-Marzooqi, F. H., and Sztriha, L. (1998). Public awareness and attitudes towards epilepsy in the United Arab Emirates. *Seizure, 7*, 219-222.

Beran, R. G., and Read, T. (1983). A survey of doctors in Sydney, Australia: Perspectives and practices regarding epilepsy and those affected by it. *Epilepsia, 24*, 79-104.

Birbeck, G. (2006). Interventions to reduce epilepsy-associated stigma. *Psychology, Health and Medicine, 11*, 364-366.

Birbeck, G. L., Chomba, E., Atadzhanov, M., Mbewe, E., and Haworth, A. (2006). Zambian teachers: What do they know about epilepsy and how can we work with them to decrease stigma? *Epilepsy and Behavior, 9*, 275-280.

Bishop, M., and Boag, E. M. (2006). Teachers' knowledge about epilepsy and attitudes toward students with epilepsy: Results of a national survey. *Epilepsy and Behavior, 8*, 397-405.

Bishop, M., and Slevin, B. (2004). Teachers' attitudes toward students with epilepsy: Results of a survey of elementary and middle school teachers. *Epilepsy and Behavior, 5*, 308-315.

Bagley, C. (1972). Social prejudice and the adjustment of people with epilepsy. *Epilepsia, 13*, 33-45.

Caixeta, J., Fernandes, P. T., Bell, G. S., Sander, J. W., and Li, L. M. (2007). Epilepsy perception amongst university students: A survey. *Arquivos De Neuro-Psiquiatria, 65 Suppl 1*, 43-48.

Canger, R., and Cornaggia, C. (1985). Public attitudes toward epilepsy in Italy: Results of a survey and comparison with U.S.A. and West German data. *Epilepsia, 26*, 221-226.

Carod-Artal, F. J., and Vazquez-Cabrera, C. B. (2007). An anthropological study about epilepsy in native tribes from Central and South America. *Epilepsia, 48*, 886-893.

Caveness, W. (1949). A survey of public attitudes toward epilepsy. *Epilepsia, B4*(1), 19-26.

Caveness, W. (1954). A survey of public attitudes toward epilepsy, 1954. *Epilepsia, 3*, 99-102.

Caveness, W. F. (1960). Trend in public attitudes toward epilepsy over the past decade. *Epilepsia, 1*, 385-393.

Caveness, W. F., and Gallup, G. H. (1980). A survey of public attitudes toward epilepsy in 1979 with an indication of trends over the past thirty years. *Epilepsia, 21*, 509-518.

Caveness, W. F., Merritt, H. H., and Gallup, G. H. (1969). A survey of public attitudes toward epilepsy in 1969 with an indication of trends over the past twenty years. *Epilepsia, 10*, 429-440.

Caveness, W. F., Merritt, H. H., and Gallup, G. H. (1974). A survey of public attitudes toward epilepsy in 1974 with an indication of trends over the past twenty-five years. *Epilepsia, 15*, 523-536.

Caveness, W. F., Merritt, H. H., and Gallup, G. H. and Ruby, E. H. (1965). A survey of public attitudes toward epilepsy in 1964, with an indication of trends over the past fifteen years. *Epilepsia, 6*, 75-86.

Chaplin, J. (2005). Vocational assessment and intervention for people with epilepsy. *Epilepsia, 46 Suppl 1*, 55-56.

Choi-Kwon, S., Park, K. A., Lee, H. J., Park, M. S., Lee, C. H., Cheon, S. E., et al. (2004). Familiarity with, knowledge of, and attitudes toward epilepsy in residents of Seoul, South Korea. *Acta Neurologica Scandinavica, 110*, 39-45.

Chung, M. Y., Chang, Y. C., Lai, Y. H., and Lai, C. W. (1995). Survey of public awareness, understanding, and attitudes toward epilepsy in Taiwan. *Epilepsia, 36*, 488-493.

Coelho, T. (2006). The key to ending stigma. *Epilepsy and Behavior, 8*, 3-4.

Danesi, M. A., and Adetunji, J. B. (1994). Use of alternative medicine by patients with epilepsy: A survey of 265 epileptic patients in a developing country. *Epilepsia, 35*, 344-351.

Dantas, F. G., Cariri, G. A., Cariri, G. A., and Ribeiro Filho, A. R. (2001). Knowledge and attitudes toward epilepsy among primary, secondary and tertiary level teachers. *Arquivos De Neuro-Psiquiatria, 59*(3-B), 712-716.

Daoud, A., Al-Safi, S., Otoom, S., Wahba, L., and Alkofahi, A. (2007). Public knowledge and attitudes towards epilepsy in Jordan. *Seizure, 16*, 521-526.

de Boer, H. M. (2005). Overview and perspectives of employment in people with epilepsy. *Epilepsia, 46*, 52-54.

Demirci, S., Dönmez, C. M., Gündoğar, D., and Baydar, Ç L. (2007). Public awareness of, attitudes toward, and understanding of epilepsy in Isparta, Turkey. *Epilepsy and Behavior, 11*, 427-433.

Diamantopoulos, N., Kaleyias, J., Tzoufi, M., and Kotsalis, C. (2006). A survey of public awareness, understanding, and attitudes toward epilepsy in Greece. *Epilepsia, 47*, 2154-2164.

Diehl, L. W. (1975). Changes in popular attitudes toward epilepsy in the federal republic of Germany and the USA. In D. Janz (Ed.) *Epileptology: Proceedings of the Seventh International Symposium on Epilepsy,* (pp. 97-100). Stuttgart, Georg Thieme Verlag.

Diehl, L. W., and Hauck, G. (1975). Changes in public attitudes toward epilepsy in the federal republic of Germany since 1967. *Der Nervenarzt, 46*, 519-524.

DiIorio, C. A., Kobau, R., Holden, E. W., Berkowitz, J. M., Kamin, S. L., Antonak, R. F., et al. (2004). Developing a measure to assess attitudes toward epilepsy in the US population. *Epilepsy and Behavior, 5*, 965-975.

Ekermo, C. (1975). What it means to have epilepsy: Emotional experience and social reality. In D. Janz (Ed.) *Epileptology: Proceedings of the Seventh International Symposium on Epilepsy,* (pp. 91-96). Stuttgart, Georg Thieme Verlag.

Elliott, J., and Shneker, B. (2008). Patient, caregiver, and health care practitioner knowledge of, beliefs about, and attitudes toward epilepsy. *Epilepsy and Behavior, 12*, 547-556.

Elliott, J. O., Moore, J. L., and Lu, B. (2008). Health status and behavioral risk factors among persons with epilepsy in Ohio based on the 2006 behavioral risk factor surveillance system. *Epilepsy and Behavior, 12*, 434-444.

Ellison, R. E., Guvener, A., Feksi, G., Placentia, M., and Shorvon, S. A. (1989). A study of approaches to anti-epileptic drug treatment in four countries in the developing world. In: J. Manelis, E. Bental, J.N. Loeber, F.E. Dreifuss, (Eds.), *Advances in Epileptology—XVIIth Epilepsy International Symposium*, New York, Raven Press.

Fernandes, P. T., Cabral, P., Araujo, U., Noronha, A. L., and Li, L. M. (2005). Kids' perception about epilepsy. *Epilepsy and Behavior, 6*, 601-603.

Fernandes, P. T., Noronha, A. L., Araujo, U., Cabral, P., Pataro, R., de Boer, H. M., et al. (2007). Teachers perception about epilepsy. *Arquivos De Neuro-Psiquiatria, 65 Suppl 1*, 28-34.

Fernandes, P. T., Noronha, A. L., Sander, J. W., Bell, G. S., and Li, L. M. (2007). Training the trainers and disseminating information: A strategy to educate health professionals on epilepsy. *Arquivos De Neuro-Psiquiatria, 65 Suppl 1*, 14-22.

Fernandes, P. T., Salgado, P. C., Noronha, A. L., de Boer, H. M., Prilipko, L., Sander, J. W., et al. (2007). Epilepsy stigma perception in an urban area of a limited-resource country. *Epilepsy and Behavior, 11*, 25-32.

Finke, M. (1981). Public attitudes toward epilepsy in the federal republic of Germany. trends from 1967 to 1978 *Der Nervenarzt, 52*, 581-584.

Fong, C. Y., and Hung, A. (2002). Public awareness, attitude, and understanding of epilepsy in Hong Kong special administrative region, China. *Epilepsia, 43*, 311-316.

Frith, J. F., Harris, M. F., and Beran, R. G. (1994). Management and attitudes of epilepsy by a group of Sydney general practitioners. *Epilepsia, 35*, 1244-1247.

Gambhir, S. K., Kumar, V., Singhi, P. D., and Goel, R. C. (1995). Public awareness, understanding and attitudes toward epilepsy. *The Indian Journal of Medical Research, 102*, 34-38.

Gomes, M. D. (2000). Doctors' perspectives and practices regarding epilepsy. *Arquivos De Neuro-Psiquiatria, 58*(2A), 221-226.

Gouvier, W. D., Brown, L. M., Prestholdt, P. H., and Hayes, J. S. (1995). A survey of common misconceptions about epilepsy. *Rehabilitation Psychology, 40*(1), 51-59.

Gunadharma, S. (2004). Public awareness, understanding and attitude towards epilepsy in Bandung, Indonesia. *Neurology Asia, 9*(S1), 133-134.

Gutteling, J. M., Seydel, E. R., and Wiegman, O. (1986). Previous experiences with epilepsy and effectiveness of information to change public perception of epilepsy. *Epilepsia, 27*, 739-745.

Hauck, G. (1968). The attitude of the population on epilepsy in the United States and Germany. *Der Nervenarzt, 39*, 181-183.

Hawley, S. R., Paschal, A. M., Ablah, E., St. Romain, T., Liow, K., and Molgaard, C. A. (2007). Initial perspectives from Midwestern neurologists: Epilepsy patients' barriers and motivators for seeking treatment. *Epilepsia, 48*, 1920-1925.

Hayes, S. M., Melin, J. D., Dupuis, M., Murray, S., and Labiner, D. M. (2007). Assessing the true learning needs of health care professionals in epilepsy care. *Epilepsy and Behavior, 11*, 434-441.

Helde, G., Brodtkorb, E., Brathen, G., and Bovim, G. (2003). An easily performed group education programme for patients with uncontrolled epilepsy - A pilot study. *Seizure, 12*, 497-501.

Helgeson, D. C., Mittan, R., Tan, S. Y., and Chayasirisobhon, S. (1990). Sepulveda epilepsy education: The efficacy of a psychoeducational treatment program in treating medical and psychosocial aspects of epilepsy. *Epilepsia, 31*, 75-82.

Herranz Fernandez, J. L., Lastra Martinez, L. A., Gonzalez Gonzalez, A., Capa Garcia, L., Granda Alonso, C., Moustafa, I., et al. (1990). Knowledge and attitude of professors concerning epilepsy. Evaluation of a survey conducted on 4,099 professors of Cantabria. *Anales Espanoles De Pediatria, 33*, 523-527.

Hills, M. D., and MacKenzie, H. C. (2002). New Zealand community attitudes toward people with epilepsy. *Epilepsia, 43*, 1583-1589.

Howe, G. W., Feinstein, C., Reiss, D., Molock, S., and Berger, K. (1993). Adolescent adjustment to chronic physical disorders - I. Comparing neurological and non-neurological conditions. *Journal of Child Psychology and Psychiatry, and Allied Disciplines, 34*, 1153-1171.

Hsieh, L., and Chiou, H. (2001). Comparison of epilepsy and asthma perception among preschool teachers in Taiwan. *Epilepsia, 42*, 647-650.

Iivanainen, M., Uutela, A., and Vilkkumaa, I. (1980). Public awareness and attitudes toward epilepsy in Finland. *Epilepsia, 21*, 413-423.

Institute of Medicine (U.S.). Committee on Nervous System Disorders in Developing Countries. (2001). *Neurological, psychiatric, and developmental disorders: Meeting the challenge in the developing world.* Washington, DC: National Academy Press. pp. 179-216.

Ismail, H., Wright, J., Rhodes, P., and Small, N. (2005). Religious beliefs about causes and treatment of epilepsy. *The British Journal of General Practice, 55*, 26-31.

Ismail, H., Wright, J., Rhodes, P., Small, N., and Jacoby, A. (2005). South Asians and epilepsy: Exploring health experiences, needs and beliefs of communities in the north of England. *Seizure, 14*, 497-503.

Jacoby, A., Baker, G. A., Steen, N., Potts, P., and Chadwick, D. W. (1996). The clinical course of epilepsy and its psychosocial correlates: Findings from a U.K. community study. *Epilepsia, 37*, 148-161.

Jacoby, A., Gorry, J., and Baker, G. A. (2005). Employers' attitudes to employment of people with epilepsy: Still the same old story? *Epilepsia, 46*, 1978-1987.

Jacoby, A., Gorry, J., Gamble, C., and Baker, G. A. (2004). Public knowledge, private grief: A study of public attitudes to epilepsy in the United Kingdom and implications for stigma. *Epilepsia, 45*, 1405-1415.

Jensen, R., and Dam, M. (1992). Public attitudes toward epilepsy in Denmark. *Epilepsia, 33*, 459-463.

Kabir, M. :. I., Z., Abubakar, S., Kabir, Z. S., and Farinyaro, A. U. (2005). Knowledge attitude, and beliefs about epilepsy among adults in a Northern Nigerian urban community. *Annals of African Medicine, 4*, 107-112.

Kale, R. (1997). Bringing epilepsy out of the shadows. *British Medical Journal, 315*, 2-3.

Kaleyias, J., Tzoufi, M., Kotsalis, C., Papavasiliou, A., and Diamantopoulos, N. (2005). Knowledge and attitude of the Greek educational community toward epilepsy and the epileptic student. *Epilepsy and Behavior, 6*, 179-186.

Kankirawatana, P. (1999). Epilepsy awareness among school teachers in Thailand. *Epilepsia, 40*, 497-501.

Katzenstein, J. M., Fastenau, P. S., Dunn, D. W., and Austin, J. K. (2007). Teachers' ratings of the academic performance of children with epilepsy. *Epilepsy and Behavior, 10*, 426-431.

Keulers, B. J., Welters, C. F., Spauwen, P. H., and Houpt, P. (2007). Can face-to-face patient education be replaced by computer-based patient education? A randomised trial. *Patient Education and Counseling, 67*, 176-182.

Kim, M. K., Cho, K. H., Shin, S. J., and Kim, S. J. (1994). A study of public attitude toward epilepsy in Kwang-Ju area. *J Korean Neurol Assoc, 12*, 410-427.

Kim, M. K., Kim, I. K., Kim, B. C., Cho, K. H., Kim, S. J., and Moon, J. D. (2003). Positive trends of public attitudes toward epilepsy after public education campaign among rural Korean residents. *Journal of Korean Medical Science, 18*, 248-254.

Kobau, R., DiIorio, C. A., Anderson, L. A., and Price, P. H. (2006). Further validation and reliability testing of the attitudes and beliefs about living with epilepsy (ABLE) components of the CDC epilepsy program instrument on stigma. *Epilepsy and Behavior, 8*, 552-559.

Kobau, R., Zahran, H., Grant, D., Thurman, D. J., Price, P. H., and Zack, M. M. (2007). Prevalence of active epilepsy and health-related quality of life among adults with self-reported epilepsy in California: California health interview survey, 2003. *Epilepsia, 48*, 1904-1913.

Kobau, R., Zahran, H., Thurman, D. J., Zack, M. M., Henry, T. R., Schachter, S. C., et al. (2008). Epilepsy surveillance among adults-19 states, Behavioral Risk Factor

Surveillance System, 2005. *MMWR. Surveillance Summaries: Morbidity and Mortality Weekly Report. Surveillance Summaries CDC, 57*, 1-20.

Koss, J. D. (1990). Somatization and somatic complaint syndromes among Hispanics: Overview and ethnopsychological perspectives. *Transcultural Psychiatry, 27*, 5-29.

Krämer, G. (2003). Einstellung der bevölkerung zur epilepsie in der schweiz 2003. *Epileptologie, 20*, 145-148.

Krauss, G. L., Gondek, S., Krumholz, A., Paul, S., and Shen, F. (2000). "The scarlet E": The presentation of epilepsy in the English language print media. *Neurology, 54*, 1894-1898.

Krishnamoorthy, E. S., Satishchandra, P., and Sander, J. W. (2003). Research in epilepsy: Development priorities for developing nations. *Epilepsia, 44 Suppl 1*, 5-8.

Lai, C. W., Huang, X. S., Lai, Y. H., Zhang, Z. Q., Liu, G. J., and Yang, M. Z. (1990). Survey of public awareness, understanding, and attitudes toward epilepsy in Henan province, China. *Epilepsia, 31*, 182-187.

LaMartina, J. M. (1989). Uncovering public misconceptions about epilepsy. *Journal of Epilepsy, 2*, 45-48.

Le, Q. C., Dinh, D. T., and Jallon, P. (2006). Survey of public awareness, attitudes, and understanding toward epilepsy in Nhan Chinh, Hanoi, Vietnam, in 2003. *Epilepsy and Behavior, 8*, 176-180.

Lee, Y., Kim, S. S., Lim, J. G., Yi, S. D., and Park, Y. C. (1997). Knowledge and attitude toward epilepsy in some Taegu-Kyungbook residents. *J Korean Neurol Assoc, 15*, 257-266.

Lee, S. A. (2005). What we confront with employment of people with epilepsy in Korea. *Epilepsia, 46 Suppl 1*, 57-58.

Li, L. M., Fernandes, P. T., Noronha, A. L., Marques, L. H., Borges, M. A., Borges, K., et al. (2007). Demonstration project on epilepsy in Brazil: Outcome assessment. *Arquivos De Neuro-Psiquiatria, 65 Suppl 1*, 58-62.

Lim, K. M., Tan, L. P., Lim, K. T., and Tan, C. T. (1999). Survey of public awareness, understanding and attitudes toward epilepsy among Chinese in Malaysia. *Neurol J Southeast Asia, 4*, 31-36.

Madsen, L. P. (1996). Danish primary school teachers' knowledge about epilepsy in children. *Ugeskrift for Laeger, 158*, 1977-1980.

Martiniuk, A. L., Speechley, K. N., Secco, M., Campbell, M. K., and Donner, A. (2007). Evaluation of an epilepsy education program for grade 5 students: A cluster randomized trial. *Epilepsy and Behavior, 10*, 604-610.

Mason, C., Fenton, G. W., and Jamieson, M. (1990). Teaching medical students about epilepsy. *Epilepsia, 31*, 95-100.

Matuja, W. B., and Rwiza, H. T. (1994). Knowledge, attitude and practice (KAP) towards epilepsy in secondary school students in Tanzania. *The Central African Journal of Medicine, 40*, 13-18.

May, T. W., and Pfafflin, M. (2002). The efficacy of an educational treatment program for patients with epilepsy (MOSES): Results of a controlled, randomized study. modular service package epilepsy. *Epilepsia, 43*, 539-549.

Mbewe, E., Haworth, A., Atadzhanov, M., Chomba, E., and Birbeck, G. L. (2007). Epilepsy-related knowledge, attitudes, and practices among Zambian police officers. *Epilepsy and Behavior, 10*, 456-462.

McLin, W. M., and de Boer, H. M. (1995). Public perceptions about epilepsy. *Epilepsia, 36*, 957-959.

Mecarelli, O., Li Voti, P., Vanacore, N., D'Arcangelo, S., Mingoia, M., Pulitano, P., et al. (2007). A questionnaire study on knowledge of and attitudes toward epilepsy in schoolchildren and university students in Rome, Italy. *Seizure, 16*, 313-319.

Mielke, J., Adamolekun, B., Ball, D., and Mundanda, T. (1997). Knowledge and attitudes of teachers towards epilepsy in Zimbabwe. *Acta Neurologica Scandinavica, 96*, 133-137.

Millogo, A., and Siranyan, A. S. (2004). Knowledge of epilepsy and attitudes towards the condition among schoolteachers in Bobo-Dioulasso (Burkina Faso). *Epileptic Disorders, 6*, 21-26.

Mirnics, Z., Czikora, G., Zavecz, T., and Halasz, P. (2001). Changes in public attitudes toward epilepsy in Hungary: Results of surveys conducted in 1994 and 2000. *Epilepsia, 42*, 86-93.

Moross, H. (1974). Social-psychiatric aspects of epilepsy. Special reference to the south African national epilepsy league (SANEL). *South African Medical Journal, 48*, 1035-1037.

Murthy, J. M. K. (2003). Some problems and pitfalls in developing countries. *Epilepsia, 44 Suppl 1*, 38-42.

Naeem, F., Ayub, M., Kingdon, K., Mujtaba, M., Zaidi, Q. A., Bhatti, F., et al. (2007). A survey of knowledge and attitude of the general public towards epilepsy in Lahore, Pakistan. *Journal of Pakistan Psychiatric Society, 4*, 96.

Ndour, D., Diop, A. G., Ndiaye, M., Niang, C., Sarr, M. M., and Ndiaye, I. P. (2004). A survey of school teachers' knowledge and behaviour about epilepsy, in a developing country such as Senegal. *Revue Neurologique, 160*, 338-341.

Ndoye, N. F., Sow, A. D., Diop, A. G., Sessouma, B., Sene-Diouf, F., Boissy, L., et al. (2005). Prevalence of epilepsy its treatment gap and knowledge, attitude and practice of its population in sub-urban Senegal an ILAE/IBE/WHO study. *Seizure, 14*, 106-111.

Njamnshi, A. K., Angwafor, S. A., Tabah, E. N., Jallon, P., and Muna, W. F. (2009). General public knowledge, attitudes, and practices with respect to epilepsy in the Batibo health district, Cameroon. *Epilepsy and Behavior, 14*, 83-88.

Noronha, A. L., Fernandes, P. T., Andrade Mda, G., Santiago, S. M., Sander, J. W., and Li, L. M. (2007). Training medical students to improve the management of people with epilepsy. *Arquivos De Neuro-Psiquiatria, 65 Suppl 1*, 23-27.

Novotna, I., and Rektor, I. (2002). The trend in public attitudes in the Czech Republic towards persons with epilepsy. *European Journal of Neurology, 9*, 535-540.

Nyame, P. K., and Biritwum, R. B. (1997). Epilepsy: Knowledge, attitude and practice in literate urban population, Accra, Ghana. *West African Journal of Medicine, 16*, 139-145.

Office of Health Economics. (1971). *Epilepsy in society.* London, England, pp. 1-35.

Ojinnaka, N. C. (2002). Teachers' perception of epilepsy in Nigeria: A community-based study. *Seizure, 11*, 386-391.

Okumura, A., and Watanabe, K. (2008). Questionnaire survey on the understanding of epilepsy among non-medical persons. *Pediatrics International, 50*, 319-321.

Olley, B. O., Osinowo, H. O., and Brieger, W. R. (2001). Psycho-educational therapy among Nigerian adult patients with epilepsy: A controlled outcome study. *Patient Education and Counseling, 42*, 25-33.

Otoom, S. A., Al-Safi, S. A., Sequeira, R. P., and Alkofahi, A. S. (2006). Knowledge of management of epilepsy in young adults in Jordan. *Epilepsy and Behavior, 9*, 349-354.

Pala, I., and Vankar, G. K. (1997). Epilepsy and teachers: A survey. *Indian Journal of Pediatrics, 64*, 211-214.

Pandian, J. D., Santosh, D., Kumar, T. S., Sarma, P. S., and Radhakrishnan, K. (2006). High school students' knowledge, attitude, and practice with respect to epilepsy in Kerala, Southern India. *Epilepsy and Behavior, 9*, 492-497.

Park, S. J., Jeong, X. J., Kim, M. K., Cho, K. H., Choi, J. S., and Kim, S. J. (1996). Public attitude toward epilepsy in Chonnam rural areas. *J Korean Neurol Assoc, 14*, 389-407.

Paschal, A. M., Hawley, S. R., Romain, T. S., Liow, K., Molgaard, C. A., Sly, J., et al. (2007). Epilepsy patients' perceptions about stigma, education, and awareness: Preliminary responses based on a community participatory approach. *Epilepsy and Behavior, 11*, 329-337.

Peltzer, K. (2001). Perceptions of epilepsy among black students at a university in South Africa. *Curationis, 24*, 62-67.

Price, V., Murphy, S. O., and Cureton, V. Y. (2004). Increasing self-efficacy and knowledge through a seizure education program for special education teachers. *The Journal of School Nursing, 20*, 43-49.

Prpic, I., Korotaj, Z., Vlasic-Cicvaric, I., Paucic-Kirincic, E., Valerjev, A., and Tomac, V. (2003). Teachers' opinions about capabilities and behavior of children with epilepsy. *Epilepsy and Behavior, 4*, 142-145.

Radhakrishnan, K., Pandian, J. D., Santhoshkumar, T., Thomas, S. V., Deetha, T. D., Sarma, P. S., et al. (2000). Prevalence, knowledge, attitude, and practice of epilepsy in Kerala, South India. *Epilepsia, 41*, 1027-1035.

Rajbhandari, K. C. (2004). Epilepsy in Nepal. *The Canadian Journal of Neurological Sciences, 31*, 257-260.

Ramasundrum, V., Mohd Hussin, Z. A., and Tan, C. T. (2000). Public awareness, attitudes and understanding towards epilepsy in Kelantan, Malaysia. *Neurol J Southeast Asia, 5*, 55-60.

Rambe, A. S., and Sjahrir, H. (2002). Awareness, attitudes and understanding towards epilepsy among school teachers in Medan, Indonesia. *Neurol J Southeast Asia, 7*, 77-80.

Reno, B. A., Fernandes, P. T., Bell, G. S., Sander, J. W., and Li, L. M. (2007). Stigma and attitudes on epilepsy a study: With secondary school students. *Arquivos De Neuro-Psiquiatria, 65 Suppl 1*, 49-54.

Rose, A.W., Peace, L. and McBride, M. (1955). On changing social conceptions of epilepsy. *Epilepsia, c4*, 99-107.

Hicks, R.A., and Hicks, M.J. (1991). Attitudes of major employers toward the employment of people with epilepsy: A 30-year study. *Epilepsia, 32*, 86-88.

Kobau, R., and Price P. (2003). Knowledge of epilepsy and familiarity with this disorder in the U.S. population: Results from the 2002 HealthStyles survey. *Epilepsia, 44*, 1449-1454.

Ross, C. E., and Wu, C. (1995). The links between education and health. *American Sociological Review, 60*, 719-745.

Rusch, N., Angermeyer, M. C., and Corrigan, P. W. (2005). Mental illness stigma: Concepts, consequences, and initiatives to reduce stigma. *European Psychiatry, 20*, 529-539.

Rwiza, H. T., Matuja, W. B., Kilonzo, G. P., Haule, J., Mbena, P., Mwang'ombola, R., et al. (1993). Knowledge, attitude, and practice toward epilepsy among rural Tanzanian residents. *Epilepsia, 34*, 1017-1023.

Sands, H., and Zalkind, S. S. (1972). Effects of an educational campaign to change employer attitudes toward hiring epileptics. *Epilepsia, 13*, 87-96.

Sanya, E. O., Salami, T. A., Goodman, O. O., Buhari, O. I., and Araoye, M. O. (2005). Perception and attitude to epilepsy among teachers in primary, secondary and tertiary educational institutions in middle belt Nigeria. *Tropical Doctor, 35*, 153-156.

Scott, R. A., Lhatoo, S. D., and Sander, J. W. (2001). The treatment of epilepsy in developing countries: Where do we go from here? *Bulletin of the World Health Organization, 79*, 344-351.

Seidenberg, M., and Berent, S. (1992). Childhood epilepsy and the role of psychology. *The American Psychologist, 47*, 1130-1133.

Senanayake, N., and Abeykoon, P. (1984). Epilepsy in Sri Lanka: Public awareness and attitudes. *The Journal of Tropical Medicine and Hygiene, 87*, 61-66.

Seneviratne, U., Rajapakse, P., Pathirana, R., and Seetha, T. (2002). Knowledge, attitude, and practice of epilepsy in rural Sri Lanka. *Seizure, 11*, 40-43.

Shafiq, M., Tanwir, M., Tariq, A., Kasi, P. M., Zafar, M., Saleem, A., et al. (2007). Epilepsy: Public knowledge and attitude in a slum area of Karachi, Pakistan. *Seizure, 16*, 330-337.

Shafiq, M., Tanwir, M., Tariq, A., Saleem, A., Zafar, M., and Khuwaja, A. K. (2008). Myths and fallacies about epilepsy among residents of a Karachi slum area. *Tropical Doctor, 38*, 32-33.

Shorvon, S. D., and Farmer, P. J. (1988). Epilepsy in developing countries: A review of epidemiological, sociocultural, and treatment aspects. *Epilepsia, 29 Suppl 1*, 36-54.

Sirven, J. I., Lopez, R. A., Vazquez, B., and Van Haverbeke, P. (2005). Que es la epilepsia? Attitudes and knowledge of epilepsy by Spanish-speaking adults in the United States. *Epilepsy and Behavior, 7*, 259-265.

Slikkerveer, L. J. (1982). Rural health development in Ethiopia. Problems of utilization of traditional healers. *Social Science and Medicine, 16*, 1859-1872.

Smeets, V. M. J., van Lierop, B. A. G., Vanhoutvin, J. P. G., Aldenkamp, A. P., and Nijhuis, F. J. N. (2007). Epilepsy and employment: Literature review. *Epilepsy and Behavior, 10*, 354-362.

Snape, D., Wang, W., Wu, J., Jacoby, A., and Baker, G. A. (2009). Knowledge gaps and uncertainties about epilepsy: Findings from an ethnographic study in china. *Epilepsy and Behavior, 14*, 172-178.

Spatt, J., Bauer, G., Baumgartner, C., Feucht, M., Graf, M., Mamoli, B., et al. (2005). Predictors for negative attitudes toward subjects with epilepsy: A representative survey in the general public in Austria. *Epilepsia, 46*, 736-742.

Spatt, J., Langbauer, G., and Mamoli, B. (1998). Subjective perception of seizure precipitants: Results of a questionnaire study. *Seizure, 7*, 391-395.

Stores, G. (1975). Teaching medical students about epilepsy. *Developmental Medicine and Child Neurology, 17*, 518-519.

Sturniolo, M. G., and Galletti, F. (1994). Idiopathic epilepsy and school achievement. *Archives of Disease in Childhood, 70*, 424-428.

Sue, S. (1988). Psychotherapeutic services for ethnic minorities. *American Psychologist, 43*, 301-308.

Sue, S., and Zane, N. (1987). The role of culture and cultural techniques in psychotherapy. *American Psychologist, 42*, 37-45.

Tekle-Haimanot, R., Abebe, M., Forsgren, L., Gebre-Mariam, A., Heijbel, J., Holmgren, G., et al. (1991). Attitudes of rural people in central Ethiopia towards epilepsy. *Social Science and Medicine, 32*, 203-209.

Tellez-Zenteno, J. F., Patten, S. B., Jette, N., Williams, J., and Wiebe, S. (2007). Psychiatric comorbidity in epilepsy: A population-based analysis. *Epilepsia, 48*, 2336-2344.

Thacker, A. K., Verma, A. M., Ji, R., Thacker, P., and Mishra, P. (2008). Knowledge awareness and attitude about epilepsy among schoolteachers in India. *Seizure, 17*, 684-690.

Thorbecke, R. (1987). Public attitudes toward epilepsy in the Federal Republic of Germany, 1984. In Wolf, P., Janz, D., Dam, M. and Dreifuss, F.E. (Eds.) *Advances in Epileptology: XVIth Epilepsy International Symposium* (pp. 739-743). New York: Raven Press.

Tiamkao, S., Aaauevitchayapat, N., Arunpongpaisal, S., Chaiyakum, A., Jitpimolmard, S., Phuttharak, W., et al. (2005). Knowledge of epilepsy among teachers in Khon Kaen province, Thailand. *Journal of the Medical Association of Thailand, 88*, 1802-1808.

Tidman, L., Saravanan, K. and Gibbs, J. (2003). Epilepsy in mainstream and special educational primary school settings. *Seizure, 12*, 47-51.

Tran, D. S., Odermatt, P., Singphuoangphet, S., Druet-Cabanac, M., Preux, P. M., Strobel, M., et al. (2007). Epilepsy in Laos: Knowledge, attitudes, and practices in the community. *Epilepsy and Behavior, 10*, 565-570.

Troxell, J. (1997). Epilepsy and employment: The Americans with disabilities act and its protections against employment discrimination. *Medicine and Law, 16*, 375-384.

Tuan, N. A., Cuong, L. Q., Allebeck, P., Chuc, N. T., and Tomson, T. (2007). Knowledge attitudes and practice toward epilepsy among adults in BaVi, Vietnam: First report from the population-based EPIBAVI study. *Epilepsia, 48*, 1914-1919.

U.S. Department of Health and Human Services (2005). *Quick guide to health literacy.* Retrieved June 27, 2007 from Office of Disease Prevention and Health Promotion Web site: http://www.health.gov/communication/literacy/quickguide/Quickguide.pdf.

Varma, N. P., Sylaja, P. N., George, L., Sankara Sarma, P., and Radhakrishnan, K. (2007). Employment concerns of people with epilepsy in Kerala, South India. *Epilepsy and Behavior, 10*, 250-254.

Watts, A. E. (1989). A model for managing epilepsy in a rural community in Africa. *British Medical Journal, 298*, 805-807.

Weiss, M. G., and Ramakrishna, J. (2006). Stigma interventions and research for international health. *Lancet, 367*, 536-538.

Win, N. N., and Soe, C. (2002). Public awareness, attitude and understanding toward epilepsy among Myanmar people. *Neurol J Southeast Asia 2002, 7*, 81-88.

Wong, V., Chung, B., and Wong, R. (2004). Pilot survey of public awareness, attitudes and understanding towards epilepsy in Hong Kong. *Neurology Asia, 9*, 21-27.

Wu, K. N., Lieber, E., Siddarth, P., Smith, K., Sankar, R., and Caplan, R. (2008). Dealing with epilepsy: Parents speak up. *Epilepsy and Behavior, 13*, 131-138.

Young, G. B., Derry, P., Hutchinson, I., John, V., Matijevic, S., Parrent, L., et al. (2002). An epilepsy questionnaire study of knowledge and attitudes in Canadian college students. *Epilepsia, 43*, 652-658.

Zielinska, A., Klos, E., and Talarska, D. (2005). Youth's knowledge and attitude to epilepsy. *Roczniki Akademii Medycznej w Bialymstoku, 50 Suppl 1*, 99-101.

Zielinski, J. J. (1974). *Epidemiology and medical-social problems of epilepsy in Warsaw. (Final report on research program No. 19-P-58325-F-01 DHEW. Social and rehabilitation services).* Washington, DC: U.S. Government printing office. pp. 1-253.

In: Social Epileptology
Editors: J. Pinikahana and C. Walker
ISBN 978-1-60876-228-6

Chapter 10

EMPLOYMENT AND EPILEPSY

Ramon Edmundo D. Bautista*[*,1] and Logan A. Crews[2]
[1]Comprehensive Epilepsy Program,
University of Florida Health Sciences
Center/Jacksonville, Jacksonville, Florida, USA
[2]College of Pharmacy, University of Florida,
Gainesville, Florida, USA.

ABSTRACT

Epilepsy is a common neurologic condition that affects up to 1% of the population. Despite advances in medical care a significant number of individuals with epilepsy remains unemployed. The estimated lost income due to under- or unemployment is staggering and is estimated to be as high as 86% of the total cost of the disease.

Poor seizure control is the primary reason for the lack of employability among epilepsy patients. However, individuals with epilepsy also have numerous medical and psychiatric co-morbidities that may encumber their participation in work-related activities.

As a group, epilepsy patients remain poorly educated, under-trained and lack the necessary experience needed to compete in the workplace. This lack of education has been associated with the age of seizure onset and the extent of seizure control. Many of these patients end up settling for unskilled manual labor, earn limited income, and place themselves at greater risk for injury.

Individual attitudes also play an important role in influencing employment status among epilepsy patients. A lack of belief in the importance of work for personal growth and development as well as an increased fear of workplace discrimination are associated with lack of employment among epilepsy patients regardless of seizure control. Some epilepsy patients and their families have an overriding fear of losing their disability support and these payments actually serve as a disincentive to finding work.

While there has been some progress in educating society about epilepsy, social stigma and workplace discrimination towards individuals with epilepsy is still prevalent in many parts of the world, making it difficult for epilepsy patients to find work. In many

[*] Correspondence: Dr Ramon Edmundo D. Bautista, Associate Professor of Neurology. University of Florida Health Sciences Center/Jacksonville. Tele: (904) 244-9190. Fax:(904) 244-9493. Email: ramon.bautista@jax.ufl.edu

respects, employer attitudes towards epilepsy determine whether these individuals are accepted into the workplace. Despite the intent of the Americans with Disabilities Act and the Disability Discrimination Act to protect individuals with disabilities from workplace discrimination, the subjective nature of the hiring and retention process at work continues to limit the employment opportunities for epilepsy patients. Compounding this problem is the lack of an adequate public transportation system that hinders workplace accessibility.

Despite these challenges, the results from various vocational rehabilitation programs, especially those directed towards the epilepsy population, are encouraging and have actually resulted in increased employment. Enhancing employment and work productivity among epilepsy patients remains an important societal challenge. Developing effective strategies to increase their employability will not only help improve their quality of life but may also decrease the cost burden of this disease.

INTRODUCTION

Epilepsy is a common neurologic condition that affects up to 1% of the population [1]. Given the current therapies available, a significant number has reasonably controlled seizures. It is estimated that with currently available antiepileptic medications, up to 90 % of epilepsy patients have controlled seizures [2,3]. For patients whose seizures are not controlled on medications, treatment options such as epilepsy surgery and use of the vagus nerve stimulator may result in good seizure control [4,5]. Despite these good clinical outcomes, more than 25% of individuals with epilepsy remain unemployed [6,7], a figure that is significantly higher than anticipated on the basis of adequate seizure control. In general, the unemployment rate for persons with epilepsy is more than twice the national average [8]. Across many studies, the inability to work has been repeatedly cited as a major concern of individuals with epilepsy [3,9,10]. The potential loss of manpower by not utilizing the economic potential of individuals with epilepsy is devastating. The indirect cost of epilepsy (income lost due to under- or unemployment) is estimated to be as high as 86% of the total cost of the disease or over $10 billion per year [11]. In this review, we examine the various factors, both individual and societal, that contribute to the persistent underemployment of the epilepsy population. We also look at the utility of vocational rehabilitation and job placement programs in their attempts to integrate epilepsy patients into society. Lastly, this review provides useful insights into future initiatives to increase the participation of individuals with epilepsy in the workplace and encourage their continuing assimilation into society.

CLINICAL AND PSYCHOSOCIAL VARIABLES AFFECTING EMPLOYMENT

Across different studies, inadequate seizure control has consistently been the main factor associated with unemployment in the epilepsy population. A postal survey of 1709 members of the British Epilepsy Association living in England and Wales was performed to obtain demographic, clinical, and employment-related information [12]. Using Principal Component Analysis, lower seizure frequency and less severe seizures were among the variables associated with good employment history. Another survey performed on 385 individuals with epilepsy living in Sweden showed that individuals with uncontrolled seizures were significantly less likely to be employed and more likely to receive a disability pension [13]. These individuals were also more likely to experience epilepsy-related stigma and work limitations. The importance of seizure control in determining employability was highlighted in another study performed in the U.K. [14]. The results of this study showed that the employment rates of individuals with well-controlled seizures were similar to the general population (79% for men and 64% for women). In fact, of the 494 individuals included in the study, only 4% of unemployed men and 3% of unemployed women gave their epilepsy as the reason for not working.

Other studies that have established the importance of good seizure control as a prerequisite for employment have focused on the epilepsy surgery population. In a study of 32 individuals with refractory epilepsy who underwent cortical resection, post-surgery employability was strongly associated with improved seizure control [15]. A related study of 151 surgical patients [16] showed that early and successful epilepsy surgery was vital in improving or maintaining one's employment status. A third study [17] of 94 patients who underwent epilepsy surgery also showed that employment rates significantly differed according to seizure control. In that study, 80% of patients who became seizure-free post-surgery subsequently became employed compared to 53% of those who continued to have 10 or less seizures a year. In contrast, only 27% of patients who had more than 10 seizures a year or who were not considered good surgical candidates were employed.

Aside from the need for adequate seizure control, other challenges encountered by epilepsy patients that affect their productivity include the various medical co-morbidities associated with their condition. Compared to the general population, individuals with epilepsy have a higher rate of cancer, arthritis, heart disease, strokes, severe headaches, lower back pain, neck pain, and asthma [18]. Studies comparing epilepsy patients to matched cohorts found that they were more likely to experience accidents, especially seizure-related ones that commonly result in burns, abrasions, and other injuries [19-21]. However, another study found that non-seizure related accidents were actually lower in patients with epilepsy, probably due to the increased caution epilepsy patients naturally exhibit [22].

Cognitive and behavioral issues can also affect the productivity of epilepsy patients. The link between epilepsy, depression, and other cognitive effects has been well established [18,23,24]. There are various neurobiological and psychological theories that explain the association between epilepsy and mood disorders. These include the site of seizure origin, feelings of learned helplessness, sexual dysfunction, the continuing need for secrecy, as well as a myriad of educational and employment problems these individuals continue to face [25]. Some studies estimate that up to 80% of individuals with epilepsy suffer from depression and a significant number of them remain untreated [26]. The use of antiepileptic medications has also been linked to cognitive and behavioral problems that include memory impairment, aggression, depression, irritability, and disturbances in attention [25]. Individual productivity is also adversely affected by these cognitive and physical side effects making it much more difficult for epilepsy patients to secure employment.

A significant proportion of the epilepsy population lacks the education, training and job experience needed to obtain employment in many fields. Decreased educational attainment and poor employment history has been consistently linked with one another. Some studies indicate that in certain populations, less than 50% of epilepsy patients actually complete a high school education [27,28]. And in a survey conducted among 250 individuals with epilepsy in Kerala, India, only 25% of those with low educational levels were employed compared to 51.2% of those who had a higher education [29].

Some studies also indicate that the age of seizure onset influences the level of education of individuals with epilepsy. In a study by Koponen and colleagues that compared the social functioning of 22-25 year old Finnish epilepsy patients to healthy age- and gender- matched controls [30], only 39% of individuals with seizure onset before 7 years of age had a college level education compared to 52% of those with later onset seizures. In a study of individuals with epilepsy living in the Netherlands, those who were diagnosed to have seizures on or before 18 years of age generally achieved a lower level of education. There was no relation between schooling achievement and the onset of epilepsy after 18 years of age [31]. However, other studies did not show this association. [29].

The value of education as a means to obtaining work in this population is so vital that even becoming seizure free is oftentimes no guarantee of finding employment. Among those who became seizure free after epilepsy surgery, work experience prior to surgery and the ability to obtain further education after surgery were important factors that were necessary in order to find work post-operatively [32]. However, because many epilepsy patients are less likely to receive an adequate education or training, most end up being unskilled manual laborers [33]. Unfortunately, some of these jobs involve tasks, such as heavy lifting, that put these individuals at physical risk if they were to experience a seizure. Thus, although epilepsy patients may be willing to work, their limited education usually makes them either unqualified or decreases their competitiveness in the job market.

The psychological and social difficulties individuals with epilepsy encounter when obtaining an education was highlighted in the earlier referenced study [30] that found that while performance in the matriculation examination of those with epilepsy was not significantly different compared to healthy controls, significantly fewer epilepsy patients went on to obtain a college-level degree. Compared to the epilepsy group, more healthy controls thought that their university studies had gone well. The authors concluded that despite passing the matriculation examination, those with epilepsy appeared to have poorer social relations and coping skills compared to healthy controls, and these adversely affect their educational experience.

Individual patient attitudes towards work also determine their willingness and desire to find employment. While the research in this area is relatively sparse, certain trends can be established. Compared to employed epilepsy patients, those who were unemployed felt that they had to be "normal" before they could work. These individuals also believed that they did not have an adequate-enough education and that they would be unable to obtain transportation to and from work. They also thought that working increased the risk of injury to themselves and their coworkers and that their families did not want them to work outside of the home. Lastly, these patients believed that their seizures would negatively affect their performance at work. Concerns about taking their medications on time and arriving to work on time were also expressed by unemployed patients. These patients were also concerned that they would lose their external income support if they worked and would not be able to manage without it [34]. In a related study, psychosocial factors such as the lack of belief in the importance of work for personal growth and fulfillment and the perceived fear of workplace discrimination were factors that were independently associated with lack of employment among epilepsy patients, regardless of their state of seizure control [28].

SOCIETAL STIGMA AND EMPLOYMENT

In many respects, the acceptance of those with epilepsy into the workplace mirrors society's ongoing stigma towards these individuals. Stigma is defined as the loss of societal standing due to the possession of a particular attribute, such as a medical condition, that is regarded as undesirable [35]. This loss of societal standing is typically beyond the limitations imposed by the medical condition itself. Stigma among epilepsy patients can be either "felt" (when patients are ashamed of their condition and fearful of encountering actual stigma) or "enacted" (the actual experience of discrimination). According to Scrambler [36], while a significant number of individuals with epilepsy experiences felt stigma, only a few can recount actual experiences of discrimination. However, it is this felt stigma that influences patient behaviors such as the non-disclosure of their disorder in social gatherings and in the workplace.

While studies that examined epilepsy-related stigma within a given population cannot be directly compared with one another due to differing study methodologies, patient demographics, and study periods, it is clear that societal stigma towards individuals with epilepsy, particularly in the area of employment, continues to exist. The degree of stigma varies across different societies with western-oriented cultures generally displaying an increased acceptance of individuals with epilepsy who are employed.

In 1979, the American Institute of Public Opinion Poll performed a survey of adults in the United States [37] that indicated that up to 79% of respondents believed that individuals with epilepsy should be employed. Interestingly, this figure had been trending upwards during the previous 30 years that the survey was conducted beginning with a low of 45% in 1949. Another survey conducted 4 years later by the Italian Institute of Public Opinion [38] on 1,043 individuals showed that 70% of respondents believed that persons with epilepsy should be employed.

The results of these two studies are in contrast to a more recent survey conducted in 1988 on over 1,200 individuals residing in the Henan Province in China [39]. In that study, more than half of the respondents believed that individuals with epilepsy should not be employed in jobs similar to those without epilepsy. Another recent study published in 2000 [40] described a door-to-door survey performed in Kerala, India of 1,118 individuals from households without epilepsy to assess their knowledge, skills and attitudes towards the disease. Of those surveyed, 40% believed that individuals with epilepsy could not be properly educated or employed. In a telephone interview conducted as recently as 2002 on 1,000 healthy individuals living in Seoul. Korea [41] to gauge their knowledge and perceptions of epilepsy, up to 87.4% of respondents agreed to working with persons with epilepsy but only 37.5% were willing to hire someone with the condition. At around the time of this study, another direct survey was performed on 1,694 members of the general public in the United Kingdom to assess their attitudes towards epilepsy [42]. Ninety-four percent of respondents agreed that those with epilepsy could be as successful as others in their chosen career.

The degree of social stigma towards individuals with epilepsy in certain regions in the African continent was described in a paper published by Jilek-Aall and colleagues in 1997 [43]. Interestingly, this paper also reflects the relation between societal progress and the acceptance of individuals with epilepsy. The authors documented the perceptions towards epilepsy of villagers living in the neighboring villages of Mahenge and Ruaha located in

Tanzania. Many of the more traditional notions of epilepsy continued to exist in the less developed Ruaha, including the existence of the vengeful epilepsy spirit (*kifafa*). The notion that epilepsy is contagious was still prevalent among the village people resulting in an inordinate amount of social restriction and isolation imposed on those with the condition. In contrast, those residing in more developed Mahenge had progressive and tolerant views of epilepsy resulting in the increased acceptance and societal integration of individuals with this disorder.

Social stigma towards individuals with epilepsy is not limited to cultures and races. Certain demographic profiles are more likely to show bias against epilepsy patients. In general, more unfavorable opinions of having individuals with epilepsy in the workplace can be found among the elderly, those who reside in rural areas, are less educated and have lower levels of employment themselves [37,41,44,45].

Despite the work-related stigma related to epilepsy that continues to exist, many studies have shown that the degree and severity of stigma has been decreasing over time, likely a result of increased public education and understanding of the disease. The study of Caveness referred to earlier [37] already showed that over a 30 year period (1949-1979) there was a significant increase in the public's acceptance of employment for epilepsy patients. A similar trend was reported in a study conducted in the South Moravian region of the Czech Republic. In that study, Novotna and colleagues [46] conducted a survey of 235 individuals in 1997 to determine their attitudes towards epilepsy. This study was then compared to an earlier survey of 387 individuals that was performed in the same region in 1981 [47]. The results of these two studies showed that in 1987, 74% of respondents believed that individuals with epilepsy should be employed in jobs like other people. This was a significant improvement from the 1981 survey wherein only 42% of those surveyed shared this belief. A third study conducted in Hungary [48] compared the results of a survey performed on 1,000 individuals in 2000 to a similar one conducted in 1994. In the 1994 survey, 55% of respondents believed that people with epilepsy could not be employed like other people. In contrast, by 2000, only 38% of respondents shared this view.

Epilepsy and the Workplace

There remains a widespread concern that individuals with epilepsy consistently under-perform and are a burden in the workplace. However, published studies tell a different story. MacIntyre [49] collected data from 29 work physicians on nearly 150,000 workers employed in various industries in the United Kingdom. One hundred and seventy-seven of these workers (0.12%) had epilepsy and were employed in relatively heavy industries. Eighty-nine percent of these workers were able to function without any difficulties although a third required a job change or modification. Interestingly, the accident frequency rate among epilepsy workers was 0.06% which was less than the average accident frequency rate of 1.92% seen in 29 companies that employed over 1,000 workers. It is estimated that approximately one hour of work is lost for every thousand hours worked by individuals with active epilepsy [50]. Another study [51] examined the work performance of 45 epilepsy workers of the British Steel Corporation and matched them for age, sex, and occupation with 38 healthy controls. Nineteen of the epilepsy workers were classified as being moderately to severely disabled. However, there was no relation between seizure severity and job type. Although there was more reluctance among epilepsy workers to do shift work, there was no significant difference between the epilepsy and control groups with regards to overall sickness and accident records. Also, using a 5-point merit scale, there was no difference in the job performance between these groups. In fact, a position paper released by the Employment Commission of the International Bureau for Epilepsy [52] states that "*the vast majority of jobs are suitable for people with epilepsy*" and that "*when a person with epilepsy possesses the right qualifications and experience, job suitability should normally be assumed*".

Employer attitudes are a major factor that determines whether an individual with epilepsy is employed. Several studies have examined employer attitudes towards epilepsy and the hiring of those with the condition. In a study by John and McLellan [53], a survey was sent to 26 companies in the Southampton area in the United Kingdom. The results of the survey indicated that employers tended to underestimate the prevalence of epilepsy and overestimated the frequency of seizures. More than half of employers believed that epilepsy was generally associated with reduced intelligence and a quarter of them believed that they did not have any available jobs for individuals with epilepsy. Interestingly, this reluctance was not associated with the type of employment but rather with the size of the business. Smaller-sized companies were less likely to have any work available for those with epilepsy and this reluctance was comparatively less for individuals with diabetes, heart disease and chronic bronchitis. As will be discussed later on, the reluctance of small-sized business to hire individuals with epilepsy is likely related to certain provisions of the Disability Discrimination Act. In another study [54], the author interviewed individuals who were involved in the hiring of personnel in 5 large organizations in the United Kingdom to determine their attitudes towards epilepsy. Similar to the above study, none of the employers interviewed were aware of how common epilepsy was, or of the employment difficulties facing individuals with epilepsy. In a more recent study [55], a postal survey was conducted among 204 United Kingdom-based companies representing the 14 economic regions and a wide range of industries. Twenty six percent of respondents knowingly employed individuals with epilepsy in their company while 16% did not believe that any position in their company could be filled by someone with epilepsy. Twenty-one percent of employers thought having epilepsy would be a major issue when considering a prospective employee for a position. Forty-two percent thought that hiring an individual with epilepsy would increase employer liability insurance costs. Similar to other studies, and also likely influenced by the Disability Discrimination Act in the United Kingdom that exempted smaller businesses from its provisions at the time of this study, a higher proportion of jobs in larger business was regarded as suitable for individuals with epilepsy compared to smaller companies. Lastly, the type of industry also influenced the number of jobs deemed suitable for those with epilepsy with public service employers reporting to have a greater proportion of jobs suitable for those with epilepsy compared to those in retail and manufacturing.

The difficulty of changing employer attitudes towards the hiring of individuals with epilepsy was best exemplified in a work by Sands and Alkind [56]. In their study, they measured the attitudes towards epilepsy of executives in Reading and Lancaster, Pennsylvania before and after conducting a high saturation educational campaign on epilepsy aimed at employers of the control city (Lancaster). Despite the campaign, there was no significant change in the attitudes of employers towards individuals with epilepsy. Only less than a third of respondents would recommend hiring someone with epilepsy. Around 44% of respondents did not believe that employer bias influenced the non-hiring of individuals with epilepsy and 70% did not believe that their personal attitudes towards those with epilepsy would ever change.

Despite the continuing employer barriers to productivity, a series of surveys done by Hicks and Hicks [57] from 1956-1986 of the 100 largest employers in the San Francisco Bay Area actually showed an increase in both the number of employers who knowingly hired individuals with epilepsy and in the number of jobs filled by individuals with the disorder. In 1956 only 79% of employers indicated that they had jobs that could be filled by individuals with epilepsy and only 21% knowingly hired these workers. In contrast, by 1986 all respondents had jobs that could be filled by workers with epilepsy and 95% stated that their company knowingly hired them.

Currently, in the United States, individuals with epilepsy cannot enter military service (except for certain non-combat positions) unless they have been seizure-free for at least five years and are no longer taking seizure medications. Also, these individuals cannot be employed in jobs that make them directly responsible for public safety. These occupations include that of being an airline pilot, bus driver, train operator, or air traffic controller. Safety concerns also limit the availability of jobs that involve operating dangerous machines, being a police officer, a firefighter, or driving a vehicle. Whether or not individuals with epilepsy can engage in such work usually depends on their individual qualifications and degree of seizure control [58].

In addition to dealing with employer anxieties towards working with individuals with epilepsy, it is important to also deal with co-workers' concerns. In one study [59], 3 different vignettes illustrating hypothetical cases of a co-worker suffering from depression, multiple sclerosis and epilepsy were presented to a group of individuals. These vignettes were followed by 8 identical questions meant to assess the respondents' level of comfort of dealing with co-workers with these conditions. The study showed that dealing with a co-worker with epilepsy caused more anxiety compared to one having multiple sclerosis or depression. In particular, respondents worried more about the sudden, unpredictable behavior displayed by those with epilepsy. And although half of the respondents felt comfortable providing first aid to a co-worker with depression or multiple sclerosis, only 30% were comfortable providing first aid to those with epilepsy.

LEGISLATION, EPILEPSY AND WORK

For the majority of human history, existing laws were blatantly prejudiced against those with epilepsy and only served to worsen the existing societal stigma towards these individuals. One of the earliest known laws relating to individuals with epilepsy involved in the slave trade in ancient Babylonia can be found in the Code of Hammurabi (circa 2250 BC). Article 278 of the Code states that "*if a man sells a male or female slave, and the slave has not completed his month, and the bennu fever falls upon him, he (the purchaser) shall return him to the seller and he shall receive the money which he paid*" [60]. Many scholars believe that the term "bennu fever" refers to convulsive seizures of individuals possessed by *Bennu*, deputy of the moon-god *Sin* [61].

Even as recently as 1956, 18 states within the United States still had laws that provided for the eugenic sterilization of individuals with epilepsy [62]. In the United Kingdom, a law prohibiting people with epilepsy from marrying was not repealed until 1970 [63] while in the United States the last state repealed its law forbidding marriage to individuals with epilepsy only in 1980 [62].

The first federal law in the United States that prohibited discrimination against individuals with epilepsy was the Rehabilitation Act of 1973. However the scope of this bill was limited to programs conducted by Federal agencies, those receiving Federal financial assistance, Federal employment, and to employment practices of Federal contractors [64].

Because of widespread public education and awareness, comprehensive laws have now been passed in various nations that aim to protect the rights of workers with disability. These include the United States' Americans with Disabilities Act (ADA) of 1990 and the Disability Discrimination Acts (DDA) in Australia (1992) and the U.K. (1994) [55]. These Acts make it unlawful for most employers to discriminate against qualified individuals on the basis of their disability. It also obligates them to provide reasonable accommodation to disabled individuals, unless it can be shown that such accommodations lead to undue hardship. Examples of reasonable accommodations include, but are not limited to, installing safety guards on pieces of machines or rubber mats, installing carpets to cover concrete floors in work areas, scheduling consistent day work shifts for individuals whose seizures are worsened by rotating shifts, and providing flame-retardant clothing and safety helmets [65].

In its original form, the provisions of the ADA applied only to private firms with 25 or more employees. However, as of 1994, this was broadened to include firms with 15 or more employees. Other important provisions of the ADA include the fact that employers may not inquire about an applicant's medical condition nor require the applicant to take a medical examination before making a conditional job offer. The diagnosis of epilepsy does not permit an employer to withdraw a job offer from an applicant unless it can be shown that the applicant cannot perform the essential functions of a job without posing a direct threat to safety. Lastly, the ADA requires that employers keep confidential any information regarding the medical condition of their workers [66].

It appears that some plaintiffs with epilepsy have been able to use the ADA to their benefit [67]. West and colleagues [68] examined the database of ADA Title 1 allegations maintained by the U.S. Equal Employment Opportunity Commission (EEOC) between July 1992 and September 2003. Their study identified 5,232 unduplicated, closed records with an allegation basis of epilepsy, representing around 3% of all cleansed data. Most respondents were companies with less than 200 employees. There was an overrepresentation of disability-related allegations in Southern states and these comprised 45.2% of all cases. The majority of allegations occurred post-hire and were in the areas of job retention (discharges, lay-offs) and inadequate working conditions (disciplinary actions, wages, harassment) while only a quarter of allegations were related to hiring practices. Interestingly, only 30% of allegations were determined by the EEOC to be of merit and were ruled in the plaintiffs' favor.

The ability of the Disability Discrimination Act in the United Kingdom to close the employment gap between those with and without disabilities has not been established. Pope and Bambra [69] compared the employment rate of individuals with disability using the General Household Survey from 1990-2002. Their study indicated that although the employment rate for disabled people during the 7 years prior to the DDA was slightly higher compared to the period following the Act, the difference was not significant. Furthermore, the average difference in the employment rates between the non-disabled and the disabled group actually increased post-DDA enactment.

Several reasons have been given to account for the inability of the DDA to fully protect the working rights of the disabled [70]. These include the fact that under the DDA, individuals have to prove that they are disabled and the law does not cover individuals who were discriminated because they were wrongly perceived to be disabled. The DDA provisions only apply to individuals with long term disabilities that have a substantial impact on their lives and exclude those on short term disability or whose degree of impairment produce a relatively trivial impact on their quality of life. Individuals such as general practitioners may not be fully familiar with DDA terminologies and standards yet are often asked to evaluate the risks of a given disability within an individual's work environment, even though they may not be qualified to do so. Also, the employment provisions of the DDS do not apply to certain entities such as businesses with fewer than 15 employees, as well as the fire service, armed forces, and police department. Lastly, employers are not required to specify the essential functions of a job beforehand resulting in difficulties for job seekers who are gauging their suitability for a particular type of work.

Driving and Work

Any review on the relationship between epilepsy and employment would be incomplete without a discussion on the subject of driving. In several regions worldwide, especially in the more industrialized areas, driving is often an integral part of life. For many, driving is a vital part of one's job description while for others, the ability to drive significantly increases work accessibility. It is not surprising then that both driving and work are important and contemporaneous concerns of many individuals with epilepsy [3,9,10,71].

Individual state and international laws restrict the ability of those with epilepsy to drive [72-74]. In the United States, individual state driving laws mandate the required seizure-free interval restriction, the exceptions based on mitigating factors, the medical review interval, and physician liability [75]. Permission to drive is premised on a defined period of seizure freedom and undergoing medical care. In some countries such as Argentina individuals with epilepsy are completely banned from driving [76] while others like Slovenia require a seizure-free period for 2 years without the use of any antiepileptic drug [77]. In Japan, driving laws for individuals with epilepsy have been recently relaxed. Whereas it was previously illegal for anyone with epilepsy to drive, as of 2002, Japanese law only required that individuals be seizure free for 2 years before being granted a driver's license [78].

Unfortunately, a significant number of individuals with epilepsy with incompletely controlled seizures continue to drive. In a survey of 307 epilepsy patients followed at a Level 4 Epilepsy Center [79], 20% of respondents who had at least 1 seizure a year admitted to driving. Disturbingly, 24% of those with daily seizures admitted to drive. Despite the low employment rate in this population, being employed and not receiving disability income were the major reasons these patients continued to drive. The implications of this study are similar to an earlier one [80] that found that driving was a necessary part of the work description in 9 of 21 individuals with epilepsy who had a motor-vehicle accident due to seizures. Among those with epilepsy, having a driver's license is associated with employment [81] and probably because of the fear of losing their license and livelihood, there is a tendency for individuals with epilepsy to underreport their seizures to their physicians [82,83].

Despite the various programs that exist to help integrate those with epilepsy into the workforce [84] and the progress made due to the ADA of 1990, the lack of a reliable public transportation system in most U.S. cities has been acknowledged as one of the main barriers that prevent the full integration of disabled individuals into the workplace [85].

Vocational Training and Job Placement Programs for Individuals with Epilepsy

Over the past decades, vocational training and job placement programs have assisted individuals with epilepsy in improving their employment readiness while at the same time helping them to find and maintain a job. High-quality vocational rehabilitation evaluation usually includes detailed neuropsychological, psychosocial, medical, and vocational assessments. These evaluations are important when developing an effective and individualized rehabilitation plan by uncovering subtle deficiencies that may be masked by good adaptive skills and by addressing the individual's internal psychological status as well as their adjustments to social networks. Training and work restrictions are then individualized taking into account one's functional limitation while avoiding blanket provisions and restrictions [86].

The published results of vocational rehabilitation in individuals with epilepsy have generally been mixed. While this may be due to the different vocational rehabilitation techniques employed, this may also have been influenced by societal and employer attitudes towards epilepsy at the time of the study. Freeman and Gayle [87] surveyed 47 individuals with epilepsy who received training at the Maryland State Division of Vocational Rehabilitation. Thirty-one of those surveyed completed training at the time of the survey while 12 were still in training. The rest dropped out of the program. Of those who completed training, 17 (55%) obtained a job within 6 months of training and 15 were still employed at the time of the survey. Carroll [88] described the experiences of 45 individuals with epilepsy in Ireland who underwent a 6-month training designed to help them develop their social and communication skills as well as basic skills in art, drama, home management, woodwork, decorating, and leatherwork. Their program resulted in a 60% placement rate for trainees with epilepsy, versus a 72% placement rate for those without the disorder. Equally important, 40% of those with epilepsy were still employed one year later.

In the United States, some tertiary epilepsy programs such as the University of Washington Regional Epilepsy Center have an in-house Vocational Services Program to assist individuals with epilepsy with their vocational needs. The Vocational Services Program has been in place since 1975 and offers a wide range of services that include neuropsychological and vocational assessment, jobsite and accommodation consultation, specialized placement and post-placement support. An important feature of this program is its goal of incorporating each patient's individual seizure-related information when performing vocational planning and determining job placement. Of the 106 individuals who comprised the first batch of enrollees into the program, 47.2% were in competitive employment within 18 months after entering the program while 19.8% dropped out of the program [89].

In 1976, the Epilepsy Foundation of American developed the Training and Placement Services (TAPS) in several cities across the United States in order to increase employment opportunities for individuals with epilepsy. The program focused on employer education as well as a wide spectrum of employment services that include vocational counseling and training as well as job placement. TAPS provided scheduled follow-ups up to one year after job placement. From 1977-1979, around 60% of those enrolled in TAPS were placed in competitive employment at a savings to society of $2,007 per TAPS-placed client per year [90]. Unfortunately, this program has been discontinued [91].

The state of epilepsy-related vocational rehabilitation varies across different countries. Gomes [92] examined the outcomes of 15 individuals with epilepsy who attended a vocational rehabilitation program in Brazil. Vocational rehabilitation did not appear to significantly improve the employment prospects of these individuals, and this was thought to be due to the patients' low level of education, poor seizure control and coexisting psychosocial problems.

In certain countries in Europe, state-mandated vocational rehabilitation exists for individuals with epilepsy and other disabilities. Patients are evaluated by the Department of Vocational Rehabilitation and formal training usually takes 3 years [93]. Several training centers exist in Germany, one of which, the Bethel Epilepsy Center, focuses primarily on the vocational training of individuals with epilepsy [94]. Another European vocational training program is the Transnational Epilepsy Training Project that was set up by England, Ireland, Scotland and the Netherlands in order to train individuals with epilepsy and assist them in finding employment [95]. However, despite the best of intentions, completion of these training programs do not necessarily guarantee successful placement in open employment [93].

In some countries such as the Netherlands and Germany, sheltered employment also exists for individuals who through their disability are not considered competitive for the open job market. In these centers, individuals with epilepsy make up between 10-15% of employees [93]. The use of sheltered employment has not widely been adapted nor has it significantly impacted the work status of individuals with epilepsy.

In general, those who received help at epilepsy-specialized vocational rehabilitation centers had significantly higher rates of job placement when compared with those who received vocational placement services at general rehabilitation state agencies. Those who received help at general centers had placement rates that ranged from 9-21%, while those who received help at specialized centers had rates that were upwards of 40%. There were also fewer dropouts among individuals who attended specialized programs. And although data was limited, it appears that the mean salary of those who underwent vocational training at specialized epilepsy centers were higher than those trained at general vocational centers [96].

Neuropsychological evaluation can also predict those who respond to vocational rehabilitation services. Among 46 adult outpatients who were referred to the University of Washington Regional Epilepsy Center for vocational services, the Wechsler Adult Intelligence Scale (WAIS) Digit Symbol subtest and the name-writing procedure from the neuropsychological battery by Dodrill were the best discriminators of later employability. These findings indicate that hand speed and dexterity are important skills for entry into the job market, as well as good attention span, visual acuity, and scanning capabilities [97].

A past history of psychological and addiction treatment and the number of months an individual with epilepsy was employed in the last 2 years prior to admission into the program were the main variables that distinguished those who obtained unsubsidized employment from those who were program drop-outs. On the average, those who were successfully employed had 12 months of work experience before enrolling in the vocational rehabilitation program. In contrast, those who dropped out of the program were employed for an average of 7 months before entering vocational rehabilitation. As far as the reasons for job loss was concerned, emotional and attitudinal difficulties on the job were the main reasons, followed by the lack of job-relevant skills and job lay-offs due to economic reasons. Interestingly, the presence of seizures on the job was not a main cause for job termination and occurred in only 1 of 20 cases of job loss [89].

QUO VADIMUS: IMPROVING EMPLOYMENT OPPORTUNITIES FOR INDIVIDUALS WITH EPILEPSY

In this review, we focused on the state of employment for individuals with epilepsy and highlighted the various reasons for the persistent lack of employability in this population. Our review shows that despite the advances in health care, legislation, and public acceptance, individuals with epilepsy remain at a serious disadvantage when it comes to finding and maintaining work.

This review highlights the importance of good seizure control as the primary variable that affects the employability of individuals with epilepsy. This was seen among the general epilepsy population [12,13,99] and among the subgroup of patients who have undergone epilepsy surgery [15-17]. In fact, in some advanced Western cultures, individuals with epilepsy who have good seizure control believe that they can be as successful in their careers compared to those without the disease [42].

While there is no current study that relates the occurrence of mood disorders in the epilepsy population to a lack of work productivity, it is well established that individuals suffering from depression have a decreased probability of employment and a greater number of missed days due to illness [98]. This lack of productivity is even higher in whose individuals who have both major depression and chronic disorders compared to those who have major depression alone [99]. The importance of early diagnosis and treatment of mood disorders in the epilepsy population cannot be underemphasized. Aside from improving an individual's quality of life [100,101], proper treatment should also contribute to increased work productivity.

The role of public awareness, education, and continuing legislation in support of individuals with epilepsy has also led to their acceptance into society and increased accessibility into the workplace. The latter half of the 20th century has already seen a steady decrease in the amount of social stigma attached to epilepsy [37]. The increased acceptance of individuals with epilepsy in society has also extended into the workplace with more and more employers acknowledging their work contributions [57]. Legislation such as the Americans with Disabilities Act of 1990 has undoubtedly helped increase workplace accessibility for these individuals. However, even recent data have shown that the acceptance of individuals with epilepsy both in society and in the workplace is less prevalent in developing societies [39-41]. Despite education and awareness, the road to full public acceptance of individuals with epilepsy continues to be slow and arduous [56]. Therefore the campaign in behalf of those with the disorder should be further intensified and should take on global proportions.

There is also a need to develop standards that define precisely the work capabilities and limitations of individuals with epilepsy in the workplace. It is reasonable to think that depending on the type of work, and primarily as a safety concern, some industries may need to impose more stringent restrictions on its workers with epilepsy [55]. However, these restrictions have not been standardized and are still based on the individual judgment and perceptions of the employer [53-55].

These work standards should provide employers and companies with objective guidelines when developing the job descriptions of these individuals. These guidelines should also address the legitimate concerns of employers such as the legal and financial ramifications of hiring workers with epilepsy. The concept that the majority of individuals with epilepsy can work and become equally productive as those without the condition is one that should be eventually accepted by all.

When considering ways to improve workplace accessibility, the issue of driving and transportation to work should be addressed, especially in societies that heavily rely on commuting. This especially affects those individuals whose seizures are reasonably but not completely controlled. Job placement programs do not routinely address the need for a reliable public transportation system to enhance the productivity of persons with epilepsy. It cannot be overemphasized that the lack of a reliable public transportation system in many parts of the United States remains a hindrance preventing the full assimilation of individuals with epilepsy into the workplace [85].

In this digital age, it may be possible to harness the power of the internet and other modern technologies that make working from home a reality and lessen the dependency on transportation. One way to enhance workplace accessibility, at least for some individuals with epilepsy, is via telecommuting. Though the use of this tool in this population has not yet been studied, it is conceivable that this technology offers individuals with epilepsy new workplace opportunities that overcome their own physical limitations [102,103].

This review also indicates that individual motivation and work values also influence the employability of individuals with epilepsy [28,34]. Work motivation is defined as "a set of energetic forces that originate both within as well as beyond an individual's being, to initiate work-related behavior and to determine its form, direction, intensity and duration" [104]. Work motivation is a "psychological process that results from the interaction between the individual and the environment" [105]. Future studies are needed to determine ways to improve the work motivation of those with epilepsy. In part, work motivation may be related to the coping mechanisms of those with this condition. Previous studies have shown that adaptive coping styles such as the use of learned resourcefulness, global problem solving, and self-efficacy improve psychosocial well-being while a patient focus on an external locus of control (the belief that outcomes are determined by outside forces beyond one's control) results in increased depression and lower self-esteem [106]. While coping mechanisms are influenced by clinical variables such as seizure control [107], finding ways to improve epilepsy patients' coping mechanism may result in increased work motivation. A related issue which needs to be addressed is that of disability benefits. In a study of over 22,000 individuals who participated in the Veterans Health Administration compensated work therapy program, it was shown that those who received disability benefits had lower rates of participation in vocational rehabilitation programs and were less likely to be competitively employed [108]. This finding was also seen in other disease states [109,110]. It is important to determine whether this finding extends to individuals with epilepsy and to develop measures that prevent this from becoming a work disincentive.

Lastly, there is a need to make vocational rehabilitation and job placement programs more widespread and accessible to those with epilepsy. The number of vocational rehabilitation and job placement programs geared specifically to the needs of those with epilepsy is relatively small and the vast majority of individuals with epilepsy do not have access to such programs.

This is unfortunate because the limited data available indicates that these programs have been successful in enhancing employability in this population [87-89]. There is a need to reproduce the results of successful epilepsy rehabilitation programs around the world, and to standardize the services offered by successful rehabilitation programs by focusing on services and rehabilitation techniques that have been shown to be effective. For instance, it has already been shown that epilepsy-specific vocational rehabilitation programs are more successful than general programs in the areas of job placement, job retention, and earning capacity [96]. In other disease states, the use of an "empowerment" oriented approach in vocational rehabilitation wherein an individual is given an active role in goal setting and achievement has been effective in improving job retention [111].

Given the current state of healthcare, there is also a need to include economic evaluation when assessing the success of epilepsy vocational rehabilitation programs. Economic evaluation has already been used as one of the measures in assessing vocational programs in other disease states [112,113].

CONCLUSION

Perhaps more than any other disorder, our understanding of epilepsy has long been confined to the realm of the supernatural and its sufferers ostracized and shunned as victims of demons and other ungodly spirits.

Only in the past century has epilepsy been accepted as a medical condition, the treatment of which resides in the sphere of medicine and science. The advances in the treatment of epilepsy during the past century have been nothing short of phenomenal. And because the majority of individuals with seizures can be adequately treated with current technologies, we can now focus on other equally important outcomes of care. In fact, among the various neuroscience disciplines, the field of epileptology is one of the first to incorporate formal quality of life evaluations in the assessment of care [114].

The complete integration of individuals with epilepsy into the workplace represents yet another step in their quest for complete integration and acceptance into society. It is encouraging to see how much progress made over the past decades; however as this review indicates, so much more remains to be accomplished. By continuing on this road, we provide both hope and strength to those afflicted with the condition.

Acknowledgment

The authors would like to thank Nader Antonios, M.D. for his critical review of the manuscript.

References

[1] Hauser WA. Epidemiology of epilepsy. *Advances in Neurology* 1978;19:313-319.
[2] Kadir ZA, Chadwick DW. Principles of treatment of epilepsy. *Drugs Today* 1999;35:35- 41.
[3] Fisher RS, Vickrey BG, Gibson P et al. The impact of epilepsy from the patient's perspective I. Descriptions and subjective perceptions. *Epilepsy Research* 2000;41:39-51.
[4] Cascino GD. Epilepsy: contemporary perspectives on evaluation and treatment. *Mayo Clinic Proceedings* 1994;69:1199-1211.
[5] Benbadis SR, Tatum WO. Advances in the treatment of epilepsy. *American Family Physician* 2001;64:91-98.
[6] Bishop M, Allen C. Employment concerns of people with epilepsy and the question of disclosure: report of a survey of the Epilepsy Foundation. *Epilepsy and Behavior* 2001;2:490-495.
[7] Callaghan N, Crowley M, Goggin T. Epilepsy and employment, marital, education and social status. *Irish Medical Journal* 1992;85:17-19.
[8] So EL, Penry JK. Epilepsy in adults. *Annals of Neurology* 1981;9:3-16.
[9] Taylor DC, McMackin D, Staunton H, Delanty N, Philips J. Patient's aims for epilepsy surgery: desires beyond seizure freedom. *Epilepsia* 2001;42(5):629-633.
[10] Moran NF, Poole K, Bell G et al. Epilepsy in the United Kingdom: seizure frequency and severity, anti-epileptic drug utilization and impact on life in 1652 people with epilepsy. *Seizure* 2004;13:425-433.
[11] Begley CE, Famulari M, Annegers JF et al. The cost of epilepsy in the United States: an estimate from population-based clinical and survey data. *Epilepsia* 2000;41:342-351.
[12] Collins JA, Chappell B. Correlates of employment history and employability in a British epilepsy sample. *Seizure* 1994;3:255-262.
[13] Chaplin JE, Wester A, Tomson T. Factors associated with the employment problems of people with established epilepsy. *Seizure* 1998;7(4):299-303.
[14] Jacoby A. Impact of epilepsy on employment status: findings from a UK study of people with well-controlled epilepsy. *Epilepsy Research* 1995;21:125-132.
[15] Augustine EA, Novelly RA, Mattson RH et al. Occupational adjustment following neurosurgical treatment of epilepsy. *Annals of Neurology* 1984;15(1):68-72.
[16] Lendt M, Helmstaedter C, Elger CE. Pre- and post operative socioeconomic development of 151 patients with focal epilepsies. *Epilepsia* 1997;38(12):1330-1337.
[17] Kellett MW, Smith DF, Baker GA, Chadwick DW. Quality of life after epilepsy surgery. *Journal of Neurology, Neurosurgery and Psychiatry* 1997;63:52-58.

[18] Strine TW, Kobau R, Chapman DP, Thurman DJ, Price P, Balluz LS. Psychological distress,comorbidities, and health behaviors among U.S. adults with seizures: results from the 2002 National Health Interview Survey. *Epilepsia* 2005;46(7):1133-1139.

[19] Cornaggia CM, Beghi M, Moltrasio L, Beghi E. Accidents at work among people with epilepsy. Results of a European prospective cohort study. *Seizure* 2006;15:313-319.

[20] Souza KT, Guerreiro MM, Guerreiro CA. Accident risk in patients with epilepsy. *Arquivos de Neuro-psiquiatria* 2008;66:175-178.

[21] van den Broek M, Beghi E for the RESt-1 Group. Accidents in patients with epilepsy: type, circumstances, and complications: a European cohort study. *Epilepsia* 2004; 45(6):667-672.

[22] Neufeld MY, Chistik V, Kogan E, Korczyn AD. Physically traumatic events in patients with epilepsy compared with non-epileptic subjects. *Seizure* 2000;9:595-597.

[23] Mensah SA, Beavis JM, Thapar AK, Kerr M. The presence and clinical implications of depression in a community population of adults with epilepsy. *Epilepsy and Behavior* 2006;8:213-219.

[24] Ettinger A, Reed M, Cramer J. Depression and comorbidity in community-based patients with epilepsy or asthma. *Neurology* 2004;63:1008-1014.

[25] Barry JJ, Lembke A, Gisbert PA, Gilliam F. Affective disorders in epilepsy. In: Ettinger AB, Kanner AM, editors. *Psychiatric Issues in Epilepsy*, Second Edition. Philadelphia: Lippincot Williams and Wilkins;2007.

[26] Kanner AM, Palac S. Depression in epilepsy: a common but often unrecognized comorbid malady. *Epilepsia and Behavior* 2000;1:37-51.

[27] Herodes M, Oun A, Haldre S, Kaasik A. Epilepsy in Estonia: a quality-of-life study. *Epilepsia* 2001;42(8):1061-1073.

[28] Bautista RED, Wludyka P. Factors associated with employment in epilepsy patients. *Epilepsy and Behavior* 2007;10:89-95.

[29] Varma NP, Sylaja PN, George L, Sankara SP, Radhakrishnan K. Employment concerns of people with epilepsy in Kerala, South India. *Epilepsy and Behavior* 2007;10:250-254.

[30] Koponen A, Seppala U, Eriksson K et al. Social functioning and psychological well-being of 347 young adults with epilepsy only- population-based, controlled study from Finland. *Epilepsia* 2007;48:907-912.

[31] Shackleton DP, Kasteleijn-Nolst Trenite DG, de Craen AJ, Vandenbroucke JP, Westendorp RG. Living with epilepsy: long-term prognosis and psychosocial outcomes. *Neurology* 2003;61:64-70.

[32] Reeves AL, So EL, Evans RW et al. Factors associated with work outcomes after anterior temporal lobectomy for intractable epilepsy. *Epilepsia* 1997;38(6):689-695.

[33] Elwes RD, Marshall J, Beattie A, Newman PK. Epilepsy and employment: a community based survey in an area of high unemployment. *Journal of Neurology, Neurosurgery and Psychiatry* 1991;54:200-203.

[34] Clarke BM, Upton ARM, Castellanos C. Work beliefs and work status in epilepsy. *Epileps and Behavior* 2006;9:119-125.

[35] Goffman E. Stigma: notes on the management of spoiled identity. New Jersey:Prentice Hall; 1963.

[36] Scrambler G, Hopkins A. Social class, epileptic activity, and disadvantage at work. *Journal of Epidemiology and Community Health* 1980;34:129-133.

[37] Caveness WF, Gallup GH Jr. A survey of public attitudes towards epilepsy in 1979 with an indication of trends over the past thirty years. *Epilepsia* 1980;21(5):509-518.

[38] Canger R, Cornaggia C. Public attitudes toward epilepsy in Italy: results of a survey and comparison with U.S.A. and West German data. *Epilepsia* 1985;26(3):221-226.

[39] Lai CW, Huang XS, Lai YH, Zhang ZQ, Liu GJ, Yang MZ. Survey of public awareness, understanding, and attitudes toward epilepsy in Henan Province, China. *Epilepsia* 1990;31(2):182-187.

[40] Radhakrishnan K, Pandian JD, Santhoshkumar T, et al. Prevalence, knowledge, attitude, and practice of epilepsy in Kerala, South India. *Epilepsia* 2000;41(8):1027-1035.

[41] Choi-Kwon S, Park KA, Lee HJ, et al. Familiarity with, knowledge of, and attitudes toward epilepsy in residents in Seoul, South Korea. *Acta Neurologica Scandinavica* 2004;110:39-45.

[42] Jacoby A, Gorry J, Gamble C, Baker GA. Public knowledge, private grief: a study of public attitudes to epilepsy in the United Kingdom and implications for stigma. *Epilepsia* 2004;45(11):1405-1415.

[43] Jilek-Aall L, Jilek M, Kaaya J, Mkombachepa L, Hillary K. Psychosocial study of epilepsy in Africa. *Social Science and Medicine* 1997;45(5):783-793.

[44] Chung MY, Chang YC, Lai YH, Lai CW. Survey of public awareness, understanding, and attitudes toward epilepsy in Taiwan. *Epilepsia* 1995;36(5):488-493.

[45] Gambhir SK, Kumar V, Singhi PD, Goel RC. Public awareness, understanding and attitudes toward epilepsy. *The Indian Journal of Medical Research* 1995;102:34-38.

[46] Novotna I, Rektor I. The trend in public attitudes in the Czech Republic towards persons with epilepsy. *European Journal of Neurology* 2002;9:535-540.

[47] Rektor I, Svejdova M, Sirek J. [Social problems of epileptics at the present time. Results of a poll in the South Moravia region]. *Casopis Lekaru Ceskych* 1983;122:179-185.

[48] Mirnics Z, Czikora G, Zavecz T, Halasz P. Changes in public attitudes towards epilepsy in Hungary: results of surveys conducted in 1994 and 2000. *Epilepsia* 2001;42(1):86-93.

[49] MacIntyre I. Epilepsy and employment. Community Health 1976;7:195-204.

[50] Risch F. We lost every game--but. *Rehabilitation Record* 1968;9:16-18.

[51] Dasgupta AK, Saunders M, Dick DJ. Epilepsy in the British Steel Corporation: an evaluation of sickness, accident and work records. *British Journal of Industrial Medicine* 1982;39:145-148.

[52] Employment Commission of the International Bureau for Epilepsy. Employing people with epilepsy: principles for good practice. *Epilepsia* 1989;30(4):411-412.

[53] John C, McLellan DL. Employers' attitudes to epilepsy. *British Journal of Industrial Medicine* 1988;45:713-715.

[54] Cooper M. Epilepsy and employment-employer's attitudes. Seizure 1995;4:193-199.

[55] Jacoby A, Gorry J, Baker GA. Employers' attitudes to employment of people with epilepsy: still the same old story? *Epilepsia* 2005;46:1978-1987.

[56] Sands H, Zalkind SS. Effects of an educational campaign to change employer attitudes toward hiring epileptics. *Epilepsia* 1972;13:87-96.

[57] Hicks RA, Hicks MJ. Attitudes of major employers toward the employment of people with epilepsy: a 30-year study. *Epilepsia* 1991;32:86-88.

[58] Gumnitt RJ. *Living Well With Epilepsy*. New York, New York: Demos Medical Publishing LLC, 1997.
[59] Harden CL, Kossoy A, Vera S, Nikolov B. Reactions to epilepsy in the workplace. *Epilepsia* 2004;45(9):1134-1140.
[60] Harper RF. *The Code of Hammurabi King of Babylon about 2250 B.C.* Chicago: University of Chicago Press; 1904.
[61] Stohl M. *Epilepsy in Babylonia*. The Netherlands: Brill Publishers, 1993.
[62] McLin WM, de Boer HM. Public perceptions about epilepsy. *Epilepsia* 1995;36(10):957- 959.
[63] Parsonage M. Historical overview of the legislative aspect of epilepsy. In: Canger R, Loeber JN, Castellano F, editors. Epilepsy and society: realities and prospects. *Amsterdam:Excerpta Medica;* 1988:227-230.
[64] Epilepsy Foundation of America. *The Americans with Disabilities Act: a guide to provisions affecting persons with seizure disorders.* Maryland: The Epilepsy Foundation of America;1992.
[65] Fraser RF, Bruyere SM. "Working effectively with employees who have epilepsy" 2001. Available at: *http://works.bepress.com/susanne_bruyere/31*. Accessed on October 16, 2008.
[66] Questions and answers about epilepsy in the workplace and the Americans with Disabilities Act (ADA) [online]. Available at: *http://www.eeoc.gov/facts/epilepsy.html*. Accessed August 22, 2008.
[67] Lehman C. EFA commentary: epilepsy, employment and the ADA: a status report. *Journal of Epilepsy* 1995;8:264-265.
[68] West MD, Dye AN, McMahon BT. Epilepsy and workplace discrimination: population characteristics and trends. *Epilepsy and Behavior* 2006;9:101-105.
[69] Pope D, Bambra C. Has the Disability Discrimination Act closed the employment gap? *Disability and Rehabilitation* 2005;27(20):1261-1266.
[70] Delany L, Moody JE. Epilepsy, employment and the Disability Discrimination Act. Does legislation make a difference? *Seizure* 1999;8:412-420.
[71] Martin R, Vogtle L, Gilliam F, Faught E. What are the concerns of older adults living with epilepsy? *Epilepsy and Behavior* 2005;7:297-300.
[72] Fisher RS, Parsonage M, Beaussart M et al. For the Joint Commission on Drivers' Licensing of the International Bureau for Epilepsy and the International League Against Epilepsy. Epilepsy and driving: an international perspective. *Epilepsia* 1994;35(3):675-684.
[73] Ooi WW, Gutrescht JA. International regulations for automobile driving and epilepsy. *Journal of Travel Medicine* 2000;7:1-4.
[74] Krauss GL, Ampaw L, Krumholz A. Individual state driving restrictions for people with epilepsy in the US. *Neurology* 2001;57:1780-1785.
[75] State Driving Laws. Available at: *http://www.epilepsyfoundation.org/living/wellness/transportation/drivinglaws.cfm. Accessed August 2*, 2008.
[76] Casas Parera I, Barreiro de Madariaga L, Gimeno A, Lehkuniec E. *Epilepsy and driving in Argentina. A new proposal. Medicine* (B Aires) 2003;63(3):249-255.
[77] Groselj J. Epilepsy and driving license regulations in Slovenia. *Medicine and Law* 1997;16(2):289-294.

[78] Inoue Y, Ito M, Kurihara M, Morimoto K. Epilepsy and driving in Japan. *Epilepsia* 2004;45(12):1630-1635.

[79] Bautista RED, Wludyka P. Driving prevalence and factors associated with driving among epilepsy patients. *Epilepsy and Behavior* 2006;9:625-631.

[80] Stanaway L, Johnson RH, Lambie DG. Epilepsy and driving. *The New Zealand Medical Journal* 1983;96(735):525-528.

[81] Sillanpaa M, Shinnar S. Obtaining a driver's license and seizure relapse in patients with childhood-onset epilepsy. *Neurology* 2005;64:680-686.

[82] Salinsky MC, Wegener K, Sinnema F. Epilepsy, driving laws, and patient disclosure to physicians. *Epilepsia* 1992;33:469-472.

[83] Darymple J, Appleby J. Cross sectional study of reporting of epileptic seizures to general practitioners. *British Medical Journal* 2000;320:94-97.

[84] From the Epilepsy Foundation: employment for people with epilepsy: the hardest nut. *Epilepsy and Behavior* 2001;2:379-380.

[85] Schelly C, Sample P, Spencer K. The American with Disabilities Act of 1990 expands opportunities for persons with developmental disabilities. *The American Journal of Occupational Therapy* 1992;46(5):457-460.

[86] Seidenberg M, Clemmons DC. Maximizing School Functioning and the School-to-Work Transition. In: Engel J, Pedley TA, editors. *Epilepsy: A Comprehensive Textbook.* Philadelphia: Lippincott-Raven Publishers;1997:2203-2210.

[87] Freeman JM, Gayle E. Rehabilitation and the client with epilepsy: a survey of the client's view of the rehabilitation process and its results. *Epilepsia* 1978;19:233-239.

[88] Carroll D. Employment among young people with epilepsy. Seizure 1992;1:127-131.

[89] Fraser RT, Clemmons D, Trejo W, Temkin NR. Program evaluation in epilepsy rehabilitation. *Epilepsia* 1983;24:734-746.

[90] Anderson RA. Training and Placement Services: An Employment Services Model Program for Persons with Epilepsy. In: Dam M, Gram L, Penry JK, editors. *Advances in Epileptology: XIIth Epilepsy International Symposium.* New York:Raven Press;1981:245-251.

[91] Fraser RT. Employment for people with epilepsy. To the Editor. *Epilepsy and Behavior* 2002;3(2):201-203.

[92] Gomes MDM. Client with epilepsy in a work Brazilian rehabilitation center. *Arquivos de Neuro-Psiquiatrica* 2000;58(2-A):227-232.

[93] Thorbecke R, Fraser RT. The Range of Needs and Services in Vocational Rehabilitation. In: Engel J, Pedley TA, editors. *Epilepsy: A Comprehensive Textbook. Philadelphia*: Lippincott-Raven Publishers;1997:2211-2226.

[94] Pfafflin M: Bethel, Bielefeld, Germany: Epilepsiezentrum Bethel Epilepsy Centre, Bethel. *Seizure* 2003;12:S4-S8.

[95] deBoer HM, Aldankamp AP, Bullivant F et al. The transnational epilepsy training project. *International Journal of Adolescent Medicine and Health* 1994;7(4):325-335.

[96] Fraser RT, Trejo W, Blanchard W. Epilepsy rehabilitation: evaluating specialized versus general agency outcome. *Epilepsia* 1984;7:325-335.

[97] Fraser RT, Clemmons DC, Dodrill CB, Trejo WR, Frellove C. The difficult-to-employ in epilepsy rehabilitation: predictors of response to an intensive intervention. *Epilepsia* 1986;27:220-224.

[98] Simon GE, Ludman EJ, Unutzer J, Operskalski BH, Bauer MS. Severity of mood symptoms and work productivity in people treated for bipolar disorder. *Bipolar Disorders* 2008;10(6):718-725.

[99] Egede LE. Major depression in individuals with chronic medical disorders: prevalence, correlates and association with health resource utilization, lost productivity and functional disability. *General Hospital Psychiatry* 2007;29(5):409-416.

[100] Boylan LS, Flint LA, Labovitz DL et al. Depression but not seizure frequency predicts quality of life in treatment-resistant epilepsy. *Neurology* 2004;62:258-261.

[101] Johnson EK, Johnson JE, Seidenberg M et al. The relative impact of anxiety, depression, and clinical seizure features on health-related quality of life in epilepsy. *Epilepsia* 2004;45:544-550.

[102] Trent JT, Smith AL, Wood DL. Telecommuting: stress and social support. *Psychological Supports* 1994;74(3 Pt 2):1312-1314.

[103] Yancer DA, Moe YK. Telecommuters: the work force of the future. *The Journal of Nursing Administration* 1995;25(7-8):52-59.

[104] [104] Pinder CC. Work Motivation in Organizational Behavior. New Jersey:Prentice Hall;1998.

[105] Latham GP, Pinder CC. Work motivation theory and research at the dawn of the twenty-first century. *Annual Review of Psychology* 2005;56:485-516.

[106] Livneh H, Wilson LM, Duchesneau A, Antonak RF. Psychosocial adaptation to epilepsy: the role of coping strategies. *Epilepsy and Behavior* 2001;2:533-544.

[107] Piazzini A, Ramaglia G, Turner K et al. Coping strategies in epilepsy: 50 drug-resistant and 50 seizure-free patients. *Seizure* 2007;16:211-217.

[108] Drew D, Drebling CE, Ormer AV et al. Effects of disability compensation on participation in and outcomes of vocational rehabilitation. *Psychiatric Services* 2001;52(11):1479-1484.

[109] Straaton KV, Maisiak R, Wrigley JM, White MB, Johnson P, Fine PR. Barriers to return to work among persons unemployed due to arthritis and musculoskeletal disorders. *Arthritis and Rheumatism* 1996;39:101-109.

[110] Rabkin JG, McElhney M, Ferrando S, Van Gorp W, Lin SH. Predictors of employment of men with HIV/AIDS: a longitudinal study. *Psychosomatic Medicine* 2004;66:72-78.

[111] Varekamp I, Verbeek JHAM, van Dijk FJH. How can we help employees with chronic diseases to stay at work? A review of interventions aimed at job retention and based on an empowerment perspective. *International Archives of Occupational and Environmental Health* 2006;80:87-97.

[112] Cope DN. The effectiveness of traumatic brain injury rehabilitation: a review. *Brain Injury* 1995;9(7):649-670.

[113] Schene AH, Koeter MWJ, Kikkert MJ, Swinkels JA, McCrone P. Adjuvant occupational therapy for work-related major depression works: randomized trial including economic evaluation. *Psychological Medicine* 2007;37:351-362.

[114] Devinsky O, Vickrey BG, Cramer J et al. Development of the quality of life in epilepsy inventory. *Epilepsia* 1995;36:1089-1104.

In: Social Epileptology
Editors: J. Pinikahana and C. Walker

ISBN 978-1-60876-228-6

Chapter 11

EPILEPSY AND PHYSICAL EXERCISE: HOW MUCH IS TOO MUCH?

Ricardo Mario Arida*[*1], Fulvio Alexandre Scorza[2] and Esper Abrão Cavalheiro[2]

[1]Department of Physiology - Universidade Federal de São Paulo. Escola Paulista de Medicina.

[2]Department of Neurology and Neurosurgery – Universidade Federal de São Paulo/Escola Paulista de Medicina

ABSTRACT

Epilepsy is a common disease found in 1-2% of the population, affecting people from all ages. The most common risk factors for epilepsy are cerebrovascular diseases, brain tumours, alcohol, traumatic head injuries, malformations of cortical development, genetic inheritance and infections of the central nervous system. Unfortunately, persons with epilepsy have previously been discouraged from participation in physical activity and sports for fear of inducing seizures or increasing seizure frequency. However, this overprotective attitude has been slowly changing in light of more recent data on this subject. Despite a shift in medical recommendations toward encouraging rather than restricting participation, the stigma remains and persons with epilepsy continue to be less active than the general population. Most studies have suggested that adults with epilepsy have lower rates of physical fitness. For this purpose, clinical and experimental studies have analyzed the effect of physical exercise on epilepsy. Although there are rare cases of exercise-induced seizures, exercise benefits individuals with epilepsy in many ways including improved seizure control, mood, and quality of life. The majority of physical activities or sports are safe for people with epilepsy to participate in with special attention to adequate seizure control, close monitoring of medications, and preparation of family or physical educators. This chapter is designed to show the risks and benefits of physical activity in person with epilepsy, discusses sports in which epileptics may participate, and describe the positive effect of physical exercise in experimental models of epilepsy.

[*] Corresponding Address: Prof. Ricardo Mario Arida, Rua Botucatú 862, Vila Clementino, ZIP Code: 04023-900. São Paulo, Brazil

OVERVIEW OF EPILEPSY

Epilepsy is a one of the most common neurological disorder problem worldwide. In developed countries, the incidence of epilepsy is around 50 per 100 000 people per year, and is higher in infants and elderly people (Duncan et al., 2006). Epidemiological studies suggest that between 70 and 80% of people developing epilepsy will go into remission, while the remaining patients continue to have seizures and are refractory to treatment with the currently available therapies (Sander, 1993, Kwan and Sander, 2004). The most common risk factors for epilepsy are cerebrovascular diseases, brain tumours, alcohol, traumatic head injuries, malformations of cortical development, genetic inheritance and infections of the central nervous system (Halatchev, 2000). In resource-poor countries, endemic infections, such as malaria and neurocysticercosis seem to be major risk factors (Duncan et al., 2006). Moreover, temporal lobe epilepsy (TLE) is the commonest form of partial epilepsy, probably affecting at least 40% of all patients with epilepsy (Babb, 1999) and is the most common form of drug-refractory epilepsy (Engel, 1993). Individuals affected with TLE typically have comparable clinical description, including an initial precipitating injuring such as *status epilepticus* (SE), head trauma, encephalitis or childhood febrile seizures (Fisher et al., 1998; Cendes, 2002). There is usually a latent period of several years between this injury and the appearance of the chronic TLE characterized by spontaneous recurrent seizures (SRS) originating from temporal lobe foci and learning and memory impairments (Devinsky, 2004; Detour et al., 2005).

Clinically, the epilepsies are characterized by spontaneous, recurrent epileptic seizures, which are caused by partial (focal) or generalized paroxysmal discharges in the brain. Seizures are the manifestation of abnormal hypersynchronous discharges of cortical neurons. The clinical signs or symptoms of seizures depend on the location of the epileptic discharges in the cortex and the extent and pattern of the propagation of the epileptic discharge in the brain (Dichter, 1994).

Seizures and epilepsy are currently divided into two groups: partial and generalized. Partial or focal seizures have clinical or EEG evidence of local onset, usually in a region of one hemisphere, and may spread to other parts of the brain during a seizure. Generalized seizures essentially begin simultaneously in both cerebral hemispheres.

Partial seizures are subclassified into three groups: simple partial seizures, complex partial seizures, and partial seizures secondarily generalizing to clonic and/or tonic seizures. Simple partial seizures are associated with preservation of consciousness and usually with unilateral hemispheric involvement. Complex partial seizures are associated with alteration or loss of consciousness and usually with bilateral hemispheric involvement. A partial seizure can progress to secondary generalization, i.e., to a generalized tonic-clonic seizure that proceeds directly from either a simple partial seizure or a complex partial seizure. Primarily generalized seizures are subclassified mainly by the presence or different patterns of convulsive movements (Loscher, 1997; Chang and Lowenstein, 2003). The generalized seizures include: a) generalized tonic-clonic seizures (grand mal), b) absence seizures (petit mal), c) myoclonic seizures, d) atonic seizures, e) clonic seizures, and f) tonic seizures. Further description of these seizure types is beyond the scope of this chapter and can be reviewed elsewhere (Fisher et al., 2005).

Epilepsy and Exercise: Human's Studies

Historical Information

Although the positive effect of physical exercise on general health is well established, persons with epilepsy are often excluded from participation in physical activities. This is surprising because for many high-risk patients such as those with coronary heart disease and diabetes, physical exercise has proved quite beneficial. This reluctance of both patients and physicians is due to fear that exercise might make the epilepsy worse, predispose to injury, or that fatigue resulting from exercise may precipitate further seizures (Bjorholt et al., 1990).

The question whether people with epilepsy can engage in physical fitness programmes, recreational or competitive sports, particularly collision or contact, has been debated for many years. Historically, it has long been thought that regular activity is beneficial for convulsive disorders. The prominent epileptologist W.G. Lennox wrote: "Physical and mental activity seems to be an antagonist of seizures" (Lennox, 1960). Medical recommendations likely arise from a lack of clear guidelines. The attitude towards restriction and protection of the person with epilepsy has, however, changed dramatically in the last decades and general recommendations have been lately reviewed. For instance, in 1968, the American Medical Association Committee on Medical Aspects of Sports advised that people with epilepsy not controlled by medication should avoid not only collision sports but also non contact sports (American Medical Association Committee on the Medical Aspects of Sports: Convulsive disorders and participation in sports and physical education, 1968; American Academy of Pediatrics Committee on Children with Handicaps: The epileptic child and competitive school athletics, 1968). In 1974, the Committee revised its instance, describing that epileptics with rational seizure control should be allowed to play any sport except activities in which chronic head trauma may occur (American Medical Association Committee on the Medical Aspects of Sports: Epileptics and contact sports, 1974). In 1983, the American Academy of Pediatrics allowed for further individual consideration and said, "epilepsy *per se* should not exclude a child from hockey, football, basketball and wrestling" (American Academy of Pediatrics Committee on Children with Handicaps and Committee on Sports Medicine: Sports and the child with epilepsy, 1983). The International League against epilepsy recommended in 1997 that the only prohibited sports for athletes with epilepsy are skydiving and scuba diving (Commission of Pediatrics of the International League Against Epilepsy: Restrictions for children with epilepsy, 1997).

In order to give satisfactory advice about sports it is essential to understand the factor in sport that could affect the epileptic disorder. Thus, it is rather difficult to indicate the specific effects of epilepsy will have on sports participation and to draw general conclusions. In general, the literature now suggests that once a patient's seizures are well controlled, he or she should lead an active life and participate in sports and other physical activities.

Epilepsy and Physical Activities Participation

Studies have been designed to study the relationship between epilepsy and exercise comparing physical and social activities among persons with epilepsy based on questionnaires and/or clinical studies (Roth et al., 1994; Steinhoff et al., 1996) as well as to assess physical fitness by using standardized tests of physical exercise (Steinhoff et al., 1996; Jalava and Sillanpaa, 1997). Interestingly, only few studies in humans have analyzed the effect of an aerobic exercise program in people with epilepsy. For instance, a study conducted by Nakken and coworkers reported that 4 weeks of physical training program at an intensity of 60% of VO2max for 45 min a day, did not change the average frequency of seizures (Nakken et al., 1990). Aerobic physical program in woman with intractable epilepsy decreased the number of seizures during the exercise period (Eriksen et al., 1994). Another study which investigated this subject showed no impact of seizure frequency after 12 weeks of physical exercise program (McAuley et al., 2001).

Another important point to be considered is the low degree of participation in physical activity among people with epilepsy (Denio et al., 1989; Nakken et al., 1999; Roth et al., 1994). In a study of people with epilepsy in Norway only 23% participated in organized physical activity (Bjorholt et al., 1990). Despite the fact that several epidemiological studies have been performed on this subject, these patient samples may not be directly applicable to developing countries. A study conducted by Arida e coworkers (2003), analyzed the degree of participation in physical activities among Brazilian people with epilepsy. Although only 15 percent of patients were qualified as active, that is, exercised regularly, more than half of the patients participated in physical activities once or twice per week or on the weekends. Other factors than exercise-induced seizures, such as lack of training facilities, problems with transportation, low motivation, medication and lack of qualified instructors have been noted as important explanatory factors (Bjorholt et al., 1990).

Risks of Sports Participation

Several investigations have analyzed the magnitude of risk for the person with epilepsy in certain activities. The general opinion is that these risks are determined by the occurrence of a seizure while the patient is participating in sport. The risk from injury due to a sudden fall without warning has been addressed in a few studies. Aisenson (1948) found that over a period of 16 years children with epilepsy had no higher rate of injury during daily activities than children who had never had a seizure. However, there is a potential hazard of falling during a seizure, so several sports must be avoided by patients who have regular seizures.

It is conceivable that seizures might be injurious during certain sport activities. Studies have also looked into the risk of injury in water sports because of the known increased risk of drowning due to seizures. Pearn et al (1978) found that 4 of 140 immersion accidents were caused by seizures over a 5-year period in Hawaii. They reported that no children died and that the accident rate was similar to that in general population. Conversely, Kemp and Sibert (1993) identified 4 children who drowned in the United Kingdom in just a 1-year period. It is generally recommended that water sports may be permitted with appropriated precautions. A review of those studies would suggest that this risk could be further reduced when performed with direct supervision.

Concerning contact sports, in general, there is no evidence that repetitive minor head trauma will worsen the frequency and/or severity of epilepsy. In fact, contact sports, especially football, are common activities for children and adolescent boys, so their prohibition can have critical consequences (Livingston and Berman, 1973). Some contact sports have been contraindicated to persons with epilepsy. However, repetitive minor head injury in athletic competition has failed to show any consistent association with epilepsy (Van Linschoten et al., 1990). Berman (1984) concluded after a study of 301 children with blunt head injury and nine with prior epilepsy that a history of epilepsy does not indicate a predisposition to a seizure after a blunt head injury. Although boxing has been a sport to be avoided among people with epilepsy, a study has shown no severe abnormalities on EEG or neuroimaging in 47 Swedish amateur boxers when compared to soccer and field athletes (Haglung and Bergstrand, 1990). In these lines, there is epidemiological evidence that head injury causes epilepsy, but the association is only significant for severe head injury (Annegers et al., 1998). Participation in contact sports is common, yet there are very few cases of seizure occurrence or exacerbation. The above information suggests that the risk of contact sports in epilepsy is minimal and not significant enough to warrant routine restrictions. Therefore, the decision for a person with epilepsy to participate in sports is concerned whether the benefit outweighs the risk. The risk-benefit for a person with epilepsy is dependent on the sport activity considered, the type of seizure that might occur as well as the probability that a seizure will occur during the sport. Table 1 summarizes some sport activities with their restrictions to people with epilepsy.

Table 1. Recommendations on some sport activities for persons with epilepsy (van Linschoten et al., 1990)

Activities to be avoided
Scuba diving
Parachuting
High altitude climbing
Gliding
Hand-gliding
Aviation
Motor-racing
Boxing
Activities requiring precautions or supervision
Water-skiing
Swimming
Canoeing
(Wind) surfing
Sailing
Activities requiring knowledge of seizure type and sports
Cycle racing
Skating
Horse-riding
Gymnastics

Mechanism by Which Exercise Can Inhibit Seizures

The particular way in which physical activity supplies protection against seizures remains uncertain. An initial theory is that acidosis serves as a protective mechanism by increasing seizure threshold (Gotze et al., 1967). Briefly, short, intensive physical activity increases serum lactate content and causes metabolic acidosis. It has been known that acidosis reduces the irritability of the cortex (Gibbs et al., 1940). Enzymes controlling brain GABA concentrations appear to be influenced by pH changes. Acidosis increases and alkalosis decreases GABA concentration. The optimum pH of the enzymes transaminase and decarboxylase are such that acidosis increases the GABA concentration in the brain and alkalosis lowers it. Exercise may decrease the pH of the blood, leading to changes in the effectiveness of enzymes involved in GABA metabolism, resulting in an increase in GABA concentration in the brain, which produces a natural anticonvulsant effect.

Other hypotheses have been proposed. Researches on brain electrical activity have shown that abnormal discharges disappear in most individuals during physical activity but return at rest (Gotze et al., 1967; Kuijer, 1980). Thus, it has been noted that fewer seizures occur during both mental and physical activity compared with periods of rest (Cordova, 1993). Additionally, it is hypothesized that during exercise, vigilance and alert are increased, factors that have long been known to decrease seizure frequency (Kuijer, 1980). Another hypothesis relates the ß-endorphins released during exercise. Endorphins produced during exercise may function as a natural anticonvulsant because β-endorphins tend to inhibit epileptiform discharges (Albrecht, 1986).

Mechanism by Which Exercise Can Induces Seizures

It is import to highlight some factors that could cause seizures during sports and exercise, although they are merely speculative. Fatigue is one such issue. Physical and especially psychic stress is generally accepted as factors that precipitate seizures (Temkin and Davis, 1984). In competitive sports this stress could induce seizures in stress-sensitive patients (McLaurin, 1973; Cordova e col., 1993). Hypoxia, hyperhydration and hypoglycaemia are other possible considerations. Hypoxia does not occur during normal sporting activities, although it may occur in climbing or alpine skiing at high altitude (> 2000m)(Boucharlat e col., 1973; MacLaurin, 1973). Hyperhydration can result from a great ingestion of water or from an extreme loss of sodium (during swimming or prolonged physical exercise such as marathon running and triathlon) and is a well known factor in provoking seizures. Overingestion of isotonic or hypotonic liquids may lead to hyponatraemia (Bennett and Wagner, 1983; Noakes e col., 1984). Hypoglycaemia can occur during long distance running, cycling or swimming, especially when regular liquid and food intake is reduced (French, 1983). Hyperthermia is also known to trigger seizures. Prolonged exercise (marathon, triathlon) at high temperatures and under humid conditions puts people at risk (Millington, 1985; van Willigen, 1988). One factor that is raised frequently, but inappropriately, is that of hyperventilation. Because hyperventilation in the laboratory may provoke epileptiform discharges on EEG and even seizures, especially absence some have erroneously believed that increased ventilation during exercise may cause seizures (Esquivel e col., 1991).

However, increased ventilation during physical training is a compensatory homeostatic mechanism; the respiratory alkalosis of induced hyperventilation does not occur (Wasserman e col. 1973).

Psychological Benefits of Exercise on Epilepsy

Epilepsy patients suffer considerable lack of physical fitness that is likely to impact their general health and quality of life (Steinhoff et al., 1996). Exercise is well known to improve health and quality of life in the general population and this is true for those with epilepsy as well. Several factors such as cognitive, emotional and behavioral conditions, ability to work, social functioning, family stability, self-esteem, stigma, and adjustment to seizures seem to be especially crucial to the quality of life of patients with epilepsy (Devinsky, 1996; Kellett, et al., 1997). Some studies have implicated seizure frequency as having a significant impact on quality of life, with a particularly strong effect on physical role functioning (Leidy, et al., 1999). Some reports show a low degree of participation in physical activities among persons with epilepsy (Bjorholt, et al., 1990; Denio et al., 1989). The notion that physical activity might provoke seizures or make patients prone to injuries represents an obstacle for some individuals with epilepsy who wish to live an active life (Roth et al., 1994). In addition to seizures themselves, worries about the reaction from others to seizures also contributed to the stressful nature of epilepsy. The amount of patients that fear they can feel embarrassed after having a seizure while exercising or afraid that exercise might lead to health problems has been considerably elevated. In addition, co-morbidity such as depression and general emotional distress are common in people with epilepsy (Blumer, et al., 1998). In this line, regular physical exercise has received considerable attention as a mechanism for enhancing resistance to negative effects of psychosocial stress in healthy adult populations. Physical exercise is generally accepted as contributing to general health and well-being (Bouchard, 1990), positive changes in life style (Shepard, 1990), improved mood, life quality (Folkins and Sime, 1981) and reduction of anxiety and depressive symptoms (Martinsen et al., 1985), together with increased ability to cope with stress (Steptoe et al., 1989). Single sessions of moderate aerobic exercise can provide acute mood benefits (Roth et al., 1989) and exercise programs reduce depression (Griest et al., 1979).

A number of evidences demonstrates that people with epilepsy would receive similar benefits from physical activity. For instance, in a study, which examined physical exercise, stressful life experiences, and depression in adults with epilepsy, found that active subjects had significantly lower levels of depression than inactive subjects, as well as better psychosocial adjustment (Roth et al., 1994). Similarly, Eriksen et al. study on intractable epilepsy in women found that a regular exercise programme improved psychosocial functioning and quality of life (Eriksen et al., 1994). Nakken et al. (1990) also noted that after a 4-week exercise intervention, individuals with epilepsy had an improved mental state and became more sociable. Roth et al. (1994) found that seizure frequency was positively correlated with depression. Therefore, it can be concluded that patients with epilepsy experience emotional problems as a result of their disease, which decreases their quality of life.

Antiepileptic Drugs and Exercise

Antiepileptic drugs (AEDs) are the most common therapy for epilepsy and seizures. However, most have side effects that cause fatigue and lethargy, which are obstacles for some active people with epilepsy. Other side effects such as blurred or double vision, concentration difficulty, and impaired coordination, fatigue, drowsiness, dizziness, or gastrointestinal upset can influence physical performance of people with epilepsy and also account for the decrease in total sports activity. To this point some questions need to be addressed: Does exercise affect drug metabolism, absorption and serum drug concentration? What are the adverse effects of AEDs, and do they affect physical performance?

It has been reported that physical training has a liver enzyme-inducing effect, increasing with increasing physical fitness (Frenkl et al., 1980). Nevertheless, it is not well known whether physical training affect serum levels of certain AEDs (Nakken et al., 1990; Eriksen et al., 1994). Indeed, serum AED levels of people participating in regular exercise programs should be monitored closely, especially in the first few months of training. Some persons with epilepsy have been warned against exercise due to fears that it might alter AED metabolism and result in seizures due to reduced serum AED concentrations. In a study conducted by Wong and Wirrell (2006), children receiving three or more AEDs presented a significant negative correlation with sports participation. The possible explanation suggested by the authors was that children who had taken more AEDs were considered more "vulnerable" and therefore participated less in activities. In a Norwegian study (Nakken et al., 1990), 21 adult inpatients who had active epilepsy (at least one seizure per month for the previous year) took part in a 4-week exercise program at a minimum of 60% of their maximal aerobic capacity for 45 minutes a day, 6 days a week. This training program did not significantly change AED levels and did not reduce seizure frequency. But until further studies are done, serum levels of liver enzymes should be closely observed. In a review of drugs to avoid in athletes, Henderson (1998) does not list AEDs specifically. No studies have been published that show a relationship between AEDs and athletic performance.

Morbidity and Mortality in Epilepsy

Limited data on psychiatric and somatic morbidity in people with epilepsy have been reported in various studies. A recent cross-sectional study, however, revealed that people with epilepsy have double the risk of psychiatric disorders and an increased risk of the following somatic disorders: neurodegenerative conditions, particularly dementias, Alzheimer's disease, and Parkinson's disease; cardiovascular disorders; cerebrovascular disorders; upper gastrointestinal hemorrhages; fractures; pneumonia; chronic lung diseases; diabetes; and brain tumors. Eczema, osteoarthritis, rheumatoid arthritis, and extracranial tumors did not occur more frequently (Gaitatzis et al., 2004). Thus, studies suggest that people with epilepsy are at increased risk of developing comorbid conditions and at increased risk of dying prematurely.

It is reliably established that mortality in epilepsy is increased compared to an age-matched general population (Cockerell et al., 1994; Hauser et al., 1980). People with epilepsy are two- to three-fold increase to die prematurely than those without epilepsy and the most common epilepsy-related category of death is sudden unexpected death in epilepsy (SUDEP) (Tomson et al., 2005). SUDEP is defined as sudden, unexpected, witnessed or unwitnessed, nontraumatic and nondrowning deaths in patients with epilepsy, with or without evidence of a seizure and excluding documented *status epilepticus*, in which post mortem examination does not reveal a toxicological or anatomical cause of death (Nashef, 1997). Information concerning risk factors for SUDEP is conflicting, but potential risk factors include: age, early onset of epilepsy, duration of epilepsy, uncontrolled seizures, seizure frequency, seizure type and antiepileptic drugs number (Stollberger and Finsterer, 2004). The exact pathophysiological causes of SUDEP is unknown, but it is very probable that cardiac arrhythmia during and between seizures play a potential role (Stollberger and Finsterer, 2004).

Preventative measures other than medical and surgical therapies could be useful in the prevention of SUDEP (Scorza et al., 2008). Among these factors, physical activity may play an interesting role (Scorza et al., 2008; Arida et al., 2008a/b). Considerable evidence from animal and clinical studies indicates that physical activity reduces seizure frequency, as well as lead to improved cardiovascular and psychological health in patients with epilepsy (Arida et al., 2008a).

It is important to point out that the risk of injury or death does not appear to be higher in people with epilepsy who participate in organized sports or just exercise regularly. For instance, in 1948, Aisenson reviewed the records of 960 patients engaged in full athletic programmes over a period of 16 years in order to compare the incidence of potentially serious injuries in convulsive and non- convulsive children. The accident rate in people with epilepsy was similar to non- epileptic controls. Fischer and Daute, (1988) who more recently examined this issue, found comparable data to Aisenson study.

In view of the discussion above, information is lacking not only to support the beneficial outcome of exercise in seizure reduction but also to understand the mechanisms by which exercise protects the epileptic brain. In this sense, animal studies have been performed for this purpose.

EPILEPSY AND EXERCISE: ANIMALS' STUDIES

Animal Models of Epilepsy

Animal models for seizures and epilepsy have played a fundamental role to the understanding of the physiological and behavioral changes associated with human epilepsy. They allow us to determine the nature of injuries that might contribute to the development of epilepsy, to observe and intercede in the disease process subsequent to an injury preceding to the onset of spontaneous seizures, and also to study the chronically epileptic brain in detail, using physiological, pharmacological, molecular, and anatomical techniques.

As described above, temporal lobe epilepsy (TLE) is the commonest form of partial epilepsy. Animal models constitute one of our most valuable tools to better understand the pathophysiology of TLE. Between many animal models of TLE, we will focus on two specific models of epileptogenesis that were used to understand the mechanisms by which physical exercise interfere in epilepsy: the Kindling model and the Pilocarpine model (for review see Goodman, 1998).

Kindling Model

Since its introduction in 1969 (Goddard et al., 1969), kindling has become one of the most widely used animal model of epilepsy (Sato et al., 1990). Kindling can be induced by repeated administration of a subconvulsive stimulus administered through a bipolar electrode implanted into a limbic structure such as the amygdala, hippocampus, entorhinal cortex or other brain areas. Over a period of several stimulation days, the animal displays both behavioral and electrographic seizures that spread to become secondarily generalized. In rats stimulated in the amygdala, the initial stimulus often elicits focal paroxysmal activity (i.e., so called "after discharges") without apparent clinical seizure activity. Subsequent stimulations induce the progressive development of seizures, generally evolving through the following stages: 1- immobility, facial clonus, eye closure, twitching of the vibrissae, 2- head-nodding, 3- unilateral forelimb clonus, 4- rearing, 5- rearing and falling accompanied by secondary generalized clonic seizure (Racine, 1972). The behavior observed in stages 1 and 2 mimics that found in human complex partial (limbic or temporal lobe) seizures; the behavior in the latter three stages would be consistent with complex partial seizures evolving to generalized motor seizures. An animal is usually considered being fully kindled after it displays several (e.g., at least 3) stage 5 seizures.

Pilocarpine Model

The pilocarpine model of epilepsy reproduces the main features of human TLE in rats and mice. The pilocarpine model as well as the kainic acid model are probably the most commonly studied chemical-inductive models for TLE. As extensively described by Turski et al. (1983a/1984), a single high dose of pilocarpine (300-380 mg/kg, ip.), a potent muscarinic cholinergic agonist originally isolated from the leafless of South America shrubs, acutely induces sequential behavioral and electrographic changes indicative of sustained epileptic activity, resulting in widespread damage to the forebrain in both rats and mice. The initial alterations comprise akinesia, ataxia, facial automatisms and head tremor. After 15-25 min those changes evolve to motor limbic seizures with rearing, forelimb clonus, salivation, intense masticatory movements and fall. Such fits recur every 2-8 min and lead to *status epilepticus* within 50-60 min after pilocarpine administration that last for up 12 hours, rendering the animals prostate or critically ill. The first 24 h taken by those manifestations, when the lethality rate reaches 30%, has been called acute period. After a silent period, (seizure-free phase) that varies from 4 to 44 days (mean 14,8±3,0 days) all surviving animals start exhibiting the spontaneous recurrent seizures which characterize the chronic period, varying from 2 to 15 seizure episodes per month (mean of 2-3 seizures per week). Behaviorally, a spontaneous seizure is characterized by facial automatisms, head nodding, forelimb clonus, rearing and fall (Cavalheiro et al., 1991; Leite et al., 1990). The behavioral analysis of this model was detailed reviewed posteriori (Arida et al., 1999). Morphological analysis of the brain after pilocarpine-induced *status epilepticus* lead to cell loss in the hippocampal subfields CA1 and CA3 and in the hilus of dentate gyrus, in the septum, olfactory tubercle, amygdala, piriform cortex, neorcortex, and thalamic nuclei (Turski et al., 1983/1986). Supragranular sprouting of the mossy fibers is also observed, starting as early as

4 days after SE and increases with time reaching a plateau by 100-day survival (Mello et al., 1993).

Effect of Physical Exercise in Experimental Models of Epilepsy

Experimental studies have also demonstrated a positive effect of physical exercise in animals with epilepsy (Arida et al., 1998/1999/2003/2004). The first study relating the effect of physical exercise on epilepsy used the kindling model (Arida et al., 1998). To assess the acute effect of exercise on kindling evolution, animals were submitted to a daily bout of aerobic exercise which consisted of 40 min running on the treadmill at 20 meters per min. One minute post-exercise, animals were kindling stimulated. To the chronic effect of exercise, animals were submitted to an aerobic exercise program (45 sessions of 40 min running on a treadmill at 20 meters per min, 7 days per week). After this period of training, they were submitted to 40 min running at the same speed and kindling stimulated one min post-exercise. The number of stimulations required to reach stage 5 was statistically higher for the chronic exercise group when compared to the acute exercise group and control group. The number of stimulations required to reach stage 5 in the acute exercise group was higher but not statistically different from the control group. Thus, the acute and chronic exercise groups spent a longer time and a shorter afterdischarge (AD) duration during stage 1 than the control group.

Some factors could probably be contributing to this effect. Several lines of evidence show that brain neurotransmission is influenced by exercise. For instance, an increase in noradrenaline levels in whole brain has been reported (Brown and Van Huss, 1973, De Castro and Duncan, 1985). It's well known that among catecholamines, noradrenaline has a tonic inhibitory effect on kindling development but not on kindling state (Westerberg, 1984). Bortolotto and Cavalheiro (1986) observed that the depletion of noradrenaline induced by DSP4 facilitated the propagation of epileptiform activity and the rate of hippocampal kindling. Evidence in favor of changes in synthesis and metabolism of catecholamines during exercise and the inhibitory involvement of this neurotransmitter system in the amygdala kindling support the hypothesis that the effect of chronic exercise on brain catecholamines can contribute to retard the kindling development.

A subsequent study, using the pilocarpine model of epilepsy, evaluated the effect of an aerobic physical program on seizure frequency (Arida et al., 1999). After the first spontaneous recurrent seizure animals were submitted to an aerobic exercise program of 45 sessions on a treadmill, 7 days per week at the intensity of 60% VO_{2max}. A reduced frequency of seizures in trained animals with epilepsy was observed. In this study, only two animals presented 3 seizures each during 3600 Hs of exercise and 2 animals presented 1 seizure, 1 min post-exercise.

Further investigations were performed to better clarify the factors that may interfere on this process. A study evaluated, using local cerebral metabolic rates for glucose (LCMRglu), whether physical training modifies the functional activity in rats with epilepsy (Arida et al., 2003). LCMRglu was measured by the quantitative [^{14}C]2-deoxyglucose (2DG) method. The purpose to study the brain metabolism during the interictal phase (between seizures) was that all animals present seizures at rest and not during exercise (Arida et al., 1999). The hypothesis that animals with epilepsy submitted to a physical training would exhibit a marked metabolic alteration in the interictal phase was, however, not confirmed. It was observed an increase in interictal LCMRglu in inferior colliculus and auditory cortex in the trained rats with epilepsy when compared to rats with epilepsy. A study conducted by Vissing et al. (1996) demonstrated a higher local cerebral glucose utilization in the auditory and visual cortex during exercise, suggesting that these changes are not related directly to the exercise per se, but to a higher mental alertness in exercise than in resting rats. Since physical activity does need a certain level of alertness, the increased attention and vigilance observed during physical activity could reduce the number of seizures (Kuijer, 1980). The increased metabolic rate in these structures could explain a lower seizure number in trained rats with epilepsy in the present and previous work (Arida et al., 1999).

An electrophysiological study was carried out to study the effect of aerobic exercise on "in vitro" hippocampal electrophysiological parameters observed in rats submitted to the pilocarpine model of epilepsy (Arida et al., 2004). Trained rats with epilepsy exhibited a reduction in population spikes when compared with nontrained rats (monitored by extracellular field potentials recorded from CA1 area).

Another study evaluated the occurrence of structural changes in hippocampal formation of trained rats with epilepsy by means of an immunohistochemical approach. Markers of the GABAergic system, such as calcium-binding proteins; parvalbumin and calbindin have been extensively used in different models of epilepsy to visualize morphological changes occurring in the brain (Sloviter, 1989; Freund et al., 1991). They represent effective and sensitive markers of hippocampal cells [77] and in particular, of a population of inhibitory interneuron(Celio, 1990). In these lines, animals with epilepsy were submitted to voluntary or forced exercise, trained acutely or chronically. Both voluntary and forced exercise, lead to prominent changes in the staining of parvalbumin in the dentate gyrus from control rats and rats with epilepsy (Arida et al., 2007).

CONCLUSION

On the basis of the available data in literature, seizures occurring during exercise are infrequent. Furthermore, generalizations about persons with epilepsy can never be made. The majority of people with epilepsy can participate in regular exercise with a very small risk of exacerbating their seizures. Every patient is unique concerning the type, frequency, severity and impact of his or her seizures. A good insight into the patients' history regarding accidents caused by seizure, periods of freedom from seizures, drug compliance is required. To this point, more studies are necessary to confirm the beneficial effects of exercise on epilepsy. The existing clinical data on the impact of exercise on patient outcomes have limitations. There is a lack of prospective studies, studies using appropriate controls, studies examining behavioral aspects, and studies using a comprehensive approach in an outpatient setting. Experimental studies in animal models of epilepsy have strengthened the positive effects of exercise in human's studies. Although the question of impact of physical exercise on epilepsy remains unsolved, people with epilepsy should have the same benefits as others from the positive effects on maximal aerobic and work capacity, body weight, and self-esteem (Nakken et al., 1990). In these lines, it appears justifiable that physicians should encourage most persons with epilepsy to participate in regular physical activities.

References

Aisenson MR. Accidental injuries in epileptic children. *Pediatrics* 1948; 2:85-8.

Albrecht H., Endorphins, sport, and epilepsy: getting fit or having one, *NZ Med. J.* 1986; 99:915.

American Medical Association Committee on the Medical Aspects of Sports: Convulsive disorders and participation in sports and physical education. *JAMA* 1968; 206:1291.

American Academy of Pediatrics Committee on Children with Handicaps: The epileptic child and competitive school athletics. *Pediatrics* 1968; 42:700-2.

American Medical Association Committee on the Medical Aspects of Sports: Epileptics and contact sports. *JAMA*, 229: 820-82, 1974.

American Academy of Pediatrics Committee on Children with Handicaps and Committee on Sports Medicine. Sports and the child with epilepsy. *Pediatrics* 1983;72:884-5.

Annegers JF, Hauser WA, Coan SP, et al. A population-based study of seizures after traumatic brain injuries. *N Engl J Med* 1998; 338:20-4.

Arida RM, Vieira AJ, Cavalheiro EA. Effect of physical exercise on kindling development. *Epilepsy Res.* 1998; 30:127-32.

Arida RM, Scorza FA, Peres CA, Cavalheiro EA. The course of untreated seizures in the pilocarpine model of epilepsy. *Epilepsy Res 1*999;34:99-107.

Arida RM, Scorza FA, Santos NF, Peres CA, Cavalheiro EA. Effect of physical exercise on seizure occurrence in a model of temporal lobe epilepsy in rats. *Epilepsy Res* 1999; 37:45-52.

Arida RM, Scorza FA, Albuquerque M, et al. Evaluation of physical exercise habits in Brazilian patients with epilepsy. *Epilepsy and Behav* 2003; 4:507-10.

Arida RM, Fernandes MJS, Scorza FA. Preti SC, Cavalheiro E.A. Physical training does not influence interictal LCMRglu in pilocarpine-treated rats with epilepsy. *Physiol. Behav* 2003;79:789-94.

Arida RM, Sanabria ERG, Silva AC, Faria LC, Scorza FA, Cavalheiro EA. Physical training reverts hippocampal electrophysiological changes in rats submitted to the pilocarpine model of epilepsy. *Physiol. Behav.* 2004a; 83:165-71.

Aridan RM, Scorza CA, da Silva AV, Scorza FA, Cavalheiro EA. Differential effects of spontaneous versus forced exercise in rats on the staining of parvalbumin-positive neurons in the hippocampal formation. *Neurosci. Lett.* 2004b;364:135-8.

Arida RM, Scorza CA, Scorza FA, Gomes da Silva S, da Graça Naffah-Mazzacoratti M, Cavalheiro EA. Effects of different types of physical exercise on the staining of parvalbumin-positive neurons in the hippocampal formation of rats with epilepsy. Prog. Neuropsychopharmacol. *Biol. Psychiatry* 2007;31:814-22.

Arida RM, Cavalheiro EA, da Silva AC, Scorza FA. Physical activity and epilepsy: proven and predicted benefits. *Sports Med.* 2008a;38: 607-15.

Arida RM, Scorza CA, Schmidt B, de Albuquerque M, Cavalheiro EA, Scorza FA. Physical activity in sudden unexpected death in epilepsy: much more than a simple sport. *Neurosci. Bull.* 2008b;24(6):374-80.

Babb TL. Synaptic reorganizations in human and rat hippocampal epilepsy. *Adv. Neurol.* 1999;79:763-79.

Bennett HT, Wagner T. Acute hyponatremia and seizures in an infant after a swimming lesson. *Pediatrics* 1983;72:125-27.

Berman W. Sports and the child with epilepsy. *Pediatrics* 1984;74:520-21.

Bjorholt PG, Nakken KO, Rohme K, Hansen H. Leisure time habits and physical fitness in adults with epilepsy. *Epilepsia* 1990; 31:83-7.

Blumer D, Wakhlu S, Davies K, Hermann B. Psychiatric outcome of temporal lobectomy for epilepsy: incidence and treatment of psychiatric complications. *Epilepsia* 1998; 39:478-86.

Bortolotto ZA, Cavalheiro EA. Effect of DSP4 on hippocampal kindling in rats. Pharmacol. *Biochem. Behav.* 1986;24;777-79.

Boucharlat J, Maitre A, Ledru J. Sport et epilepsy de l'enfant. *Ann. Med-psychol* 1973; 131:392-401.

Bouchard C. The consensus statement. In: Exercise, fitness and health. *A consensus of current Knowledge*. (Eds C. Bouchard, R.J. Shephard, T. Stephens, J.R. Sutton, B.D. McPherson). Champaign, IL, *Human Kinetics Books*, 1990: pp. 497-510.

Brown B, Van Huss C. Exercise and rat brain catecholamines. *J Appl Physiol* 1973;34:664-69.

Cavalheiro EA, Leite JP, Bortolotto ZA, Turski WA, Ikonomidou C, Turski L. Long-term effects of pilocarpine in rats: Structural damage of the brain triggers kindling and spontaneous recurrent seizures. *Epilepsia* 1991;32:778-82.

Cendes F. Febrile seizures and mesial temporal sclerosis. *Curr. Opin. Neurol.* 2002;17:161-64.

Chang B, Lowenstein DH. Mechanisms of disease. Epilepsy. *N. Engl. J. Med.* 2003; 349:1257-66.

Cockerell OC, Johnson AL, Sander JW, et al. Mortality from epilepsy: results from a prospective population-based study. *Lancet* 1994;344:918-21.

Commission of Pediatrics of the International League Against Epilepsy: Restrictions for children with epilepsy. *Epilepsia* 1997;38:54-6.

Cordova F. Epilepsy and sport. *Australian Family Physician* 1993;22:558-62.

De Castro J, Duncan G, Operantly conditioned running: effects on brain catecholamine concentrations and receptor densities in the rat. *Pharmacol. Biochem. Behav* 1985;23:495-500.

Denio LS, Drake ME, Pakalnis A. The effect of exercise on seizure frequency. *J Med* 1989;20:171-6.

Devinsky O. Quality of life in epilepsy. In:. *The Treatment of epilepsy: principles and practice* (Ed. E. Wyllie). Baltimore, Williams and Wilkins, 1996: pp. 1243-50.

Devinsky O. Diagnosis and treatment of temporal lobe epilepsy. *Rev. Neurol. Dis.* 2004;1:2-9.

Detour J, Schroeder H, Desor D, Nehlig A. A 5-month period of epilepsy impairs spatial memory, decreases anxiety, but spares object recognition in the lithium-pilocarpine model in adult rats. *Epilepsia* 2005; 46:499-508.

Dichter MA. Emerging insights into mechanisms of epilepsy: implications for new antiepileptic drug development. *Epilepsia* 1994;35;S51-S57.

Duncan JS, Sander JW, Sisodiya SM, Walker MC. Adult epilepsy. *Lancet* 2006;367:1087-1100.

Engel J Jr. Update on surgical treatment of the epilepsies. Summary of the Second International Palm Desert Conference on the Surgical Treatment of the Epilepsies. *Neurology* 1993;43:1612-1617.

Eriksen HR, Ellertsen B, Gronningsaeter H, et al. Physical exercise in women with intractable epilepsy. *Epilepsia* 1994;35 1256-64.

Esquivel E, Chaussain M, Plouin P, et al. Physical exercise and voluntary hyperventilation in childhood absence epilepsy. *Electroenceph. Clin. Neurophysiol.* 1991;79:127-32.

Fischer A, Daute KH. Die unfallsgefahrdung anfallskraner kinder im schulsport un bei speilerischen Freizeitbeschaftigungen. *Med. Sport* 1988;28: 93-5.

Físher PD, Sperber E., Mosh, SL. Hippocampal sclerosis revisited. *Brain Dev.* 1998;20:563-73.

Fisher RS, van Emde Boas W, Blume W, Elger C, Genton P, Lee P, Engel J Jr. Epileptic seizures and epilepsy: definitions proposed by the International League Against Epilepsy (ILAE) and the International Bureau for Epilepsy (IBE). *Epilepsia* 2005;46:470-2.

Folkins CH, Sime WE. Physical fitness training and mental health. *Am Psychol* 1981;36:373-89.

French JK. Hypoglycaemia-induced seizures following a marathon. *NZ Med. J.* 1983;96:407.

Frenkl R, Gyore A, Meszaros J, et al. A study of the enzyme inducing effect of physical exercise in man. The 'training liver'. *J. Sports Med.* 1980; 20:371-6.

Freund TF, Ylinen A, Miettinen R, Pitkanen A, Lahtinen H, Baimbridge KG, Riekkinen PJ. Pattern of neuronal death in the rat hippocampus after status epilepticus. Relationship to calcium binding protein content and ischemic vulnerability. *Brain Res Bull* 1991;28:27-38.

Gaitatzis A, Carroll K, Majeed A, Sander W. The epidemiology of the comorbidity of epilepsy in the general population. *Epilepsia* 2004;45:1613-22.

Gibbs FA, Williams D, Gibbs EL. Modification of cortical frequency spectrum by changes in CO2. *J. Neurophysiol.* 1940;3:49-58.

Goodman JH. Experimental models of status epilepticus. In: Peterson, S.L., Albertson, T.E. (Eds.), *Neuropharmacological Methods in Epilepsy Research,* CRC Press, Boca Raton, pp. 95-125, 1998.

Gotze W, Kubicki St, Munter M, Teichmann J. Effect of physical exercise on seizure threshold. *Dis. Nerv. Syst* 1967;28:664-67.

Griest JH, Klein MH, Eischens RR, et al. Running for treatment of depression. *Comp. Psychiatry* 1979;20:41-54.

Halatchev VN. Epidemiology of epilepsy--recent achievements and future. *Folia Medica* (Plovdiv) 2000;42:17-22.

Haglund Y, Bergstrand G. Does Swedish amateur boxing lead to chronic brain damage? A retrospective study with CT and MRI. *Acta Neurol. Scand.* 1990;82: 297-302.

Hauser WA, Annegers JF, Elveback LR. Mortality in patients with epilepsy. *Epilepsia* 1980;21:399-412.

Henderson JM. Therapeutic drugs: what to avoid with athletes. *Clin. Sports Med.* 1998;17:229-43.

Kellett MW, Smith DF, Chadwick DW. Quality of life after epilepsy surgery. *J. Neurol. Neurosurg Psychiatry* 1997;63:52-8.

Kemp AM, Sibert JR. Epilepsy in children and the risk of drowning. *Arch. Dis. Child* 1993;68:684-5.

Kuijer A. Epilepsy and exercise, electroencephalographical and biochemical studies, in: Wada, J.A., Penry, J.K. (Eds), *Advances in Epileptology*: The 10th Epilepsy International Symposium New York, Raven Press, pp.543, 1980.

Jalava M, Sillanpaa M. Physical activity, health-related fitness, and health experience in adults with childhood-onset epilepsy: a controlled study. *Epilepsia* 1997;38:424-29.

Kwan P, Sander JW. The natural history of epilepsy: an epidemiological view. *J Neurol Neurosurg Psychiatry* 2004;75:1376-81.

Leidy NK, Elixhauser A, Vickrey B, Means E, Willian MK. Seizure frequency and the health related quality of life of adults with epilepsy. *Neurology* 1999;53:162-6.

Leite JP, Bortolotto ZA, Cavalheiro EA. Spontaneous recurrent seizures in rats: An experimental model of partial epilepsy. *Neurosc Biobehav Rev* 1990;14:511-17.

Lennox WG, Lennox MA. *Epilepsy and related disorders*. Vol. 2. Boston-Toronto: Little, Brown and Co., 1960.

Livingston SL, Berman W. Participation of epileptic patients in sports. *JAMA* 1983;224:236-8.

Loscher W. Animal models of intractable epilepsy. *Progress in Neurobiology* 1997;33:239-58.

McAuley JW, Long L, Heise J, Kirby T, Buckworth J, Pitt C, Lehman KJ, Moore JL, Reeves AL. A Prospective Evaluation of the effects of a 12-week outpatient exercise program on clinical and behavioral outcomes in patients with epilepsy. *Epilepsy Behav.* 2001;2:592-600.

McLaurin R. Epilepsy and contact sports: factors contraindicating participation. *JAMA* 1973:225:285-87.

Martinsen EW, Medhus A, Sandvik L. Effects of aerobic exercise on depression: a controlled study. *BMJ* 1985;291:109.

Mello LEAM, Cavalheiro EA, Tan AM, Kupfer WR, Pretorius JK, Babb TL, Finch DM. 1993. Circuit mechanisms of seizures in the pilocarpine model of chronic epilepsy: Cell loss and mossy fiber sprouting. *Epilepsia* 34:985-95.

Millington JT. Should epileptics scuba dive? Correspondence. *JAMA* 1985; 254:22:3182-83.

Nakken KO, Bjorholt PG, Johannessen SI, Loyning T, Lind E. Effect of physical training on aerobic capacity, seizure occurrence, and serum level of antiepileptic drugs in adults with epilepsy. *Epilepsia* 1990:31:88-94.

Nakken KO. Physical exercise in outpatients with epilepsy. *Epilepsia* 1999;405: 643-65.

Nashef L. Sudden unexpected death in epilepsy: terminology and definitions. *Epilepsia* 1997:38:6-8.

Noakes ID. Goodwin N, Raymer BL, Branken T, Taylor RKN. Water intoxication, a possible complication during endurance exercise. *Medicine and Science in Sports and Exercise* 1984;17:370-75.

Pearn J, Bart R, Yamaoka R. Drowning risks to epileptic children: a study from Havaii. *BMJ* 1978; 2(6147):1284-85.

Racine RJ. Modification of seizure activity by electrical stimulation: II, Motor seizure. *Electroenceph. Clin. Neurophysiol.* 1972:32:281-294.

Roth DL, Goode KT, Williams VL, Faught E. Physical exercise, stressful life experience, and depression in adults with epilepsy. *Epilepsia* 1994;35:1248-55.

Roth DL, Wiebe DJ, Fillingim RB, et al. Life events, fitness, hardiness, and health: a simultaneous analysis of proposed stress resistance effects. *J Pers Soc Psychol* 1989:57:136-42.

Roth DL, Goode KT, Williams VL, Faught E. Physical exercise, stressful life experience, and depression in adults with epilepsy. *Epilepsia* 1994:35:1248-55.

Sander JW. Some aspects of prognosis in the epilepsies: a review. *Epilepsia* 1993;34:1007-16.

Scorza FA, Colugnati DB, Pansani AP, Sonoda EY, Arida RM, Cavalheiro EA. Preventing tomorrow's sudden cardiac death in epilepsy today: what should physicians know about this? *Clinics* 2008:63: 389-94.

Sato M, Racine RJ, McIntyre DC. Kindling: basic mechanisms and clinical validity. *Electroenceph Clin Neurophysiol* 1990;76:459-72.

Shepard RJ. Costs and benefits of an exercising versus a nonexercising society. In: *Exercise, fitness and health* (Eds C. Bouchard, R.J. Shepard, T. Stephens, J.R. Stton, B.D. McPherson). *A consensus of current knowledge.* Champaing, IL, Human Kinetics Books, 1990: 49-60.

Sloviter RS. Calcium-binding protein (Calbindin-D28k) and parvalbumin immunocytochemistry: localization in the rat hippocampus with specific reference to the selective vulnerability of hippocampal neurons to seizure activity. *J CompNeurol* 1989:280:183-96.

Steinhoff BJ, Neususs K, Thegeder H, et al. Leisure time activity and physical fitness in patients with epilepsy. *Epilepsia* 1996;37:1221:27.

Steptoe, A., Edwards, S., Moses, J., Mathews, A. The effects of exercise training on mood and perceived coping ability in anxious adults from the general population. *J Psychosom Res* 1989;33:537-47.

Stollberger C, Finsterer J Cardiorespiratory findings in sudden unexplained/unexpected death in epilepsy (SUDEP). *Epilepsy Res* 2004; 59:51-60.

Temkin NR, Davis GR. Stress as risk factors for seizures among adults with epilepsy. *Epilepsia* 1984;25:450-56.

Tomson T, Walczak T, Sillanpaa M, Sander JW. Sudden unexpected death in epilepsy: a review of incidence and risk factors. *Epilepsia* 2005;46(Suppl 11):54-61.

Turski WA, Czuczwar SJ, Cavalheiro EA, Turski L, Kleinrok Z. Acute and long-term effects of systemic pilocarpine in rats: spontaneous recurrent seizures as a possible model of temporal lobe epilepsy. *Naunyn Schmiedebergs Arch Pharmacol* 1983a; 324:25R.

Turski L, Cavalheiro EA, Sieklucka-Dziuba M, Ikonimidou-Turski C, Czuczwar SJ, Turski WA. Seizures produced by pilocarpine: neurophatological sequelae and activity of glutamate decarboxylase in the forebrain. *Brain Res* 1986:398:37-48.

Turski L, Cavalheiro EA, Sieklucka-Dziuba M, Ikonimidou-Turski C, Czuczwar SJ, Turski WA. Seizures produced by pilocarpine: neurophatological sequelae and activity of glutamate decarboxylase in the forebrain. *Brain Res* 1986:398:37-48.

Van Linschoten R, Backx FJG, Mulder OGM, et al. Epilepsy and sports. Sports Med 1990;10:9-19.

van Willigen J. Hardlopers en doodlopers; oververhitting in een gematigd klimaat (Running and exhaustion; hyperthermia in a moderate climate). *Nederlands Tijdschrift voor Geneeskunde* 1988;132:437-40.

Vissing J, Andersen M, Diemer NH. Exercise-induced changes in local cerebral glucose utilization in the rat. *J. Cereb Blood Flow Metab* 1996;16:729-36.

Wasserman K, Wipp B, Koyal S, Beaver W. Anaerobic threshold and respiratory gas exchange during exercise. *J. Appl. Physiol.* 1973;35:236-43.

Westerberg V, Lewis J, Corcoran ME. Depletion of noradrenaline fails to affect kindling seizures. *Exp Neurol* 1984;84:237-40.

Wong J. Wirrell E. Physical activity in children/teens with epilepsy compared with that in their siblings without epilepsy. *Epilepsia* 2006;47:631-39.

In: Social Epileptology
Editors: J. Pinikahana and C. Walker
ISBN 978-1-60876-228-6

Chapter 12

ECONOMIC AND PSYCHOSOCIAL BURDEN OF EPILEPSY IN DEVELOPING COUNTRIES

Sanjeev V. Thomas*

Department of Neurology,
Sree Chitra Tirunal Institute for Medical Sciences and Technology,
Trivandrum, India

ABSTRACT

Globally there are about 50 million people with epilepsy. Epilepsy is probably the longest known disorder known to mankind and it continues to be the most common serious neurological disorder in all the continents. The incidence of epilepsy in developing countries (69/100,000) is more than in developed countries (43/100,000).In developing countries, many people regard epilepsy as a curse or possession by spirits. Some persons resort to faith healing and alternate systems of treatment. Such false beliefs and stigma interfere with optimal treatment and rehabilitation of persons with epilepsy. Several surveys have shown that the vast majority of people with epilepsy do not receive appropriate treatment. Social, economic and logistic factors contribute to the treatment gap in these countries. Frequent seizures and treatment with multiple drugs are known to impair quality of life for persons with epilepsy. In 2001, the economic burden of epilepsy in India was over USD 1.7 billion. Close to 73% of this was contributed by indirect costs due to loss of productivity from recurrent seizures. Recurrent seizures reduce the economic productivity of the affected persons and their families and increase the economic burden several times over. In India, the treatment gap of epilepsy ranges from 35% to 70%. It is possible to reduce the overall economic burden of epilepsy by better control of seizures through more effective treatment. The burden of epilepsy in India has a gender bias that leaves women more affected than men. The psychosocial consequences and stigma of epilepsy affects women more than men. Fewer women receive treatment for epilepsy when compared to men. Women with epilepsy have more difficulty finding marital partners. Antiepileptic drugs may interfere with oral contraception and impair

* Correspondence: Prof. Sanjeev V. Thomas, Department of Neurology, Sree Chitra Tirunal Institute for Medical Sciences and Technology, Trivandrum 695011. India, Telephone: +91 471 2524468; Fax: +91 471 2446433; Email; sanjeev.v.thomas@gmail.com

bone health. Prenatal exposure to antiepileptic drugs can induce malformations in a small minority of infants and possibly lead to neurocognitive impairment. Efforts to reduce the treatment gap would considerably reduce the burden of epilepsy. Focused educational programs to bring epilepsy out of the shadows, and establishment of comprehensive epilepsy care programs are important steps in this direction. The burden of epilepsy in India and several developing countries can also be reduced by focusing attention on prevention.

INTRODUCTION

Epilepsy is the most common serious neurological disorder. Our understanding of the causation of epilepsy has been oscillating between biological, supernatural, organic and psychological domains. In India the Ayurvedic system of medicine has been in existence since several centuries BC. The basic concepts of epilepsy were enunciated in the Charaka Samhita (BC 400) the oldest compilation of ancient Ayurvedic treatment. In Charaka Samhita, epilepsy is termed 'Apasmara' which means "loss of consciousness" and is described as a biological phenomenon. Later on Hippocrates, the father of modern medicine also considered epilepsy as an organic disorder. Nevertheless, in subsequent years, a supernatural causation of epilepsy became prevalent. Much of the psychosocial burden and stigma of epilepsy are directly or indirectly related to this misconcept. It was only in the early 19th century that the organic concepts of epilepsy regained scientific acceptance.

Globally there are about 50 million people with epilepsy. It is the most common serious neurological disorder on all continents. More than 85% of people with epilepsy live in developing countries, where the infrastructure to treat epilepsy remains far below optimal levels. The incidence of epilepsy in India (69/100,000) is more than in developed countries (43/100,000). In India there are more than 5.5 million people with epilepsy, and over 70% of them are not receiving any treatment [1]. Women make up more than half of the vulnerable [1]. It is predicted that in India, the number of new cases of epilepsy each year would be close to half a million. Because the rural population constitutes 74% of the Indian population, the number of people with epilepsy in rural areas will be approximately 4.1 million, three fourths of whom will not be getting any specific treatment as per the existing standard. WHO has recently estimated that globally the disability adjusted life years lost due to epilepsy are 7,613,000 out of which South East Asian countries account for 2,155,000. The economic burden of epilepsy is not adequately appreciated by health administrators or care providers.

KNOWLEDGE ATTITUDE AND PRACTICE ISSUES

Epilepsy had remained shrouded in many misconcepts for many centuries. Even today many people regard epilepsy as a curse or possession by spirits. Such false beliefs and stigma interfere with treatment and rehabilitation of persons with epilepsy. Many persons resort to faith healing and alternate systems of treatment. In North India, it is a popular belief that smelling leather shoes or onions will abort seizures, while in certain southern states people consider that contact with metal objects such as a key will abort seizures. Many persons believe that epilepsy is a psychological disorder and would be cured after marriage. This type of belief not only deters the patient from obtaining correct treatment for epilepsy but may lead to several psychosocial problems.

A survey in Pakistan revealed that a quarter of people surveyed there believed that epilepsy is caused by evil spirits, black magic or envy and that persons with epilepsy would develop impotence or cancer later in life [2]. A similar survey in Kerala State, India revealed that 44% of respondents objected to employing persons with epilepsy and another 29% considered that people with epilepsy cannot be married [3]. In both studies misconcepts were significantly more prevalent among illiterate and poorly educated people. Similar unfavourable beliefs and misconcepts are prevalent in other parts of the world. Misunderstandings and wrong attitudes to epilepsy lead to unhealthy practices in the community that ultimately paves the way to stigma. In their efforts to conceal the disease, people with epilepsy tend to avoid seeking modern medical help but rather proceed secretly to faith healers and other unscientific approaches.

Stigma of Epilepsy

Epilepsy is a highly stigmatizing disorder. It is associated with increased stigma, more frequent stressful life events and poor adjustment to epilepsy. People with epilepsy tend to have increased financial stress, vocational problems and external locus of control [4]. Stigma of epilepsy is reinforced by lack of information about the disease, discriminating attitudes of the community and fear of loss of physical and emotional control [5]. The degree to which epilepsy is stigmatized is similar to the stigma associated with AIDS according to a survey carried out in Brazil. The authors hypothesized that empowerment of patients leading to improvement of their self-esteem may shift this scale. It is likely that different societies may have different attitudes to epilepsy, depending upon their knowledge and beliefs. Jacoby and colleagues observed that many people in China and Vietnam understood epilepsy to be a chronic, not curable, but a controllable disorder. People with epilepsy in these countries experience low social status, rejection that negatively influences their quality of life [6]. When faced with seizures for the first time, most people would seek medical attention and do not attempt to hide the event. In contrast to this, people tend to hide the events, when seizures recur. [7].

Treatment Gap

One of the practical difficulties in controlling epilepsy is the disparity between the availability of treatment and actual utilization of treatment. The treatment gap is defined as the proportion of patients out of all patients with active epilepsy who are not receiving treatment. It is widely known that epilepsy can be treated successfully in more than 70% of patients. Unfortunately most patients who would otherwise have benefited from treatment do not receive treatment in India and most other developing countries. Several surveys have shown that the treatment gap in India varies from 25% - 70%. The situation in most Asian countries is not different. Social, economic and logistic factors contribute to the treatment gap in these countries. There is often a gender bias in treatment gap that results in fewer women with epilepsy receiving treatment [8].

Over 48% of patients attending an epilepsy clinic of a teaching hospital in North India discontinued treatment in a period of one year and 89% of them had recurrent relapse of seizures. The cost of medicines constituted 40% of the individual's income for those who discontinued the treatment, where as it constituted only 18% of the income for those who continued treatment. There was a significant association between the cost of medicines and risk of discontinuing treatment [9]. Frequent seizures and treatment with multiple drugs are known to impair quality of life for persons with epilepsy.

There are several possible reasons for the high treatment gap for epilepsy. They include: errors in diagnoses, lack of consistent supply of medication, many widely-held counter-productive beliefs, no or low priority within a nation's health system, limited knowledge of epilepsy in the population, attribution issues of brain disorders. The reasons for the treatment gap are likely to vary from place to place and community to community. It is important to identify and tackle the precise reasons that prevail in a community in order to reduce the treatment gap. It has recently been demonstrated that the cost of AEDs adversely influences the utilization of treatment in several countries and availability of low cost AEDs could reduce the treatment gap considerably [10].

Economic Burden

The economic burden of a disease can be evaluated from three perspectives. From a patient's perspective the out of pocket expenditure and the loss of earnings are important. From the healthcare provider's viewpoint the cost involved in the care of the patient, the demand on the health care resources including medical expertise, hospital bed, operation theatres and laboratory resources are taken in to consideration. From a community viewpoint the economic burden refers to the loss of productivity and expenses in caring for a person with epilepsy. There are several caveats when the cost of a disorder is estimated. For chronic diseases like epilepsy, the initial cost of evaluation of the disorder may be high, where as the cost involved in subsequent years, may be less when maintenance treatment is less expensive. Strictly speaking a single seizure is not considered as epilepsy and hence all the expenses involved in the evaluation of the first seizure may not be included under the cost of epilepsy. In order to make comparisons between countries, economies, different diseases and different time periods, Disability Adjusted life years (DALY) which is a unit free yardstick is generally preferred.

In 2001, the economic burden of epilepsy was over USD 1.7 billion in India[11]. Close to 73% of this was contributed by indirect cost due to loss of productivity from recurrent seizures. Direct cost accounted for 27% of the cost out of which the main component was cost of medicines. The annualized cost of laboratory services and investigations for epilepsy accounted for only 7% of the direct cost and 2% of the entire cost of epilepsy per person. The scenario prevailing in India was characterized by very high treatment gap (70%), very limited investigations and diagnostic evaluation, outright prescription of antiepileptic drugs and inadequate control of epilepsy in most patients resulting in low direct costs and relatively high indirect cost (73%). In contrast, the indirect cost in some of countries with advanced equitable health care delivery systems was as low as 33% (Switzerland) [16] and 55% (Australia)[14,15]. (see table 1)

Table 1. Annual cost (USD) per person with epilepsy in selected countries

Country/yr	Direct cost	Indirect cost	Total cost
India [11] (2001)	93	251	344
Columbia [12] (1999)	215	364	579
Indonesia [13] (1993)	292	195	487
Australia [14,15] (1992)	2,751	3,381	6,132
Switzerland [16] (1990)	9,400	5,130	15,530
UK. [17] (1990)	2,600	5,989	8,589
USA. [18] (1994)	2,971	9,418	12,389

In India and other developing countries only a small proportion of patients were undergoing investigations and appropriate treatment. Recurrent seizures reduce economic productivity of the affected persons and their families and increase the economic burden by several folds. Several studies have shown that improved control of seizures (in spite of higher direct cost) leads to lower economic burden [19]. It is possible to reduce the overall economic burden of epilepsy by better control of seizures through more effective treatment. A multicentric population based study demonstrated that by extending AED treatment coverage to 50% of primary epilepsy cases it would be possible to avert 150 - 650 DALYs per one million population. This would be equivalent to a reduction of current burden of epilepsy by 13-40% at an annual per capita cost of international dollars 0.20-1.33. Older first-line AEDs (Phenobarbitone and Phenoytoin) were most cost-effective on account of their similar efficacy but lower acquisition cost (IUS dollars 800-2,000 for each DALY averted) [20]. The economic burden of epilepsy in developing countries can be reduced significantly by scaling-up the routine availability of low-cost AEDs. Critical factors in the successful implementation of such a scaled-up level of service delivery are renewed political support and investment. appropriate training of health personnel and continuity of drug supply.

Psychosocial Burden

Most people with epilepsy have psychosocial problems. A host of psychological comorbidities have been described for people with epilepsy. There may be associated cognitive and social problems. These psychosocial problems are attributed to the impact of recurrent seizures, adverse effects of antiepileptic drugs and adverse social reactions to the disorder. Altered neurodevelopment of the brain, cognition, and behaviour; exacerbation of the comorbidities due to decades of medically intractable epilepsy; and possible acceleration of common age-associated changes also contribute to the psychosocial burden [21]. They may experience social isolation and difficulty in getting jobs. Anxiety, depression, and reduced self-esteem are observed in people with epilepsy [22].

Quality of Life

Quality of life is an important aspect of the outcome of care for epilepsy. It is only recently that researchers have started evaluating quality of life (QOL) as an outcome measure of treatment of epilepsy. The Commission on Outcome Measurement in Epilepsy identified five dimensions viz. (a) genetic and inherited characteristics; (b) biochemical,physiologic, and anatomic condition, including impairment of these systems, disease, signs, and symptoms; (c)functional status, which includes performance of the usual activities of life, such as self-care, physical activities, and work; (d) mental condition, which includes positive and negative feelings; and (e) health potential, including longevity and prognosis that influence the health status [23].

Quality of life encompasses subjects' assessments of all aspects of their experience. The long term assessment of quality of life should also include evaluation of how far the patients' aspirations and goals in life are achieved and to what extent they feel that the purpose of their life is fulfilled.

Since the attributes of quality of life are idiosyncratic, it is very difficult to develop suitable instruments to measure it. Further, the aspirations and expectations of persons with epilepsy may change over a period of time. Those persons who experience frequent seizures may regard control of seizures as their priority, but when the seizures are controlled, may develop new goals related to their social needs such as AED withdrawal or employment or marriage. There have been very few studies on the quality of life for persons with epilepsy in India.

We studied the quality of life of persons with epilepsy (n = 112) living in the Kerala State, India using an adaptation of the Quality of Life in Epilepsy (QOLIE) 31 instrument into the local Keralan language of Malayalam to measure quality of life on several subheadings. This provides a total score for the subject based on their experience in the past four weeks. [24]

We observed that their total QOL ranged from 22.6 to 94.4 (mean 68.0 ± 15.8). The score on different subscales (mean ± SD) were as follows: seizure worry (5.5±2.2), emotional well-being (8.9±2.8), energy/fatigue (7.7±2.2), cognition (18.1±6.3), medication effects (1.8±0.9), social function (16.4±4.3). The QOLIE score for those on polytherapy or having frequent seizures was significantly lower than that of those who were on monotherapy or having fewer seizures. (see table 2)

In a survey among older persons with epilepsy in Australia, it was observed that a greater perception of stigma and more frequent seizures was also strongly related to poor quality of life and reduced psychosocial function. Although more than two thirds of the sample had less than one seizure per year, it was apparent that even infrequent seizures had the facility to impair Health Related Quality of Life (HRQOL), suggesting that in older adults, the apprehension induced by even the possibility of a seizure may be sufficient to reduce HRQOL [25]. These studies indicate that QOL of people with epilepsy is influenced by several disease related characteristics such as seizure frequency, type of seizures, the number and dose of antiepileptic drugs used as well as a wide variety of psychosocial factors, cultural beliefs and stigma.

Table 2. Quality of life total scores according to demographic and current clinical characteristics

Variable	Characteristic	N	Total QOL score Mean (SD)	(P)*
Occupation	Student	20	74.3(11.2)	0.193
	Employed	48	67.9(14.2)	
	Unemployed	41	67.2(17.6)	
Epilepsy type	LRE	47	65.4(18.1)	0.035
	GE	65	71.4(11.3)	
Duration of	<10	46	70.3(14.2)	0.328
epilepsy (yrs)	10-19	38	67.3(17.6)	
	20-29	20	67.5(16.0)	
	>30	8	60.7(16.5)	
Seizure freq	< 5	64	71.5(14.1)	0.001
Engle Score	5-6	40	66.8(14.1)	
	> 6	08	50.6(21.8)	
Drug therapy	Monotherapy	83	70.7(14.9)	0.002
	Polytherapy	29	60.2(16.0)	
Anti-epileptic drugs	CBZ	48	68.2(20.0)	0.29
	PB	13	66.3(13.3)	0.45
	PHT	20	69.9(14.2)	0.84
	VPA	40	73.5(10.8)	0.13
Adverse drug reactions	No ADR	93	67.8(16.3)	0.89
	ADR present	19	67.3(13.9)	

*Statistical significance on the basis of Analysis of Variance (ANOVA).

ADR = Adverse Drug Reaction; CBZ = Carbamazepine; GE = Generalized Epilepsy, LRE = Localization-Related Epilepsy; PB = Phenobarbitone PHT = Phenytoin; QOL= Quality Of Life SD = Standard Deviation; VPA = Valproic acid.

Special Issues

Epilepsy in children brings about considerable emotional, economic and psychosocial burden on the parents in India. We observed that more than 80% of parents experienced a decline in their social activities, after the onset of epilepsy in their children. It was also observed that daily routines were significantly affected in over 75% of the parents. Parents experienced frustration (52%), hopelessness (76%) and financial difficulties (60%). The most important items of expenditure were cost of drugs or cost of travel to hospital for 54% and 36% parents respectively. The impaired emotional status and poor social adaptation were co-related with the severity of epilepsy (frequent seizures/generalized seizures/attention disorder) and low economic status of the parents [26]. In a survey in the Eastern states of India, it was observed that caregivers of students with epilepsy experienced a burden involving diverse areas of functioning particularly in the lower income groups and nuclear families [27].

The burden of epilepsy has a gender bias that leaves women more affected than men. Women in most societies are considered to be vulnerable to the adverse effects of social, economic and environmental stress. The impact of such adversities is greater in economically backward societies. The psychosocial consequences and stigma of epilepsy affects women more than men. Studies from Zambia [28] and Brazil [29] show that women with epilepsy experience more social stigma compared to men. In Zambia, their social burden far outweighed the medical burden. They revealed seizure worries, injuries, limitations in role fulfillment and social rejection [28] Persons with epilepsy found it difficult to find a marital match if they revealed their epilepsy in India [30].

Fewer women receive treatment for epilepsy when compared to men. The gender specific treatment gap is probably more in developing countries such as India than in developed countries. In a recent study we observed that fewer women attend tertiary epilepsy care centers than men. In contrast to this more women with epilepsy were seeking care from primary health centers. The gender specific treatment gap for tertiary epilepsy care was more when the subjects were living in villages and remote locations and when their family income was low [31]. Women with epilepsy have more difficulty finding marriage partners.

Antiepileptic drugs may interfere with oral contraception, A minority of women with epilepsy may have impaired sexuality [32]. Epilepsy per se may influence the sexual functions. For example the amygdala which is a mesial temporal structure which has an important function in mediating sexuality is frequently affected in temporal lobe epilepsy. Some of the antiepileptic drugs such as sodium valproate may lead to polycystic ovarian syndrome associated with obesity, hyperandrogenism and infertility. Psychosocial stressors, anxiety and stigma associated with epilepsy, can also affect the sexual life of persons with epilepsy. Pregnancy is viewed with great concern by women with epilepsy as well as their relatives. Many families believe that women with epilepsy cannot conceive or have safe pregnancies.

In fact, most women with epilepsy have normal pregnancies and deliveries. Complications of pregnancy or the necessity for Cesarean sections are not increased in women with epilepsy [33]. Prenatal exposure to antiepileptic drugs can induce malformations in a small minority of infants and possibly lead to neurocognitive impairment [34,35]. Several antiepileptic drugs like phenytoin and carbamazepine are inducers of hepatic enzymes, that increase the clearance of vitamin D and lead to osteopenia and osteoporosis. This may result in impaired bone health and higher risk of fractures in elderly women.

One of the major concerns of women with epilepsy is the risk of fetal malformations. It is observed in population-based studies and pregnancy registry-based studies that epilepsy per se does not increase the risk of fetal malformations but rather the exposure to the drugs [35,36]. Recent data indicate that the risk of major congenital malformations in the offspring of women with epilepsy is 2 to 3 times that of offspring of healthy women not exposed to antiepileptic drugs. Nevertheless, more than 90% of the infants are born healthy. The risk of malformation is higher when the mother is using polytherapy.

There are some early signals that one of the antiepileptic drugs -valproate, particularly at higher doses, is associated with excess risk of malformations when compared to other AEDs used as monotherapy. A recent consensus statement recommends that AEDs may be used in monotherapy at low doses. It is preferable to avoid valproate in women of childbearing age group and if it cannot be avoided, it should be used in low doses [37].

Prevention of Epilepsy

Neurocysticercosis, a potentially preventable disease, accounts for a substantial proportion of the partial seizures observed in India and some of the Latin American countries. Effective treatment and prevention of neurocysticercosis should go a long way to reduce the burden of epilepsy in these countries. Efforts to reduce the treatment gap would considerably reduce the burden of epilepsy. Focused educational programs to bring epilepsy out of the shadows, and establishment of comprehensive epilepsy care programs are important steps in this direction. The burden of epilepsy in India and several developing countries can be reduced by focusing attention on prevention. Post traumatic epilepsy is another potentially preventable epilepsy.

REFERENCES

[1] Sridharan r, Murthy BN. Prevalence and pattern of epilepsy in India. *Epilepsia,* 1999; 40: 631-6.

[2] Shafig R, Tanwir M, Tariq A, Saleem A, Zafar M, Khuwaja AK. Myths and falacies about epilepsy among residents of a Karachi slum area. *Tro Doc*, 2008, 38(1); 32-3.

[3] Radhakrishnan K, Pandian JD, Santhoshkumar T, Thomas SV, Deetha TD, Sarma PS, Jayachandran D, Mohamed E. Prevalence, knowleege, attitude and practice of epilepsy in Kerala, South India. *Epilepsia*, 2000; 41; 1027-35.

[4] Hermann BP, Whitman S, Wyler AR, Anton MT, Vanderzwagg R. Psychosocial predictors of psychopathology in epilepsy. *Br. J. Psychiatry*. 1990 Jan;156:98-105.

[5] Lee SA, Yoo HJ, Lee BI; Korean QoL in Epilepsy Study Group. Factors contributing to the stigma of epilepsy. *Seizure*. 2005;14:157-63.

[6] Jacoby A, Wang W, Vu TD, Wu J, Snape D, Aydemir N, Parr J, Reis R, Begley C, de Boer H, Prilipko L, Baker G. Meanings of epilepsy in its sociocultural context and implications for stigma: findings from ethnographic studies in local communities in China and Vietnam. *Epilepsy Behav*. 2008;12:286-97.

[7] Pal SK, Sharma K, Prabhakar S, Pathak A. Psychosocial, demographic, and treatment-seeking strategic behavior, including faith healing practices, among patients with epilepsy in northwest India. *Epilepsy Behav*. 2008;13:323-32.

[8] Thomas SV, Deetha TD, Nair P, Sarma SP. Fewer women receive tertiary care for epilepsy in Kerala State, India. *Epileptic Disord*. 2006 Sep;8(3):184-9.

[9] Das K, Banerjee M, Mondal GP, Devi LG, Singh OP, Mukherjee BB. Evaluation of socio-economic factors causing discontinuation of epilepsy treatment resulting in seizure recurrence: a study in an urban epilepsy clinic in India. *Seizure*. 2007;16:601-606.

[10] Chisholm D Cost-effectiveness of first-line antiepileptic drug treatments in the developing world: a population-level analysis. *Epilepsia*. 2005;46:751-9.

[11] Thomas SV, Sarma PS, Alexander M, Pandit L, Shekhar L, Trivedi C, Vengamma B Economic burden of epilepsy in India. *Epilepsia*. 2001 Aug;42(8):1052-60.

[12] Fandino Franky J, Silfvenius H. World wide disparities in epilepsy care: a Latin American outlook. *Epilepsia* 1999;40(Suppl 8):48–54.

[13] Chandra B. *Economic aspects of epilepsy in Indonesia.* In Beran RG, Pachlatko C (ed) *Cost of epilepsy.* Baden: Ciba Geigy Verlag, 1995;75–82.

[14] Banks GK, Regan KJ, Beran RG. The prevalence and direct costs of epilepsy in Australia. In Beran RG, Pachlatko C (Eds), *Cost of epilepsy: Proceedings of the 20th International Epilepsy Congress.* Baden: Ciba-Geigy Verlag, 1995;39–48.

[15] Beran RG, Banks GK Indirect costs of epilepsy in Australia. In Beran RG, Pachlatko C (Eds), *Cost of Epilepsy: Proceedings of the 20th International Epilepsy Congress.* Baden: Ciba-Geigy Verlag, 1995;49–54.

[16] Gessner U, Sagmeister M, Horisberger B. The cost of epilepsy in Switzerland. *Int J Health Sci* 1993;4:121–128.

[17] Cockerell OC, Hart YM, Sanders JWS, Shorvon SD. The cost of epilepsy in the United Kingdom: an estimation based on the results of two population based studies. *Epilepsy Res* 1994;18:249–60.

[18] Cockerell OC, Hart YM, Sanders JWS, Shorvon SD. The cost of epilepsy in the United Kingdom: an estimation based on the results of two population based studies. *Epilepsy Res* 1994;18:249–60.

[19] Tetto A, Manzoni P, Millul A, Beghi E, Garattini L, Tartara A, Avanzini G; Osservatorio Regionale per l'Epilessia (OREp). The costs of epilepsy in Italy: a prospective cost-of-illness study in referral patients with disease of different severity. *Epilepsy Res.* 2002 Feb;48(3):207-16.

[20] Chisholm D; WHO-CHOICE. Cost-effectiveness of first-line antiepileptic drug treatments in the developing world: a population-level analysis. *Epilepsia.* 2005 May;46(5):751-9.

[21] Hermann B, Seidenberg M, Jones J. The neurobehavioural comorbidities of epilepsy: can a natural history be developed? *Lancet Neurol.* 2008;7:151-60.

[22] de Boer HM, Mula M, Sander JW. The global burden and stigma of epilepsy. *Epilepsy Behav.* 2008;12:540-6.

[23] G. A. Baker, C. Camfield, P. Camfield, TJ. A. Cramer, $C. E. Elger, §A. L. Johnson,A. Martins da Silva, YH. Meinardi, C. Munari, TTE. Perucca, and $$R. Thorbecke Commission on Outcome Measurement in Epilepsy, 1994-1 997:Final Report , *Epilepsia* 1998;39:213-231.

[24] Thomas SV, Koshy S, Nair CR, Sarma SP. Frequent seizures and polytherapy can impair quality of life in persons with epilepsy. *Neurol India.* 2005 Mar;53(1):46-50.

[25] McLaughlin DP, Pachana NA, Mcfarland K. Stigma, seizure frequency and quality of life: the impact of epilepsy in late adulthood. *Seizure.* 2008 Apr;17(3):281-7. Epub 2007 Oct 23.

[26] Thomas SV, Bindu VB. Psychosocial and economic problems of parents of children with epilepsy. *Seizure.* 1999;8:66-9.

[27] BK Ray, M Ghoshal, A Senapati, PK Gangopadhyay, T Roy Assessment of burden of care amongst caregivers of students with epilepsy: A study from Eastern India *Neurology Asia* 2004;9 Suppl 1: 140.

[28] Birbeck G, Chomba E, Atadzhanov M, Mbewe E, Haworth A.The social and economic impact of epilepsy in Zambia: a cross-sectional study. *Lancet Neurol.* 2007 Jan;6(1):39-44.

[29] Fernandes PT, Salgado PC, Noronha AL, de Boer HM, Prilipko L, Sander JW, Li LM. Epilepsy stigma perception in an urban area of a limited-resource country. *Epilepsy Behav.* 2007;11:25-32.

[30] Pal SK, Sharma K, Prabhakar S, Pathak A. Psychosocial, demographic, and treatment-seeking strategic behavior, including faith healing practices, among patients with epilepsy in northwest India. *Epilepsy Behav.* 2008;13:323-32.

[31] Sanjeev V Thomas, TD Deetha, Prabhachandran Nair, Sankara P Sarma. Fewer women receive tertiary care for epilepsy in Kerala State, India. *Epileptic Disorders* 2006;8:184-9.

[32] Harden CL. Sexuality in men and women with epilepsy. *CNS Spectr.* 2006;11(8 Suppl 9):13-8.

[33] Thomas SV, Sindhu K, Ajaykumar B, Devi PB, Sujamol J.Maternal and obstetric outcome of women with epilepsy.*Seizure.* 2008 Sep 19.

[34] Thomas SV, Ajaykumar B, Sindhu K, Nair MK, George B, Sarma PS. Motor and mental development of infants exposed to antiepileptic drugs in utero. *Epilepsy Behav.* 2008 Jul;13(1):229-36.

[35] Thomas SV, Sukumaran S, Lukose N, George A, Sarma PS. Intellectual and language functions in children of mothers with epilepsy. *Epilepsia.* 2007;48:2234-40.

[36] Thomas SV, Nair RR, Jose M, Sarma PS. Risk of major congenital malformations in the offsprings of women with epilepsy is not related to family history. *Epilepsy Res.* 2008 Oct 30.

[37] Meador KJ, Pennell PB, Harden CL, Gordon JC, Tomson T, Kaplan PW, Holmes GL, French JA, Hauser WA, Wells PG, Cramer JA; HOPE Work Group. Pregnancy registries in epilepsy: a consensus statement on health outcomes. *Neurology.* 2008;71:1109-17

In: Social Epileptology
Editors: J. Pinikahana and C. Walker
ISBN 978-1-60876-228-6

Chapter 13

EPILEPSY AND MEDIA

Toba Schwaber Kerson*
Mary Hale Chase Professor in the Social Sciences
and Social Work and Social Research
Bryn Mawr College
Graduate School of Social Work and Social Research,
Bryn Mawr, Pennsylvania, USA

ABSTRACT

Media are various channels of communication that include print vehicles, publications such as newspapers and magazines, as well as vehicles related to visualizing and hearing such as radio, television and film. The newest forms of media, digital, computerized or networked information and communication technologies, have transformed all of the earlier forms. With the ascendancy of the internet, and the transformation from analog to digital modes of communication, the reach of these forms of media, and thus the ability of any outside force to control content, has become limitless. The term, itself, has been borrowed from advertising where it was first used to define different outlets for particular messages that were to be communicated to specified audiences. This is very close to Aristotle's definition of rhetoric, that is the use of the most persuasive argument for a given audience. This notion of using vehicles as particular forms of targeting defined audiences with specific messages is an important concept to carry when thinking about epilepsy and media. The themes here are not so different from depictions of other illnesses and disabilities in all forms of media including literature and art. The epilepsy community would like to exert more control over the ways in which epilepsy is depicted and perceived. In fact, it would like to show the world that most people with epilepsy lead independent and full lives with very good symptom control, and would like audiences to depictions in a responsibly informed manner. However, despite work in many directions on the part of the epilepsy community, inaccurate, negative and highly stigmatizing portrayals are still often the case. This is especially interesting when one compares these depictions with those of other illnesses such as cancer or health related behaviors such as smoking. In these areas, depictions

* Corespondence: Prof. Toba Schwaber Kerson, Bryn Mawr College, Graduate School of Social Work and Social Research, 300 Airdale Road, Bryn Mawr, Pennsylvania 19010. tkerson@brynmawr.edu

have become more realistic or have almost disappeared from mainstream presentations. In this regard, this chapter reviewed the literature in relation to depictions of epilepsy in publications, particularly newspapers, and in visual and auditory media such as music, television and film. Following that, the chapter focussed on depictions of epilepsy in film and on television, and, within that, will focus on my own research. My data set now includes more than 300 examples in 14 languages over a period of more than 100 years. Conclusions drawn from all of this work point out that epilepsy continues to be portrayed as associated with victimization, rear, secrecy, possession and violence. Often, the image of a tonic-clonic seizure is included with conditions that would not, in reality, lead to these symptoms. Seizures are depicted, most often on television, in ways that will titillate, captivate and draw the audience to watch a particular show. Overall, in fact, and despite enormous educated, sophisticated and thoughtful attempts on the part of the epilepsy community to change such depictions, little has been altered. It seems that in 2008, the image of tonic-clonic seizure remains a cliché for both titillating and terrifying an audience.

INTRODUCTION

Media are various channels of communication that include print vehicles, publications such as newspapers and magazines, as well as vehicles related to visualizing and hearing such as radio, television and film. The newest forms of media, digital, computerized or networked information and communication technologies, have transformed all of the earlier forms. With the ascendancy of the internet, and the transformation from analog to digital modes of communication, the reach of these forms of media, and thus the ability of any outside force to control content, has become limitless.

The term "media" has been borrowed from advertising where it was first used to define different outlets for particular messages that were to be communicated to specified audiences. This is very close to Aristotle's definition of rhetoric; that is the use of the most persuasive argument for a given audience. So the creation of media language is part of a communication process used to influence audience reception. In mass communication, which is one way in which to categorize the forms of media that are discussed in this chapter, this is an institutionalized process that involves production, dissemination, reception and then interpretation on a large scale. This seems always to involve multiple roles on the part of the producers that are at least public and social, and are often political and commercial as well. In each of these forms of communication, popular music, newspapers, advertising, film and television, audiences are viewed as consumers who must be entertained as well as informed.

In order to develop a holistic approach to what are referred to as media products, it is necessary first to approach them theoretically, to see mass communication as a signifying process in which there is not a fixed structure of meaning but a volatile phenomenon resulting from codes of both the producers and recipients of the message. "In fact, some instances when analyses of news discourse accuse the news reports of 'distorting' may be explained by a difference between the codes of the analyst and the codes underlying the construction of the news text." [1]

This notion of using vehicles as particular forms of targeting defined audiences with specific messages is an important concept to carry when thinking about epilepsy and media. Here, in the case of the epilepsy community, that is, those who have epilepsy, their families and friends, those representing professions and disciplines who work in epileptology and the many interest and advocacy groups that are involved, there are two prime foci or intentions – to help those with epilepsy live as symptom free as possible and to eradicate the stigma attached to the condition.

The themes here are not so different from depictions of other illnesses and disabilities in all forms of media including literature and art.[2, 3, 4] The epilepsy community would like to exert more control over the ways in which epilepsy is depicted and perceived. In fact, it would like to show the world that most people with epilepsy lead independent and full lives with very good symptom control, and would like audiences to view depictions in a responsibly informed manner. However, despite work in many directions on the part of the epilepsy community, inaccurate, negative and highly stigmatizing portrayals are still often the case. This is especially interesting when one compares these depictions with those of other illnesses such as cancer or health related behaviors such as smoking. In these areas, depictions have become more realistic and thus more positive or have almost disappeared from mainstream presentations.

In this regard, this chapter will review the literature in relation to depictions of epilepsy in newspapers, advertising and in visual and auditory media such as music, television and film. Although there is a literature on epilepsy in art and literature which certainly concerns the question of symbolic communication, those areas will not be addressed here. Rather discussion will focus on mass media through which institutionalized processes of communication including the production, dissemination, reception, and interpretation attempt to influence public sociocultural and political discourse. All forms of the mass media compete for readers, listeners, and viewers; all endeavor to capture the largest possible audience.

As one thinks about epilepsy and media it is important to remember that few people, especially few people who have not reached middle age, will even witness an actual seizure. [5, 6] In 2003, the United States Centers for Disease Control included 9 epilepsy-related items on the Porter Novelli HealthStyles survey, a mail survey that is administered to a random sample of adults. Results showed that half of those surveyed have witnessed a seizure in a real-life setting with those between 45-64 years of age more likely than those 44 years or younger. More than half of those surveyed have seen a seizure on television with those between ages 18-34 most likely. That youngest group also lacks familiarity with epilepsy. Also, most adults had not read or heard about epilepsy in the past year. For those who did read or hear about epilepsy, the most usual source was television. Even among those who currently know someone with epilepsy, less than 40% are knowledgeable about the disorder and only half agree with knowing what to do if they are around a person who has a seizure. Kobau and Price note that "exaggerated media representations can adversely influence cognitive responses, which in turn can adversely affect social attitudes [7]

One inquiry examining associations between stigma and self-management and perceptions of health care among adults with epilepsy, found that most respondents described an epileptic seizure in the stereotypical terms of a tonic-clonic seizure.[8] Unless people have direct personal involvement with someone with epilepsy, it is likely that that the tonic-clonic seizure as seen in film or on television will be the synecdoche, the part that will represent the whole of the condition of epilepsy to them. The younger that they are, the more likely this is to be true. That is true as well for depictions in all forms of mass media from popular music to newspaper and magazine articles to film and television.

THE MEANING OF STIGMA

Much of the work in the area of epilepsy and stigma commences with the definition of stigma drawn from Erving Goffman's, *Stigma: Notes on the Management of Spoiled Identity [9]* The book begins by saying that the Greeks devised the term stigma in reference to bodily signs that denoted something bad and unusual about the moral status of the referent. One was cut or burnt with signs that let the community know that the bearer was a traitor, a slave or a criminal – someone to be avoided. "Later, in Christian times, two layers of metaphor were added to the term: the first referred to bodily signs that took the form of eruptive blossoms on the skin; the second, a medical allusion to this religious allusion, referred to bodily signs of physical disorder" [10].

Goffman says further that stigma refers to an attribute that is deeply discrediting but that in order to understand it, one needs a language of relationships, not attributes. This notion is supported by Schambler (in Jacoby, et al) who says that people with epilepsy are perceived by others as creating ambiguity in their interactions, thus jeopardizing the social order by being out of control and unpredictable [11].

No matter how one defines or attempts to classify stigma, one finds the same sociological feature, an undesired differentness. That is, even if one would have been welcome in ordinary social interaction, this characteristic supersedes other attributes and interferes with interaction, discrediting the person and spoiling identity. Thus, stigmatized people may feel unsure about how they will be received. Differentness derives from society; that is, a difference doesn't matter unless it is conceptualized in that way by society.

Goffman says that this is even clearer in the case of epilepsy. "Since Hippocrates' time, those who discover they have this disorder have been assured a firmly stigmatized self by the definitional workings of society. This work still goes on even though insignificant physical impairment may be involved, and even though many medical specialists now use the term to refer to a seizure disorder only when no specific (and less stigmatizing) medical disorder can be found [12].

He also makes the point that when people with specific stigma achieve high financial, occupational or political positions, they are beseeched to represent whatever category is related to that stigma. This particular issue has been vexing for the epilepsy community because they have had difficult times finding willing spokespersons with whose representation they would feel comfortable. If one's condition is well-controlled and, therefore, can be hidden, why would one publically claim a highly stigmatized position in society?

STIGMA IN RELATION TO HEALTH CONDITIONS

"Stigma related to chronic health conditions such as HIV/AIDS, leprosy, tuberculosis, mental illness and epilepsy is a global phenomenon with a severe impact on individuals and their families, and on the effectiveness of public health programmes."[13] There are studies in regard to many specific conditions including epilepsy. One more global study, published by the British Council of Organisations of Disabled People. examined disabling imagery and the media as a way to explore the principles for medial representations of disabled people [14].

An important task of this organization and the disability rights movement is to eliminate disablist language from books, schools and the media, in general. The project, itself, was motivated by the increasing concerns of disabled people that their problems were due to institutional discrimination. Studies confirm such prejudices. For example, a study in the United States which included books, radio, the press, films and television in its media category, described four underlying dimensions that characterize current attitudes about epilepsy. [15] These dimensions relate to beliefs, risk and safety concerns, expectations about work and social role capacity, and affective responses. Some examples include individuals' thinking that people with epilepsy are unreliable or should not marry, that there were risks involved in their engaging in certain activities, that they might not be successful workers and that people might be nervous around or being alone with someone with epilepsy.

Distorted representations of the experience of disability in the media were important factors in the discriminatory process. "While the media alone cannot be held responsible for this situation its impact should not be underestimated" [16]

The study's conclusions were drawn from a detailed content analysis of previous research in the field as well as contributions from several sources including media and disability organizations and advertisers. Common medial stereotypes were the disabled person as: pitiable and pathetic, an object of violence, sinister and evil, atmosphere or curio, super cripple, an object of ridicule, their own worst and only enemy, sexually abnormal, incapable of participating fully in community life, and as normal. The author even had concerns about the latter category, usually seen in advertising in the United States (for example, including a person in a wheelchair as one of a group of people in a magazine ad), because while these might be seen as a step in the right direction, they are simply a normalization of disability, and therefore they do not address the meaning of such images to disabled people. The work ends by telling the reader to which government offices in the United Kingdom such negative stereotypes can be reported.

In a recent review article, [17] Anne Jacoby writes about studies of diverse groups of individuals from Great Britain, Brazil, Canada, Pakistan, Turkey and Laos. Most studies have revealed that the public attitude toward epilepsy and the lived experience of individuals with epilepsy heighten stigma and discrimination. A recent article on fallacies about epilepsy in Karachi reports that negative attitudes are ubiquitous. [18]

Regarding a convenience sample drawn from a Karachi slum, the authors found that the great majority thought that epilepsy was caused by evil spirits and black magic. There were findings in other studies that also reported great misunderstanding of the condition from Hong Kong, China, Vietnam and Zambia [19, 20, 21, 22] And in a report on social consequences and economic aspects of epilepsy, the World Health Organization related the following examples of misunderstandings about epilepsy in various countries.

For instance, in Cameroon it is believed that the devil invades people with epilepsy causing them to convulse; in Indonesia, it can be considered a punishment from dark and unknown forces; in Uganda and other countries, epilepsy is thought to be contagious and passed through saliva; in Swaziland, some traditional healers say that sorcery causes epilepsy.[23] Thus, stigma regarding epilepsy is hardly confined to the English speaking world.

Epilepsy in Particular Forms of Mass Media

The remainder of this article is devoted to exploring the ways in which epilepsy is described and depicted in the following forms of mass media, newspapers and advertising, popular music, film and television. Because one could argue that epilepsy in the news should be the closest to reality of any form of mass media, I begin with that. However, one must keep in mind the following: "People everywhere confuse what they read in the newspaper with news," [24] and "Once a newspaper touches a story, the facts are lost forever, even to the protagonists." [25]

Epilepsy in Newspapers

Unlike fictive representations in which one assumes that interpretations will be drawn in ways that enhance plot or character, the news is meant to witness and then to report accurately what has been witnessed. After physicians and other medical personnel seen in a clinic situation, print news media are the second most important source for the public's medical information [26], the accuracy of reporting is especially important. I found just three studies that addressed epilepsy in newspapers. In the only article that addressed epilepsy exclusively, "The Scarlet "E" The presentation of epilepsy in the English language print media," Gregory Krauss and his colleagues reviewed over 2000 English language newspapers and popular magazines searching for stories about epilepsy. [27] Using NEXIS "Allnews", they searched for all stories containing the words "epilepsy", "seizure" or "epileptic" within the headline or lead of the story. In the end, they found 210 general-interest stories with epilepsy or seizures as important themes.

Their primary goal was to look for scientific inaccuracies, that is, major scientific inaccuracies, greatly exaggerated stories about advances or treatments, stigmatization or great exaggeration about the risks of having epilepsy and/or highly inaccurate or superficial stories that left out critical data. Themes found most often were personal stories about overcoming epilepsy, new drug therapies and other interventions related to diet and surgery, and scientific advances. "Other topics, in order of frequency, were famous people with seizures, clinical reviews, misdiagnosis, new epilepsy centers, unusual types of seizures (including those linked to video games), sudden death, job discrimination, violent behavior, automobile accidents, alternative medicine, and pseudoseizures." [28] Thirty-one percent of the stories had significant inaccuracies, 14% with scientific errors, 9% with greatly overstated benefits from treatment, 5% with bias towards people with epilepsy or overstated risks of seizures. Certain stories, particularly those regarding new drug and non-drug therapies and those focusing on people dealing with epilepsy, carried a disproportionate part of these errors.

Despite information supporting an epilepsy diagnosis, most celebrities and sports superstars who had recurring seizures denied having the condition. For example, the authors discuss a National Hockey League player who had been having seizures for four years whose response to questions about his condition said "it's not epilepsy . . .there is no medical term for the ailment. [29] Also, the seizure of an athlete participating at an Olympics was called a "brief bout with sleep deprivation" [30]. Finally, terminology in these stories not only used the words "epileptic" (45%) and "fits" (10%) but to a lesser extent (6%) used supernatural or otherworldly terms such as raging demons. The overarching conclusion is that these stories contribute to damaging stereotypes held about and sometimes by people with epilepsy.

One specific conclusion that the authors drew is especially important for thinking about epilepsy and the media. They say that the media and their sources are motivated to keep alive the public's deep fears elicited by seizures. That is to say, historic misconceptions about epilepsy dovetail neatly with the goals of reporters on the one hand, and those promoting new treatments or research on the other. Both seek to heighten the drama. The reporters hope that their stories will be placed prominently in the paper, and researchers and pharmaceutical firms devote themselves to promoting new advances. What better way to achieve this sensationalism than by invoking malevolent, supernatural causes, grim prognoses, and heavenly, magical cures? Moreover, it could be argued that this otherworldly imagery conveys the experience of epilepsy in a way that is emotionally valid. [31]

Another article evaluating stigmatizing language and medical errors in neurology coverage by US newspapers used Lexis-Nexis to locate 1203 stories that focused on 11 common neurologic conditions including Alzheimer disease and other dementias, head trauma, migraine, epilepsy, stroke, Parkinson disease, brain tumor, Multiple Sclerosis, ALS and Creutzfeldt-Jacob disease.[32] In the article, stigmatizing language was defined as wording that portrays conditions as socially undesirable, less desirable, or reduced in personal work. Using Goffman's definition, the authors contended that accurate portrayals can still confer stigma or a person or group. They found that stories on epilepsy (30%) and migraine (29%) contained the highest amount of stigmatizing language. As an example, they include one quote from a reporter; "For more than a century, the Jukes clan has been presented as America's most despised family. Social science researchers have long believed they were a case study of dysfunction, a bunch of genetically linked paupers, criminals, harlots, epileptics and mental defectives, whose care had placed a huge financial burden on taxpayers", and another from a family member or other interested person, "A lot of epileptics are not going to tell you they have it because they're embarrassed or because the incidence of discrimination is huge. . . .She says Rxxxx has told her that students have been seen in the back of a classroom, imitating the dramatic motions her body made when she had the seizure 18 months ago." [33] In addition, they say, " . . . illnesses that heavily affect the lives of patients and their families and in which there are conflicts of treatment options are judged as having high news value, independent of the medical or scientific value physicians might assign the information." [34] If there is a famous person involved or the subject is one about which the public is fearful, there can be a plethora of news stories even if physicians think that the content is a little public value [35]

One additional study which includes epilepsy among other sorts of disability is a bi-national comparison of types and causes of disability as reported in major newspapers.[36] Here, a content analysis of over 400 newspaper articles in Canada and Israel was collected within a three month period. Three newspapers were selected from each country, one daily "prestige," one popular daily, and one weekend paper. The purpose was to relate the type, focus and extent of articles in both countries to the type and cause of the disability that was being addressed. Findings show that, in both countries, physical disabilities gained the most attention and positive treatment, followed by psychiatric disabilities and developmental disabilities. Although the authors mention few specific conditions, they reference studies that found that employers were "least willing to hire persons with 'invisible' disabilities such as: epilepsy, sensory disorders and psychiatric or developmental disabilities (saying that) these occasions seem to be based, at least in part, on the perceived unpredictability of their behavior, fear of the unusual or likelihood to cause problems." [37] While there were some differences between the countries' reporting, overall, newspaper coverage in both countries reinforced negative attitudes especially towards those with developmental and psychiatric disabilities. The authors report that "the mass media is a key element in this process, on the one hand reflecting prevailing norms and values and on the other hand providing information which, in turn, generated and affects public values" [38]

A recent *Los Angeles Times* on line article reviewed 24 articles that had appeared in the last 10 years in relation to epilepsy. [39]. Several were "health" articles written by physicians to provide information about the condition. In addition, one had as its focus an "epilepsy" defense in a murder, another, a car crash in which an adult son with epilepsy claimed having not remembered that his mother was in the car when he left the scene of an accident because he was having a seizure at the time (his mother was dead in the car when a rescue team found her), another referred to a case of gelastic epilepsy in which a little girl's seizures, which caused her face to grimace like "Joker," Batman's arch enemy and to have an eerie laugh, were stopped as a result of surgery, others had to do with an epilepsy drug that could block cravings for addictive drugs, and others with the news that Florence Griffith Joyner's death was related to epilepsy and not drug abuse.

At this point, it is interesting to consider the coverage of John G. Roberts, Chief Justice of the United States Supreme Court who had a seizure on July 30, 2007 at his summer home on Hupper Island in Port Clyde, Maine. He had had a similar event 14 years before while golfing. "There (was) no record of any discussion of the 1993 seizure or of Roberts's health in general during his confirmation hearings. Sen. Arlen Specter (R-Pa.) who chaired the hearings, told CNN on Monday night that senators were told about the previous episode but did not find it serious enough to ask Roberts about. Roberts has no history of serious illness." [40] Two days later, a newspaper account said that since it was Roberts' second known seizure, with the first occurring 14 years before, there was some discussion about whether he met the criteria for epilepsy and whether he should be taking medication to prevent further seizures [41]. Several prominent neurologists weighed in indicating what each thought to be indicated. On the same day, an account in the *International Herald Tribune* described the event as a "benign idiopathic seizure" which could be a sign of epilepsy [42]. Again, other prominent neurologists suggested various kinds of medical follow-up. Neither Justice Roberts nor his spokespeople commented, and there was no further discussion in the newspapers.

There was a burst of news coverage on television as well. CNN's Anderson Cooper interviewed a neurosurgeon and Jeffrey Tubin, CNN's senior legal analyst. Part of Tubin's response was, "This does strike me as a fairly serious thing and for the Supreme Court to come out with a statement within hours that he's fully recovered. That seems to be in my layman's knowledge a little premature. [43]. The story was covered on July 31 or August 1 in several additional newspapers including the *Hobart Mercury* in Australia and the *London Independent*, and then it was dropped. No account mentioned the word epilepsy in relation to Justice Roberts. I would argue that if this were a heart attack or another less stigmatized condition, there would have been more extensive and deeper coverage of the event.

Here and elsewhere, the epilepsy community is taking steps to address the sensationalism that continues to be associated with epilepsy. For example, the Scottish Epilepsy Foundation is sponsoring a contest with a 500 euro prize for the best news story related to epilepsy [44] just as the International League Against Epilepsy is sponsoring a contest with a $5,000 prize for the best films made since 2000 that are inspired by or relate to epilepsy or seizures [45] Thus, to conclude this section, epilepsy continues to be stigmatized in news coverage. In some cases, when individuals with some power in the community choose to do so, they seem to be able to limit the exposure of their condition in the news. Otherwise, it is the job of the news to sell the news whether it be in newspapers or in other forms of mass media.

Epilepsy in Advertising

With regard to advertising, there is little information related specifically to epilepsy. However, there are lessons to be learned from how others groups have set about changing advertising behavior in relation to a specific topic. In summary, it is a combination of massive interest group public pressure and government intervention that makes the difference. One great example is the way that interest groups and then the government has changed the rules for smoking ads on television and in film as one part of curbing smoking altogether [46] According to an article called "Smoking in movies: Impact on adolescent smoking," the most powerful examples are how campaigns such as the SmokeFreeMovies media campaign went about its work. [47,48] This campaign understood that industries would be very reluctant to change their behavior without the perception of massive public pressure. It placed blame directly on actors, theater owners and studio executives.

In the same way, there have been massive efforts to limit smoking on television. Beginning with the Fairness Doctrine of 1967 that required that TV stations broadcast one public service announcement for every three cigarette ads until the ban on all tobacco advertising in 1971, there was a great public health effort aimed at removing tobacco advertising from the air. This followed years in which the many popular shows such as *Topper*, *I Love Lucy* and *The Flintstones* had prime tobacco sponsors and featured the cigarettes on their shows. [49] While changing stigmatizing images is also a public health concern, it may be difficult to make the leap from one effort that aims to stop people from indulging in a practice that is absolutely guaranteed to hurt those individuals and those around them to one in which a particular group whose symptoms or degree of illness will not change as a result of a public health campaign but whose social conditions and possibilities will. To me, it is helpful to think of both efforts as part of a total public health effort.

I have personally seen only one highly inappropriate use of the word epileptic in advertising and that was in several metro stations in Paris in Winter, 2007. The subject of the billboard which stretched nearly the height of the metro station wall was, itself, an advertising agency called Australie. To advertise its services, the agency created a nonsensical acrostic spelling out Australie. The wall sized picture of an iguana standing on his hind legs said, Articulant Un Slogan Tonitruant, Raoul Amadoura L'Iguane Epileptique (Mouthing a thunderous slogan, Raoul pacifies an epileptic iguana). The ads caused an immediate response from combined forces of the French International League against Epilepsy (ILAE) chapter, Epilepsie-France, FFRE and other associations. One part of the effort was to report the billboard content to the branch of the French government that is meant to protect vulnerable citizens in several areas. The agency was forced to remove the ads and, after understanding the offensive nature of its ad, it offered to help with Epilepsy Awareness Day [50]

Obviously, one cannot draw conclusions from this little information. However, both the success of the antismoking efforts and the small example of the effort of the French epilepsy community and the government are useful thinking points.

Epilepsy in Popular Music

The only article on depictions of epilepsy in popular music contends that "popular music is arguably the most accessible and ubiquitous of the creative art forms, touching most of us on a daily basis." [51]

Author Sallie Baxendale lists bands whose names are related to epilepsy terminology including seizure, aura, déjà vu, epilepsy, the hippocampus groove and status. Although few of these bands have signed with a record label for any time period, one punk group, "The Falling Sickness," played together for 11 years and recorded three albums with Hopeless Records before disbanding in 1999. [52]

Baxendale reports that while epilepsy-related themes emerge out of some band names, it is the lyrics of the songs produced that contribute to our understanding of how epilepsy is understood in various cultures and subcultures. Studied here are a wide variety of genres including rap and jazz. One particularly provocative and negative example was written and performed by Cage, a New York rapper with a long history of drug and psychiatric problems. A portion of the lyrics of the song, "Ballad of Worms," [53] is below.

> What kind of God is this?
> Give me the hottest bitch
> Then took the life from her chest and left a pile of shit
> To numb to cum, sometimes she piss while I eat her
> I tell her, keep her head up
> Even though I gotta hold it up for her
> And she seizure when she try and get up
> . . .
> Before I tasted her lips, she dislocated her hips
> Started shaking
> Couldn't feed her no medication
> To scared to beat on her chest in fear It'd cave in
> Death waved again and each time leaves her
> In a coma, for a week, to wake up to more seizures
> But this time ain't like the rest
> I can see right through her chest
> And see her heart ain't got no f**kin beats left
> . . .
> Convulse, twisted falling to the ground
> Saliva flowing free, tasting, choking
> to the reaction of onlooker

Some mentions of epilepsy in lyrics are metaphors for sex, and, in particular, sexual orgasm and dance ecstasy. For instance, following is a portion of the lyrics in rap artist 50 Cent's song, "Like my Style" [54]

From the tellie in ten minutes I'll make you a believer
Tongue touch ya'll have ya shakin like you havin a seizure
I make hits about what I do in my leisure

Of the lyrics that the author describes, the ones that most directly address epilepsy are in a song recorded by Malevolent Creation called Epileptic Seizure [55]

Convulse, twisted
Falling to the ground
Saliva flowing free
Tasting, choking
Swallowed your tongue
Eyes roll back in your head
Frantic twitching
Multiple spasms
Legs begin to buckle
Face blue, can't breath
Trying to cry out
Your efforts are useless
Hacking vomit
Want to be free
Just don't want to be seen
Convulse .....
Consuming your pride
Cursed by this disease
Those around you panic
Onlookers start to freeze
Living in fear
Tearing your soul
No cure for this pain
This is your hell
Given at birth
Symptoms take course
Seizure taking over
Consuming.....
Convulse.....

In other lyrics, the author finds references to violence, madness, retardation, all consuming love, the elderly and several instances of what she calls, "one-offs" and I refer to in my research as "throw-aways," that is, gratuitous insertions of a word related to epilepsy or a gesture which seem not to enhance lyrics, plot or character. She cites one lyric relating to Christina the Astonishing, who lived from 1150-1224, and who after a near-death experience was said to have continued to experience severe convulsions among other symptoms in order to be able to descend into purgatory and relieve the suffering of those who remained sted there. [56] The song, by Nick Cave and the Bad Seeds follows the story line drawn from what is known of Christina's life. [57] The lyrics follow:

Christina the astonishing
Lived a long time ago

She was stricken with a seizure
At the age of twenty-two
They took her body in a coffin
To a tiny church in liege
Where she sprang up from the coffin
Just after the agnus dei
She soared up to the rafters
Perched on a beam up there
Cried the stink of human sin
Is more that I can bear

. .

She fled to remote places
Climbed towers and trees and walls
To escape the stench of human corruption
Into an oven she did crawl

. .

O christina the astonishing
Behaved in terrifying manner
Died at the age of seventy-four
In the convent of st anna.[58]

In addition, Baxandale discusses epilepsy in relation to sex and to dance, saying "although the depictions of epilepsy in other art forms generally reflect the pervasive cultural attitudes toward the condition, a lyrical license allows musical artists to employ the language, characteristics, and symptoms of epilepsy as powerful metaphors for other things, most notably sexual orgasm and dance ecstasy.[59] She reports that, in the case of dance music, lyrics suggest that catching epilepsy or getting into seizures is something desirable. She concludes by saying that "Although epilepsy has often been associated with sexual vulnerability or availability in female sufferers in other art forms, the appropriation of the language of epilepsy to represent sexual orgasm and dance trance represents a contemporary departure in the artistic representation of epilepsy-related images and associations in the 21st century."[60]

This section draws information from one article and its data and, thus, is self-explanatory. To me, it is reminiscent of the turn of the last century in France when cabaret and music hall entertainers placing themselves in such categories as "the epileptic singer" made use of the gestures related to hysteria and epilepsy that were being studied, staged and filmed by French physicians such as Charcot.[61] These gestures were being used also by the nascent French film industry in productions such as *Le Cabaret Epileptique* [62] A different view of the same placing of entertainment value on these particular gestures is found in Borgstrom's discussion of some of Charcot's work in his article, "Strike a pose: Charcot's women and the performance of hysteria at La Salpetriere." [63] There, Borgstrom argues that Charcot, Chair of Clinical Diseases at Groupe Hospitalier de La Pitié-Salpétrière and considered to be the father of modern neurology linked sexual indecency and mental unreason, hysteria and female sexual chaos in order to create his own museum of living pathology using the theater and the female patients. Borgstrom is most interested in the role that specific female patients played in Charcot's ability to create, stage and market his medical discourse on hysteria. The author says that "the nature of the hysterical attack and the technical limitations of the camera allowed Charcot's women a certain physical agency in the representation, study, and documentation of a disease otherwise governed by a male-dominated discourse. [64]" Borgstrom quotes an article in the *British Medical Journal* that condemns the French for going too far; "We must say that we regret that a work of such great scientific interest should be to English readers rendered somewhat unsavory reading by the introduction of long pages of the obscene ravings of delirious hysterical girls, and descriptions of events in their sexual history." [65] But Borgstrom argues that within the male-dominated power structure of La Salpétrière, these women created a feminine language which became the basis for the scientific iconography in the medical theater at the hospital. In the end, it is the exploitation of the gestures that have been taken from seizures and from the stage of hysteria that Charcot called hystero-epilepsy that are important in thinking about epilepsy and mass media. So, in at least two moment in time, the turns of the 20th and 21st centuries, the image of the tonic-clonic seizure has been embraced in popular song and cabaret/theater as a titillating audience experience, a marketing device.

VISUAL IMAGERY – DEPICTIONS OF SEIZURES IN FILM AND ON TELEVISION

According to Andy Warhol, "It's the movies that have really been running things in America ever since they were invented. They show you what you want to do, how to do it, when to do it, how to feel about it, and how to look how you feel about it." [66] I would add to that that, at the present, television and all of the materials available through the internet have even more influence on the viewer. Little has greater influence on memory than a visual image. The fact that the image may be distorted, erroneous and stigmatizing does nothing to quell its sway.

Ten years ago, with these notions in mind, I and my colleague, neurologist Lawrence A. Kerson began to study depictions of seizures and epilepsy in film and on television. The list of films was established by consulting the following sources: the Epilepsy Foundation of America's National Epilepsy Library, the International Movie Data Base, the Literature, Arts and Medicine Data Base, the Brown University Film Archives, many film scholars and neurologists, and a large number of people who are interested in film. The database, to which we continue to add and which presently has more than 300 items, includes every film or television show suggested by any source. In addition to the large number of films in English, there are 31 French films, 13 Hindi, 8 Italian, 7 Chinese, 3 Russian, 4 German, 2 each in Japanese and Spanish, 1 each in Bengali, Danish, Hebrew, Korean, Marati, Mongolian, and Swedish, and 10 silent films. The rest of the data set are made up of episodes of American television, as well as 9 episodes of French television series. With regard to race, nearly all of the characters with seizures are Caucasian. In all, 10 characters with seizures are black, and 23, all of whom are in South or East Asian produced films, are Asian.

As in the saturation techniques used to develop grounded theory, we continue to seek films and television shows portraying seizures and to create analytical codes and categories developed from the data, to develop middle range theories, and to sample for theory construction [67,68,69] All of the films and television shows were reviewed by a board-certified neurologist with nearly 40 years of experience in treating people with epilepsy. As part of our database, we have film clips and/or photographs of the great majority of the portrayals. We have seen all but a few of the depictions.

For the purposes of this research, in the general category of seizures, we include (1) seizures in characters who are said to have epilepsy, (2) seizures in characters who are said to have some other condition, (3) seizures related to drug or alcohol use, (4) seizures that are feigned, that is where someone pretends to have a seizure in order to deceive others or pseudoseizures, that is attacks resembling an epileptic seizure but having only psychological causes, (5) an offhand or throw away category in which, for example, someone is described as or describes himself or someone else as "having a fit." Normally, within the emission, these events have been labeled as epilepsy, as being related to epilepsy or a condition such as street drug use, but sometimes they are seen as a reaction to electrical shock such as *One Flew Over the Cuckoo's Nest,* [70] *A Beautiful Mind,* [71] *Meet the Fockers,* [72],and *The Bed Sitting Room. [73]*

Previous research has enabled us to draw the following conclusions. Audiences find images of individuals falling to the ground unconscious, arms and legs twitching and shaking, foaming at the mouth, making grunts and other primitive sounds, unaware of and having no control of the reactions of people around them, to be both thrilling and frightening. Film makers and television directors have used terrifying riveting images of tonic-clonic (grand mal) seizures throughout the history of film and television and continue to do so despite the work of epilepsy advocacy organizations [74]. Such images are purposeful, disturb and distract others in the film and the audience, heighten the moment, show dimensions of the characters' interior lives and past experiences, and are often associated with insane, violent, possessed and victimized characters suggesting that people with seizure disorders are unstable, unpredictable and without self-control [75, 76, 77, 78]

Following are some more specific results of this continuing study. Since 1900, with Melies *Le Deshabillage Impossible, [76]* epileptiform events have been shown in film, and since the 1950's with Boy in the Storm, an episode of *Medic [80]* they have appeared on television. Although these depictions continue to be used to augment understanding of character and/or to support the narrative of the production, [81] [their presence rarely reflects a contemporary scientific understanding of the condition or the ability to manage it. Rather, films and television shows continue to depict seizures in ways that are entrenched in popular myth [82] and so support the stigmatization of the illness and the need for those with the disorder and their families to conceal their diagnoses. Not only do these victimized and objectified depictions corroborate people's hiding their diagnoses, but they encourage a level of secrecy that leads to people's isolating themselves and ultimately interfere with their capacities to manage their symptoms and their lives. In fact, as the symptoms are managed more successfully, only individuals who have a close relationship with someone with a seizure disorder will likely witness a seizure. Still, either because these images are being used with greater frequency in film and especially on television, or because it has been easier for the researchers to locate recent examples, the number of times that these images appear seems to be on the rise.

We argue that while there are examples in which directors sometimes unknowingly use images that resemble seizures[[83] such as *Vampire Trailer Park* or present images that are so silly and so unreal they have to be named as epilepsy for the audience to relate image to entity such as *Les Barbouzes,*[[84] *The Twelve Chairs*, [85] *The Hollywood Knights*, [86] and *Bachke Rehna Re Baba*, [87] the image particularly of a tonic-clonic (grand mal) seizure is so easy and economical to include and so consistently horrifying and riveting that it acts like Baudrillard's concept of a simulacrum in which the copy becomes a sort of replacement reality. [88] In fact, some say that a primary effect of electronic media no matter what the content, is to substitute hyper-real representations for the reality. [89] Thus, when most young viewers now have no information about epilepsy or seizures, their images of the condition rest in fictive images of those events.

It is generally after the fact that advocates for those with seizure-disorders have condemned such images and had information about epilepsy and epilepsy advocacy groups included as part of the films' final credits (see *Kangaroo Jack* [90]and an episode of *Judging Amy,* a weekly television medical drama, called You Don't Know Me [91]); however, these instances are rare, and one does not know how effective they are. It remains important to understand how epileptiform events are used in order to think about why the images persist in the face of better knowledge about and treatment for the condition.

Previous Phases of the Study

In previous phases of this study, colleagues and I have demonstrated how, over time, directors use seizures to: (1) drive the narrative, (2) enhance the overall mood of a particular genre, (3) try to evoke specific emotional reactions in the audience, (4) support certain personality and behavioral traits of the characters having the seizures, (5) highlight qualities of other characters through the ways in which they respond to the seizures, (6) act as catalysts for other actions taken in by the audience but often not recounted when the films are discussed or reviewed, (7) enhance the voyeuristic experience of the film audience as they watch the actions of characters watching the actions of those having seizures; thus a conscious, most removed audience watches the actions of conscious spectators in the film as they watch the unconscious actions of those characters who are having the seizures. Not mutually exclusive, these categories were built and filled in order to answer the overarching questions related to the persistence of the images.

Conclusions that Colleagues and I Have Drawn Thus Far.

1) Directors have used images and descriptions of tonic-clonic (grand mal) seizures since 1900 and continue to do so despite great advocacy efforts. As was mentioned previously, the earliest film in the series is *Le Deshabillage Impossible.* In the film, a traveler spending the night at an ill finds that when he hangs his coat and hat on a peg in his room, they return to his person. The more rapidly he undresses, the more rapidly his clothes return, and the process enrages him. He rolls on the floor, then on the bed, and finally has what is named an epileptic fit.

The first example that I have found on American television is an episode called "Boy in a Storm" that was part of a 1950's series called *Medic.* [92]. Robert, played by Dennis Hopper, is a very wealthy young white 17 year old male who is described later as shy and cooperative. His parents had died in a plane crash 10 years before. Since that time, because he has epilepsy, his aunt and guardian has chosen to keep him cloistered on a large estate in order to preserve the reputation of the family. He has been having several tonic-clonic seizures a week which he describes as feeling like a big storm of lights gathered behind him that blind him, blind everything just before the seizure happens. After three weeks in the hospital during which he is evaluated and treated properly, he is having no seizures. The physician who is caring for him assures him that seizures have "nothing to do with being crazy," that they are instead an electrochemical procedure in his brain. It was simply the "narrow ignorance and stupid understanding" of his caretakers that led him to be improperly treated. As the episode concludes, the audience is assured that Robert will be educated, will find love and live a full and rich life. At the end of the episode, Richard Boone, who plays the physician and is the narrator for the series, delivers a monologue directly to the audience emphasizing that epileptics are not insane or evil. Despite the use of the word "epileptic," this is one of the most realistic and positive depictions that I have seen.

Probably the most popular film example in the data set is the horror/possession film, *The Exorcist*[[93] which was first made in 1973 and then rereleased in 2000. During the first half of the film, doctors explain that the child has temporal lobe epilepsy. Over time, they change their diagnosis to demonic possession but the discussions of epilepsy accompanied by terrifying images of the child growing a goiter, having her head spin on her neck, speaking in the voices of others and attacking several people are horrifying. To understand the kind of exposure that a film like this can have, it is helpful to review some financial statistics. *The Exorcist* was first released in 1973 at a cost of $12,000,000 and restored for another $1,000,000 for its re-release in 2000. As of July 2007, it had grossed $403,500,000 world-wide. [94] The movie is billed as a realistic film about inexplicable events. How many contemporary viewers relate this film to epilepsy?

2) These images heighten the moment, adding elements of intensity and drama. They can show dimensions of past experiences, interior lives and/or conflicts. For example, in *Cleopatra [95].* Cleopatra watches Caesar have a seizure and the audience watches her watch him, all through an enormous eye that is painted on the wall of his chamber. Cleopatra's drive for more political power and her attraction to Julius Caesar, as well as Caesar's concerns about his own power being diminished if the public learns of his epilepsy are all illustrated in this scene. In *The Andromeda Strain,* [96] the senior scientist who hides her epilepsy has a tonic clonic seizure in response to a flashing light; the response of almost everyone around her is that she has caught the andromeda strain, and they flee. In *Gods and Monsters*, [97] a speculation about the last days of James Whale, director of the famous 1930's Frankenstein films, Whale experiences what appear to be temporal lobe seizures resulting from a stroke. Symptoms include olfactory and visual hallucinations which allow the protagonist to experience himself at different times of his life and bring people who had been important to him into his present. In one scene, when as an old man he is being photographed with the equally old stars of his Frankenstein films, the camera's flash causes Whale to have a seizure in which he is simultaneously with the actors at their ages when they played the characters, at their present ages and with the monsters.

A Mongolian epic called *Khadak*, [98] set in the frozen steppes of Mongolia, tells the story of Bagi, a young nomad who is confronted with his destiny of becoming a shaman. He has the special capacity of being able to hear animals over great distances. When finding a lost sheep, Bagi has a disquieting premonition and, as part of this, has a seizure. He is cared for by a shaman who foresees is also destined to become a shaman. Bagi denies this possibility despite his grandfather's warning that one must embrace one's destiny or risk tribulation. Soon after this, a military convoy appears to announce that a plague has affected all of the animals requiring them to be quarantined and the miners to be relocated to desolate mining towns. Bagi has another seizure in the truck that is removing him and his family. This time, as part of the seizure, he sees his horse's throat being cut. Another time, although she makes no noise, he "hears" a young woman who is under an avalanche of coal in a train car. A doctor diagnoses him with epilepsy and sends him to a mental hospital. Overall, in these incidents that have the slow controlled quality of tai chi movements, we see that Bagi's seizures all have to do with visions of the "present elsewhere" that no one else can see.

3) Images are often associated with insane, violent and victimized characters suggesting that people with seizure disorders are unpredictable, uncontrolled and can be brutal. Among the many examples are *The Terminal Man, [99] La Bête Humaine*, [100] and *The Flying Camel.*[101] In a 1929 film, *To What Red Hell*, a young man kills a prostitute while he is having a seizure. Another young man is arrested for the murder. Rather than let the wrong man take the blame, the young man who committed the murder, who has always been prone to violent outbursts and who has just been told that he has had epilepsy for all of his life, kills himself leaving a letter for the judge confessing to the murder and assuring himself and the world that, although he might have done this again, he has taken an action that will prevent this from ever happening [102].

A savagely dark Italian film made in 1965 called *I Pugli in Tasca* (Fists in the Pocket), [103] is referred to as a cult film and is said by some film experts to rank as one of the greatest achievements of Italian cinema. A pocketed fist is an indication of unsuccessful repression, of a premonition of unrest, and it is the release of that unrest that we see on the part of a character called Alessandro. "The film's central gesture is the epileptic fit." [104]. It is the story of a shut-down, ill and provincial family in which the mother is blind and controlling and three of four adult children have epilepsy. One brother is also mentally challenged. Alessandro, one of the brothers with epilepsy, decides to free Augusto, his only sibling without epilepsy, of the burden of taking care of these family members for whom he is the sole provider. First, Alessandro walks his blind mother over the side of a cliff and into a ravine and then, he drowns his brother in the bathtub. His sister, Giulia, has a seizure during which she falls down a flight of stairs and becomes paralyzed and bedridden. In the final scene, Alessandro has a seizure in his sister's bedroom, calls for her to hold his head, which is what she has always done in the past, and then he has a terminal seizure keeping perfect time with the Semper Libera aria from *La Traviata.*

A final example for this theme is *El Aura*, another very dark film which was made in Argentina in 2005. It tells the story of Esteban Espinoza, an obsessional taxidermist with epilepsy and a photographic memory who is fixated on committing the perfect crime. He is passive, detached and always watching from outside of the action. There are a lot of secrets in the film and there is a lot of death. When he realizes that his wife has left him, Esteban agrees to go hunting with his friend in the Patagonia forest. He cannot allow himself to kill an animal, but finally kills a man whom he mistakes for a deer. Ironically, he finds details of a plan that the dead man had made for robbing an armored car just after it had made a major pick-up at a casino. According to Estaban, he has found the plan for the perfect crime. All goes wrong, but Esteban leaves the scene untouched, and the audience, once again, observes him being the observer. There are several mentions of his epilepsy and several seizures. As in *Gods and Monsters*, *A Matter of Life and Death*, and Oliver Parker's *Othello*, [105] the seizures give the director the opportunity to blend past, present and future and to bring the audience inside of the mind of the character. The audience is brought along towards each seizure as it is preceded by an aura. Esteban says of his seizures; "There is an aura.

Everything stops. Doors open in my head, and I know things, sounds, smells, voices, images. But there is nothing that can stop it. It feels "horrible but perfect. For those few seconds, you are free. There is no choice - nothing to decide. Everything tightens up, gets narrower, and you surrender yourself." [106]

4) More important than character development and narrative effects in relation to the person having a seizure is that of others who are reacting to the event. In these examples, a conscious, removed audience watches the actions of spectators in the film as the latter watch the unconscious actions of the characters having the seizures. The fact that the character having the seizure is unconscious for the event heightens interest relates to how the spectator is led through the film experience. Audiences continue to find images of individuals falling to the ground unconscious, limbs twitching, foaming at the mouth, making primitive sounds, unaware of the reactions of people around them, to be fascinating. This voyeuristic and titillating experience is not very different from lay interest in the films made of Charcot's hysterical and epileptic patients at the end of the 19th century. Overall, such images remain icons, holding audience attention with little effort. Examples include *Disappearing Acts,* [107] *Les Pactes des Loups,* [108] and *Kaos.*

The Lunar Cycle

Although there have been several articles about the effect of the lunar cycle on seizures, [109] Kaos is the only film that I have found dealing with moonlight or the lunar cycle. Kaos [110] is the second story in a film adapted from Pirandello stories. Called either *Moon Sickness* or *Moonstruck* in English, and set in 19th century Italy, it is the story of a farmer, Bata, who tells his new wife, Sidora, that he has seizures at the full moon and when that happens, she should lock herself in the house and not let him in and he will be fine by morning. Sidora runs home to her mother and to the man whom she did not consider sane enough for her to marry before she married her husband. Both her mother and this man come to spend the night with her at the full moon. Her mother has left the house to sleep in the barn, and the other man and she begin to make love, but he is so disturbed at Bata's terrible cries that he must go to him and hold and protect him.

In one recent study, it is reported that "Contrary to the myth, epileptic seizures are not more common during a full moon." [111] Author Selim Benbadis said in a news release, "In fact, we found the number of epileptic seizures was lowest during the full moon and highest in the moon's last quarter. . . .In the past, before physicians recognized that epilepsy was caused by processes in a person's own body, the disease's frightening seizures were associated with demonic possession and witchcraft. Some people still seem to like poetic, mysterious and irrational explanations for puzzling diseases like epilepsy."

Feigned or Pseudoseizures

The notion of consciously pretending to have a seizure in order to change the direction of the action on the part of some characters or the story itself is also a part of this theme. This category of film that of feigned or pseudoseizures. In a feigned seizure, a character consciously pretends to have and thus acts out the symptoms of a tonic-clonic seizure. One example is the film *Drugstore Cowboy*[[112] in which a young woman who is part of a gang of drug addicts pretends to have a seizure in a drug store so that the pharmacist will rush to her aid while her cronies steal drugs and run off. Another is *Angela's Ashes* in which a little boy who is known in the town to have epilepsy pretends to have a seizure in the front of the movie house, thus causing those selling and taking tickets to rush out and his friend to slip in free to see the film. [113] Both *Face Off* [114] and *The Fugitive [115]* have prisoners fake a seizure in order to escape from their jailers, and *Leap Year*,[116] a very old silent comedy, has someone fake seizures in order to discourage his girlfriends' attention.

Different from a conscious pretense that is true for a feigned seizure, a pseudoseizure involves an individual unconsciously using the symptoms of a tonic-clonic seizure for psychological reasons. An example would be *Passion d'Amore [117]* where a very unhappy young woman uses such events to protect herself, or *Priest [118]* in which a teenager has such episodes in order to protect herself from being molested by her father.

5) Seizure representations are increasing because they complement the current emphasis in film and television on violence, drug use, certain mental illnesses and extreme personality characteristics, all themes having to do with the loss of control that is a primary part of the filmic depiction of a tonic-clonic seizure. Examples here include Whacked, an episode of *CSI Miami [119] Jangwha Hongryeon, [120]* Deception, an episode of *House [121] Deceiver, [122] The X Files: I Want to Believe, [123]* and *Kong Que (Peacock).* [124] *Kong Que* is a story of three children of a middle aged couple after the Cultural Revolution that is told in three parts each from the viewpoint of one child. The girl who is free spirited, dreamy and never reaches her dreams, the younger brother is smart and scholarly but bullied because of his mentally handicapped and obese brother who runs away, and comes back years later married and living off of his wife, and the fat brother, called Fatty by everyone, who is given everything, as he believes is his due, and protected by his parents and siblings. When Fatty's siblings try to kill him with rat poison, he has no reaction as he does to nothing else but wanting to please his peers and wanting more and more food. Fatty has a seizure in the bath house where his brother has taken him. Someone gives him a trick cigarette, and just after, he falls, unconscious and frothing at the mouth.

Filmic Depictions of People Known to Have Epilepsy and Their Representations in Other Forms of Media

Several films in our series feature real-life characters who had or are thought to have had epilepsy. One thinks immediately of Julius Caesar and I refer in this chapter to the film, *Cleopatra*, and the television series, *Rome*. There are also several films about Vincent Van Gogh as well as many scholarly articles that discuss his condition, life and art. Some scholars conclude that Van Gogh had epilepsy and that, for example, his auras caused him to see and paint the way he did. Of the various films, *Lust for Life*[[125] portrays Van Gogh sitting in the garden of an asylum painting a version of Starry Night. He falls backwards, grimaces, his fists, one of which holds a large tube of mustard yellow paint, clinch. Dr. Gauchet reports Van Gogh's latest seizure to his brother, Theo, and organizes his return to the north, to Paris. "This latest seizure is the most severe and prolonged that your brother has suffered to date. As a result of constant attention and observation, he is today approaching physical recovery." Soon after Van Gogh says, "Will there be warning? Will I have time?" and he is told, in return, "About those seizures of yours, forget about them!" The book from which the film is drawn, also called *Lust for Life*, [126] makes very different use of epilepsy. In a French language film called *Van Gogh,* [127] Van Gogh describes his "fits" to his doctor. Later, Van Gogh's brother and Dr. Gauchet discuss his condition and treatment comparing his fits to those of an epileptic, and still later, Van Gogh admits to his fits being fictional.

There are two more contemporary and examples of films focused on people with epilepsy. In both cases, real life situations reported in newspapers and elsewhere provided the story lines for the films. In *Let Him Have It,* [128] Derek Bentley is shown first having been trapped in rubble after a bombing in World War II. It is after this incident that he begins to have seizures. Later he is determined to have an IQ of 66 and a mental age of 11. Derek can't read. He loves to play the song "Wheel of Fortune" over and over on his record player, but he can't remember the words. Family members try to do whatever they can to protect him. There is a scene at an army recruitment station in which Derek brings a note from his doctor saying he has epilepsy. The recruiter says they've had a few of these before and they've all turned out to be forgeries. [129] People are trying to dodge their national service. The doctor at the center says, "It's all right. We've got this equipment here to see if you are really epileptic." Derek says, "I've had the test before. I don't want to do it again." Derek has a tonic-clonic seizure during the test. Afterwards, we see his parents discussing the report. His father is distressed because he is functioning at a 4th grade level, and his mother says, "He's just no good at tests." All the while, we see Derek doing push-ups and looking very upset.

In 1953, at age 19, Derek is befriended by Chris, a 15 year old who wants to be a gangster. Desperate to please Chris, Derek steals the keys to the butcher shop, and then goes with Chris and his gang to rob a warehouse. The police come during the robbery. Derek, who has no gun, walks right over to a policeman, and calls, hollers 'Let him have it, Chris." Chris then wounds one policeman and kills another. There is a trial and the debate in court and in the newspapers is whether Derek meant "let the policeman have your gun," or "shoot the policeman." Chris had been in custody for 20 minutes before the constable was killed. Both Chris and Derek are convicted of murder and because Derek is "of age" he is ordered hanged while Chris, who did murder a policeman, is jailed for 10 years.

In the film, a guard waiting with Derek just before his hanging says, "I'll tell you what, man. The truth of this story has got to come out one day. And that one day a lot of people are going to get into trouble." The guard helps Derek to write a letter to his parents which Derek signs himself, "Lots of love, Derek Bentley." He can barely write his name.

On July 30, 1998, a British appeals court found that Bentley had been denied "that fair trial which is the birthright of every British citizen." While his parents and sister who had struggled so long to clear his name have died, his niece toasted his exoneration. The case was of national importance and one can follow the story in the *Times*, The *Manchester Guardian*, the *Telegraph*, the *Independent* and the *Mirror* as well as on the BBC website. Google lists 277,000 websites that focus on or include Derek Bentley. [130] In addition, there have been several songs written about Bentley and his case including one by Elvis Costello called "Let Him Dangle" which has as its introduction,

> Bentley said to Craig,
> Let Him Have It Chris.
> They still don't know
> What he meant by this [131]

The last subject for this section is Anneliese Michel who was diagnosed with epilepsy in a psychiatric hospital in Germany when she was 17 years old and died in 1976 at age 23 of malnutrition and dehydration as a result of a year-long exorcism first supported by the Catholic church because she was possessed by demons. Bringing charges of negligent homicide against two men of the Church and her parents, the state prosecutor maintained that her death could have been prevented even one week before she died. They were found guilty of manslaughter and given suspended sentences and probation. Two films have been made from this situation which was also reported in newspapers and about which there 185,000 results when one googles her name. [132] Of the two films, Requiem [133] is closer to the real situation. The other, *The Exorcism of Emily Rose [134]* is reset in the United States, and said to be lit like *The Exorcist,* and both are described as horror films. In the final line of his review of the latter version, Roger Ebert, weighed in with his medical opinion saying, "You didn't ask but, in my opinion, she had psychotic epileptic disorder." [135]

A popular song called Annalisa was recorded by Public Image Ltd.

> Think Im proud to be your enemy
> Take your hands off of me
> Youre worse than the thing that possessed me
> The way they should have been
> Annalisa
>
> Annalisa was 15 years old
> Stole her soul
> But I have no tears
> Even been alone
> And heard the voice
> Not your own
> Ive seen those fears
> Annalisa

On YouTube, one can also watch what are purported to be exorcisms of Anneliese Michel [136] and there is also at least one video play called Pictures of Anneliese Michel with music available on the internet. [137]. It has been reported that YouTube has now become transformed from an entertainment medium to a reference tool. [138] The journalist who is writing this article asks the question, "How far will video go as an alternative to text?" He quotes Hunter Walk, a director of product management at YouTube saying "Video is a part of the discovery process. Depending on the user and type of content, users may want to start with video or text." In November 2008, Americans conducted nearly 2.8 billion searches on YouTube. I bring this to the reader's attention to demonstrate that these images as well as the outdated and horrifying understanding of epilepsy not only continue but make full use of the range of media opportunities over which there is less and less control by any kind of governing body. The last two examples began with stories of people's lives that were reported in newspapers with all of the biases of the individual papers and the times in which they were published. From these accounts, popular songs, films and many websites were produced.

Differences Found between English Language Film and American Television

In studying the data set of 91 examples drawn from English language television shows, I have been thinking about ways in which to differentiate television portrayals from those in film including: (1) that these depictions are often part of weekly television shows, (2) the genres are different, (3) the depictions seem to be more negative over time and (4) as the numbers of channels proliferate, there is always greater competition for audience share. First, seizures are used so frequently on some shows that they might subtly influence the development of the narrative. For example, since 2005, *House* has had at least 25 episodes out of a total of 98 shows with characters portraying seizures and *Grey's Anatomy* has had at least 11 such episodes.

However, I am most interested in continuing characters who become a part of the overall narrative of the show. Four television series have used continuing characters with seizures or who say they have epilepsy, *Rome*, [139] *Deadwood, The Young and the Restless* and *Huff. Rome* has one episode in which Caesar has a seizure. In Deadwood, the good and well-meaning minister is portrayed as having seizures in three different episodes with the last being status epilepticus from which he is relieved when, at the town doc's suggestion, he is suffocated by the town boss. Believe it or not, this is meant to show the sensitive side of the boss whose brother suffered from epilepsy and was humiliated as a result. The *Huff*, [140] characterization was different because the character, called Dauri Rathburn, played by Sharon Stone, twice told those enforcing the law that she was not responsible for her actions because she had epilepsy when, in fact, she did not. She pretended to have epilepsy in order to avoid prosecution for vehicular homicide.

A most positive portrayal that I have seen was an episode called "Man Hunt" (11/3/00) on *Nash Bridges*, a police procedural. Antoine, a young police officer who had served in the Gulf War, has a seizure as he stands over a captured thief who happened to have been his sergeant in the war. The ambulance tech who has been called to the scene says, "He's fine. He had a grand mal epileptic seizure. He's fine unless he lets his prescription lapse again." Antoine says, "I've had 3 seizures in the last 10 years. If I take my meds. I'm fine." The head of his unit says, "Don't do that to my men again, and don't do it to yourself. Now go home and get some rest." Unfortunately, this episode was one of the last in the six year series, and Antoine was not featured again, but there was great potential in that character.

Christina Chaplin, a writer for the *Los Angeles Times* wrote about the incident in an article called Accurate Treatment of Epilepsy saying, "Who would have thought that a police drama would have an ongoing plot line dealing with a person with epilepsy and that it would be a positive and accurate portrayal? [141] Curious, Chaplin called the producers and found that the character was based on a friend of one of the producers. Antoine was to remain part of the show but would have few seizures because this producer wanted to keep the story real.

Also, television genres are different from film, and it is possible that the genres, themselves, be they crime, action, comedy, drama or adventure, affect the portrayals. Third, I have found that television portrayals of seizures and epilepsy have become more negative over time. I have already described the highly sympathetic character in *Medic*. This is also true for a in a double episode of *Dr. Kildare [142]* in which the character with epilepsy is smart and capable. The most contemporary depictions show less concern for the person having the seizure. The most horrific example is from an episode of *The Sopranos* called Two Tonys [143], one of the hottest shows on American television. In the final moments of the first episode of a new season, two members of the Soprano family are leaving a restaurant when the waiter comes out to complain about the paltry tip that they had left him. In response, one man hits the waiter in the head with a brick. The waiter has a tonic-clonic seizure and the family members mumble "don't these people know they're supposed to take their medicine." They shoot and kill the waiter; then they take back the money they had left to pay the bill. To them, he is a nameless, insignificant object.

Finally, the numbers of channels and shows have proliferated with television's expanded capacity to transmit. Therefore, television shows are competing for the attention of the viewer. Showing someone having a seizure seems an easy way to capture attention audience attention particularly when one is surfing channels with a remote. In fact, while there is only one example of a seizure being used before the opening credits in a film (JFK), [144] in television, there are many examples of seizures being used both before the opening credits and as parts of previews of upcoming shows. So, in my opinion, the hope is to have continuing characters in popular shows whose epilepsy is intriguing but who also educate through positive responses to well-managed treatment. Thus, I was pleased to hear that a long-time star of *The Young and the Restless* would be diagnosed with and treated for epilepsy.

The Young and the Restless (Y and R)

In 2006, Tony Coelho, President of the Epilepsy Foundation of America, announced a collaboration between CBS Television and the Epilepsy Foundation. Episodes would focus on Victor Newman whose behavior has changed since his car was hijacked. As a result of this experience, Victor has become a gentler person, even turning over control of his business to a colleague. Those around him think that is due to a new view of life, but blackouts and hallucinations lead to a diagnosis of temporal lobe seizures.

In time, Victor's and his family and friends' dealing with his epilepsy was featured in more than 20 episodes. This is the only continuing character with epilepsy that I have found on American television. *The Young and the Restless*, with a daily audience of 6,000,000, presents a different kind of opportunity than the minister on Deadwood, [145] who was killed off after a few episodes, or Antoine on *Nash Bridges* or the character on *Huff*.

Despite the collaboration between the Epilepsy Foundation of America and CBS, depictions of Victor's management of his epilepsy mirror many of the themes related to concerns about being seen as weak or treated like a child, searching for herbal and other nonmedical solutions, hoping for a quick fix through surgery, naming of seizures as paranormal and/or religious experiences, relating seizures and uncontrolled violence, and confusion of epilepsy with some kinds of psychiatric illnesses. In the first of these television episodes (7/18/06), Victor learns that he has temporal lobe epilepsy. He and his daughter have seen the doctor together, but Victor asks his daughter not to tell his wife. As a result of being more emotionally engaged and less cold, distant, and calculating, he befriends Jack Abbot who has been a bitter business enemy. While Victor's attitude changes, Jack's behavior does not. Seizing an opportunity, he convinces Victor to sign away a business interest and encourages him to stop taking his epilepsy medicine.

Victor tells Jack that he does not want to appear weak and reports that his condition has provided feelings of peace, deep understanding, paranormal visions and enlightenment. Next (7/24/06), he informs Jack, that he is no longer taking his medicine, but is leaving on a what he refers to as a retreat and that Jack is to keep this a secret. As part of this journey (8/4/06), Victor visits a friend who is blind. She is a deeply spiritual and religious person whom he hopes will guide him towards understanding his condition. Keeping epilepsy a secret from his host, Victor talks instead of visions and spiritual awakenings. One day, Victor's friend returns to find him having a seizure. Afterwards (8/7/06), he says he is afraid, then he appears to "zone out," and has aural hallucinations in which he hears music. His friend mentions that perhaps his visions are religious. Later, (8/25/06), Victor tells his son that he has stopped his medication because of harmful side effects. Home to find a better solution (8/28/06), Victor is seen slicing an apple. His cutting turns violent, and he begins to mutter about killing the man who kidnapped his daughter-in-law. In a later episode (8/31/06), Victor finds his daughter- in-law at the gym, and he decides that she needs to learn how to box. His punches turn vicious and cruel; afterwards, he remembers nothing, not even his daughter-in-law's attempts to help him. On 9/11/06, Victor decides that everyone around him is laughing at him. His aural hallucinations now consist of voices calling his name, and, as he becomes increasingly paranoid, he barricades himself inside his house with a gun. When his wife comes home to try to calm him and stabilize the situation, he doesn't recognize her and points his gun at her. A physician tells his family that this level of violence and inability to recognize people who are part of one's life is a reaction to his medication. As a result of this episode, he is admitted to a psychiatric hospital because he is a danger to himself and to others, and he is seen restrained to his bed in the psychiatric ward. In another episode (9/15/06), he opts for brain surgery in lieu of medicine. Although he claims to be cured, in the next episode, he seems to be daydreaming and is depressed. His coordination is off, and although he used to have very good fine motor skills, he is unable to glue parts of a lamp together. He tells his son that he will be using natural teas to stop his seizures. Before leaving on a business trip, his wife she tries to give Victor an electronic medical alert bracelet which Victor argues is useless because he cannot press the button before he has a seizure because he does not know when he is going to have one...She then speaks about their dog and how he barked when Victor was having a seizure...Victor yells that she knows nothing about dogs and goes for a walk. After a nap, Victor has a seizure while trying to put the dog's collar back on. In this last episode in the series that I have collected (9/26/06), Victor says that he does not wish to be treated like a child or an invalid.

If I had known more about this very long running soap opera or about the character of Victor on this #1 daytime drama on U.S. television, I might have been able to predict the evolution of the depictions of epilepsy. The following quote describes some of the events in Victor's life on the show. "In the middle the melodramatic maelstrom of "YandR" is Victor Newman, who has withstood amnesia, a heart attack, spells of temporal-lobe epilepsy, a harpoon to the genital area, a carjacking, a tell-all biography ("Ruthless!"), a conviction for bribery, an enforced stay in a psychiatric ward, nine weddings (three to the same ex-stripper), six divorces, two vasectomies, and the theft of his semen from a sperm bank by two women, only one of whom managed to impregnate herself with the plunder" [146].

Thus, I agree with Mr. Coelho that featuring a continuing character with epilepsy is a great solution to educating the public, particularly if the series will allow for educational messages regarding correct responses to seizures and the importance of conferring with one's physician in order to understand the risks in stopping a recommended treatment. Of course, the problem is that these depictions of epilepsy, of individual seizures, and of the reactions of the person with epilepsy as well as those around him are fictive creations that are used to enhance the moment and the story. This is a great start, but we will all have to continue to encourage directors to use images of seizures and epilepsy in ways that will not only enthrall but educate.

Beginning Comparisons of French Language and English Language Depictions

Now that I have amassed this series, I would like to be able to compare depictions cross culturally as well as in film and on television. [147] Since I only have a reasonably large number of French language items, my first step is a comparison of films and television shows in French as opposed to English. Painting with a very broad brush, I can say that French language depictions are very creative. *Carnage*[148] makes extraordinary use of a child's hallucinations. *Les Amants du Nil [149]* shows epilepsy through the eyes of the individual with the condition. The central character's explanations of her seizures are among the most imaginative any in the total series. She likens a seizure to being dead and then returning to life. This theme is played out in other dimensions of the film and is most closely related to *A Matter of Life and Death*, [150] an English language film in which the central character has hallucinations about a heavenly messenger's trying to bring him to heaven because he has escaped death.

The use of visual hallucinations seems to be the most original part of these or any depictions, and, of course, being brought into the mind of a character is the height of intimacy for the audience. For various reasons, the most interesting finding thus far is that almost all of the depictions in French films draw the audience toward the character while this is not generally true for depictions in English language film. Even the most violent French characters with seizures evoke great sympathy from the audience while most of those in English language films do not. Specifically, I am working with four variables: (1) negativity of portrayal, that is negative dimensions of character, poor reactions of others or bizarre treatments that would contribute to a person with seizures' being presented in a demeaning or frightening light, (2) the effects of feigned or pseudo-seizures as compared to the effects of seizures that would more likely be related to epilepsy; (3) the level of violence in the films in which seizures appeared; and (4) the use of visual, olfactory and auditory hallucinations as a means of conveying the characters' experiences of having seizures.

There are intriguing distinctions. All but five of the French films include characters with negative attributes, such as emotional disorders, including depression or drug use, and all English language films have some degree of negativity. However, within this negativity, there are differences. For example, in the silent era, all but one of the English language films are tragedies whereas the French films are comedies. While all of these films were made before 1930 and are seldom viewed today, the differences are remarkable. The comic renditions do poke fun at the epileptic condition but in very playful, jesting, silly ways. For example, *La Redingote Epileptique [151]* is about a coat that, when donned, makes one in a jerky, uncontrolled fashion and gets each of its wearers into enough trouble to pass the coat to someone else. However, in the tragic examples, a character suffers extreme sorrow or is brought to ruin often as a consequence of some inner failing or an inability to cope. In the silent English film, *The Supreme Temptation*, the woman with seizures is a French working class girl whose seizures have ruined her life and now endanger the life of the English physician whom she has married. Images differ again in films of the two languages. For example, five comedies depict silly images of exaggerated symptoms. Only once in a French film does someone feign a seizure while there are French-language portrayals of three pseudoseizures. Of 14 such examples in English-language film, there are 11 feigned seizures and three, pseudoseizures.

Thus, there is a divergence in depictions of seizures in English- and French- language film even before there are "talkies." I am considering four types of negative depictions: offensive characterizations, bizarre treatments or associations, horrific reactions by others to the seizures, or seizures feigned to move the film in negative ways. There are examples of each type in both French and English language films, but at this point, I am only prepared to say that the depictions in English language film are more extreme. In relation to violence, only one French film, *La Bête Humaine,* portrays seizures in a violent character, and his violence is understood to be non-volitional and, otherwise, separate from his character. Eight films (28%) have violent themes related to war, drug use, or gross mistreatment. The English-language series has 36 characters with seizures who carry some level of violence within themselves, and almost 80% of the films have violent themes.

Conclusions

The word "media" is borrowed from advertising where it was first used to delineate specific outlets for precise messages to be delivered to particular audiences. No matter what form the media takes, it involves mass communication which entails production, dissemination, reception and then interpretation on a large scale. The goal is to sell the product. Still, this kind of mass communication is a signifying process in which meaning and significance are variable because codes of some producers and some recipients may not agree on the messages. As a dimension of this signifying process, stigma is not an inherent attribute but rather about a devaluing or discrediting on the part of a community or society. A great deal of media discourse involves clashes over meaning and room for challengers "to offer competing constructions of reality and to find support for them from readers whose daily lives may lead them to construct meaning in ways that go beyond media imagery" [152].

At times, mass messages do not adequately support, or are, in fact, counter to the goals of the epilepsy community, to help those with epilepsy live as symptom free as possible and to eradicate the stigma attached to the condition. In the situation of epilepsy and media, at least three constituencies share the images but do not agree with the meaning, the significance or the aftermath. There are the producers of the images, the journalists, writers, producers and directors who have their specific goals of marketing and increasing their audience. There is the very large general audience who wants to be informed, entertained, enthralled, etc. whom the writers, producers, journalists want to attract. Finally, there is the epilepsy community which might be further divided into two groups, the professionals and those with direct involvement with the condition. Even though they are deeply sympathetic to the plights of those with epilepsy, I see these two groups as viewing these images differently. The professionals care that the depictions can be classified and that they be as accurate as possible. They decry what one epileptologist has called "monstrous depictions" but they seem not to take them as much to heart as those with personal involvement. It is that group who has the greatest stake who are deeply hurt and offended by the depictions.

I can only buttress this argument anecdotally. A film editor in Paris said to me, "Why be concerned about these images? They are clichés. No one takes them seriously." Over time, several epileptologists have said, "You can't even classify these. You can't count them." Innumerable people who have seen presentations, members of the very large general audience to whom all producers of word and picture are trying to appeal, say they thought that what those in the epilepsy community would call a caricature, a parody, a satirical symbol of their condition was epilepsy I have also been told especially by parents of children with epilepsy, both young and grown, that these images are unbearable to watch, the worst kinds of epithets, mocking and demeaning emblems of a serious condition. In the end, I believe that I have shown that the visual experience of a tonic-clonic seizure remains so arresting that its use is likely to continue for a long time despite continued great advances in treatment. [153, 154].

CONCLUSION

Conclusions drawn from all of this work point out that primarily through the image of a simulation of a tonic-chronic seizure, epilepsy continues to be portrayed as associated with victimization, fear, secrecy, possession, supernatural power and violence. Seizures are depicted in ways that will titillate, captivate, terrify and draw the audience.

Overall, little has been altered. Whatever the intent of the producers of the images and or written descriptions, this image, has retained its power to frighten and to alienate audiences in every part of the world while, at the same time, it trivializes and mocks this very serious condition. Whatever need society has to be tantalized by the notion of someone losing control or consciousness does not seem diminished in these times. To combat these depictions will take continued education of the public, heightened vigilance and a combined effort of epilepsy interest groups and the power of every government.

In thinking about the impact of these images, one notes that as treatments for epilepsy continue to improve, most people may never witness a seizure. Thus, fictive depictions will increasingly represent epilepsy in the minds of the public [155]. It is important to note here that the average American watches more than 28 hours of TV each week. The great stigma attached to the illness means that better treatment encourages more of those with epilepsy to keep the diagnosis a secret because they worry that disclosure will cause people to isolate them or treat them punitively [156].

Keeping the secret means that their associates do not learn about the condition and continue to think of it as related to fictive images. The hope, then, lies in finding ways to use the power of all of these forms of mass communication to inform and educate the public so that, despite the captivating qualities of these stereotyped images, their presence will be diminished.

References

[1] Schroder, K.C. (2001). Media language and communication. In *Concise Encyclopedia of Sociolinguistics.* Methrie, R. Ed. Amsterdam;New York: Elsevier. http://www.credoreference.com id=802398. (accessed 12/10/08).

[2] Jones, J. M. (2000). The falling sickness in literature. *Southern Medical Journal* 93(12): 1169-72.

[3] Schacter, S. C. (1996). Epilepsy and art. *Medical Journal of Australia* 164(4):245-8.

[4] Schacter, S.C. (2009). The visions of artists with epilepsy, implications for neuroscientists. *Epilepsy and Behavior* Jan. 14. Suppl.1:12-13. Epub 2008, Oct 31.

[5] Fiske, J. and Hartley, J. (2003). *Reading Television*. London: Routledge.

[6] Gripsrud, J. (2004). Broadcast television: The chances of its survival in a digital age. In Spiegel, L. and Olsson, J. (Eds.). *Television after television: Essays on a medium in transition* (pp. 210-223). Durham, NC: Duke University Press.

[7] Kobau, R. and Price, P. (2003). Knowledge of epilepsy and familiarity with this disorder in the U.S. population: Results from the 2002 Health-Styles survey. *Epilepsia* 44: 1149-454. I.

[8] Dilorio, C., Osborne Shafer, P., Letz R. et al. (2003). The association of stigma with self-management and perceptions of health care among adults with epilepsy. *Epilepsy and Behavior*, 4: 259-63.

[9] Goffman, E. (1963). *Stigma: Notes on the Management of Spoiled Identity*. Englewood Cliffs, NJ: Prentice-Hall.

[10] Ibid, p. 1.

[11] Jacoby, A., Gerry, J., Gamble, C. and Baker, G.A. (2004). Public knowledge, private grief: A study of public attitudes to epilepsy in the United Kingdom and implications for stigma. *Epilepsia* 45(11): 1405-1415.

[12] Van Brakel, W. H. (2006). Measuring health-related stigma – A literature review. *Psychology, Health and Medicine*: 11(3): 307-334.

[13] Ibid. p334.

[14] Barnes, C. (1992). *Disabling imagery and the Media: An exploration of the principles for medial representations of disabled people*. The British Council of Organisations of Disabled People. Halifax, England. Ryburn Publishing Limited.

[15] Dilorio, CA, Kabau, R, Holden, EW, Berkowitz, JM, Kamin, St., et al. (2004). Developing a measure to assess attitudes towards epilepsy in the US population. *Epilepsy Behavior*. 5: 965-975.

[16] Barnes, C. op cit. p10.

[17] Jacoby, Ann (2008). Epilepsy and Stigma: An Update and Critical Review. *Current Neurology and Neuroscience Reports*. 8: 339-344.

[18] Shafiq, M., et al. (2008). Myths and fallacies about epilepsy among residents of a Karachi slum area. *Seizure* 38:32-33.

[19] Qidwai, W., Alim, N., Azam, S.I. (2002). Myths and fallacies about health and disease among patients presented to family physicians at the Aga Khan University Hospital Karachi, Pakistan. *Pakistan Journal of Medical Science* 18: 287-90.

[20] Lai, C.W., Huang, X.S., Lai, Y.H. (1990). Survey of public awareness, understanding, and attitudes towards epilepsy in Hunan Province, China. *Epilepsia* 31:182-87.

[21] Jacoby, A., Wang. W., Dang Vu, T., Wu, J. Snape, D. et al., (2007). Meanings of epilepsy in its sociocultural context and implications for stigma: Findings from ethnographic studies in local communities in China and Vietnam. *Epilepsy and Behavior* 12: 286-97.

[22] Mbewe, E., Haworth, A., Atadzhanov, M., Chomba, E., Birbeck, G. L. (2006). Epilepsy-related knowledge, attitudes and practices among Zambian police officers. *Epilepsy and Behavior* 10:456-62.

[23] http://www/who.int/mediacentre/factsheets/fs166/en/ (5/18/05) (accessed 5/18/05).

[24] Leibling, A.J. (nd). *Michael Moncur's Cynical Quotations*. http:www.quotationspage.com/quote/27566.html. (accessed 12/28/08).

[25] Mailer, N. (1960). http://www.quotationspage.com/quote/Norman_Mailer. (accessed 12/28/08).

[26] Lantz, J.C., Lanier, W.L. (2002). Observations for the Mayo Clinic National Conference on Medicine and the Media. *Mayo Clinic Proceedings*. 77:1306-11.

[27] Krauss, G.L., Gondek, S., Krumholtz, A., Paul, S., and Shen, F. (2000). The Scarlet "E: The presentation of epilepsy in the English language print media. *Neurology* 54:1894-98.

[28] Ibid., p. 1895.

[29] Hutchinson, J. (3/25/95). Habspick suffers seizures. *The Montreal Gazette* E3.

[30] Flo Jo resting at home after brief bout with sleep deprivation. (4/8/96). *Business Wire.*

[31] Krauss. Op. cit. p. 1897.

[32] Caspermeyer, J.J., Sylvester, E.J., Drazkowski, J.F., Watson, G.L, and Sirven, J.I. (2006). Evaluation of stigmatizing language and medical errors in neurology coverage by US newspapers. *Mayo Clinic Proceedings* Mar: 81(3):300-306.

[33] Ibid. p. 305.

[34] Ibid. p. 304.

[35] Seale, C. (2002). *Media and Health* (pp. 93-119). Thousand Oaks, CA: Sage.

[36] Auslander, G. and Gold, N. (1999). Media reports on disability: A bi-national comparison of types and causes of disability as reported in major newspapers. *Disability and Rehabilitation* 21(9): 420-431.

[37] Ibid. p. 421.

[38] Ibid. 420.

[39] http://topics.latimes/com/health/conditions/epilepsy (accessed 11/10/08).

[40] Barnes, R. and Shear, M.D. (7/30/07). Chief justice suffers seizure; Roberts is fine, Spokeswoman says. *The Washington Post* , A1.

[41] Grady, D. and Altman, L.K. (8/1/07). Roberts facing medical option on 2nd seizure. *New York Times*, Sec. A1.

[42] Greenhouse, L. (7/31/07). U.S.Chief Justice suffers a seizure but is called 'fully recovered.' NEWS, p. 6.

[43] Cooper, A. (7/31/07). AC360° (July 31). http://www.cnn.com/2007/US/law/07/30/roberts.fall/index.html. (accessed 12/1/08).

[44] http://www.medicinewstoday.com/articles/133853.php. (accessed 12/11/08).

[45] http://ilae.org/ (accessed 12/18/08).

[46] Smoking curbs: The global picture. BBC News (1/4/08). http://news.bbc.co.uk/2/hi/3758707.stm. (accessed 12/5/08).

[47] Sargent, J.D. (2005). Smoking in movies: Impact on adolescent smoking. *Adolescent Medicine Clinics* 16: 345-370.
[48] http://www.smokefreemovies.ucsf.edu/ (accessed 11/28/08).
[49] Tobacco on Television. http://frankwbaker.com/tobacco_on_television, htm (accessed 10/5/08).
[50] Personal communication (February 25, 2008). Claire Cachera, Fondation française pour la recherche sur l'épilepsie, Paris, Fr.
[51] Baxandale, S. (2008). The representation of epilepsy in popular music. *Epilepsy and Behavior* 12(1):165-69.
[52] The Falling Sickness (1999). *Dysentery*. Hopeless Records.
[53] Cage (2002).Ballad of worms. *Eastern Conference All Stars III*. Columbia Records.
[54] 50 Cent (2008). Like my style. *50 Cent in the Future*. G Unit.
[55] Malevolent Creation. (1997). Epileptic seizure. *In Cold Blood*. Crash.Music, Inc.
[56] Baxendale, S. (2008). The intriguing case of Christina the Astonishing. *Neurology* 70(21): 2004-07.
[57] DeCantimpre, T. (2000).The life of Christina the Astonishing. (2nd ed.). Toronto: Peregrine Publishing Company.
[58] Cave, N. and the Bad Seeds. (1996). Christina the Astonishing. *Henry's Dream*. Mute U.S.
[59] Baxendale, S. The representation of epilepsy in popular music op. cit. p. 168.
[60] Ibid.
[61] Gordon, R.B. (2001). *Why the French Love Jerry Lewis: From Cabaret to Early Cinema*. Stanford, CA: Stanford University Press.
[62] *Le cabaret epileptique* (1928). Dir: Henri Gad. Pathés Frères.
[63] Borgstrom, H. (2000). Strike a pose: Charcot's women and the performance of hysteria at La Salpetriere. *Theatre Annual* 53: 1-14.
[64] Ibid. p. 7.
[65] Cited in Goetz, C. (1995).Charcot: Constructing Neurology. NY: Oxford University Press: 186.
[66] http//:wwwbrainyquote.com/quotes/authors/a/warhol. Html. (Accessed 12/17/08).
[67] Strauss A. L., and Corbin J. M. (1998). *Basics of qualitative research techniques and procedures for developing grounded theory (*2nd ed.). Thousand Oaks: Sage.
[68] Charmaz, K. (2004). Grounded theory. In Hesse-Biber, S. N. and Leavy, P. (eds.). *Approaches to Qualitative Research: A Reader on Theory and Practice*. New York: Oxford University Press.
[69] Bogdan, R. and Taylor S. J. (1998). *Introduction to qualitative research methods*. New York: Wiley.
[70] *One Flew Over the Cuckoo's Nest* (1975). Dir: Milos Forman. United Artists.
[71] *A Beautiful Mind* (2001). Dir: Ron Howard. Imagine Entertainment.
[72] *Meet the Focker* (2004). Dir: Jay Roach. Universal Pictures. 2004.
[73] *The Bed Sitting Room*. Dir: Richard Lester. Oscar Lewenstein Productions. 1969.
[74] Kerson, TS. and Kerson, L.A. (2006). Implacable images: Why epileptiform events continue to be featured in film and television. *Epileptic Disorders* 8(2): 103-113.
[75] Kerson, T.S. (2004).Spasmes epileptiformes au cinema: Feigned seizures. Centre D'Etudes Transdisciplinaires: Sociologie, Anthropologie, Histoire. Paris, France.

[76] Kerson, T.S. and Kerson, L.A. (2005). Monstrous depictions of seizures in film and television. Abstract. 26th International Epilepsy Congress Proceedings. *Epilepsia* 46, Suppl 6, 189.
[77] Kerson, J. F., Kerson, T.S., and Kerson, L.A. (1999). The depiction of seizures in film. *Epilepsia*, 40: 1163-67.
[78] Kerson, T.S., Krauss, G.L., and Kerson, L.A. (2001). Reel seizures (course). American Academy of Neurology 53rd Annual Meeting, Philadelphia, PA.
[79] *Le Déshabillage Impossible.* (1900). Dir: Georges Méliès. Pathé Frères.
[80] Boy in the Storm, (1/3/55). *Medic*, Dir: Ted Post. NBC.
[81] Kerson T. S, Kerson J. F., and Kerson L. A. (2000). She'll have a seizure maybe: Then we can watch. *Social Work in Health Care* 30:95-110.
[82] Maio, G. (2001). Die Medialen Deutungsmuster von Krankheit und Medizin. *Fortschr Neurol Psychiat* 69: 138-45.
[83] *Vampire Trailer Park* (1991). Dir: Steve Latshaw. Cinemondo.
[84] *Les Barbouzes.* (1964). Dir: Georges Lautner. S.N. Gaumont.
[85] *The Twelve Chairs.* (1970). Dir. Mel Brooks. Twentieth Century Fox.
[86] *The Hollywood Knights.* (1980). Dir: Floyd Mutrux. Casablanca Films.
[87] *Bachke Rehne Re Baba.* (2005) Dir: Govind Monan. BSK Entertainment Ltd.
[88] Baudrillard, J. (1974). *Simulacra and Simulation.* Tr. SF Glaser. Ann Arbor: Michigan.
[89] Gamson, W. A., Croteau, D., Haynes, W. and Sasson, T. (1992). Media images and the social construction of reality *Annual Review of Sociology*18: 373-393.
[90] *Kangaroo Jack.* (2003). Dir. David McNally. Castle Rock.
[91] You Don't Know Me. (2/15/05). *Judging Amy 6:12*, Dir: James Kramer, CBS.
[92] Boy in the Storm op. cit.
[93] *The Exorcist* (1973, 2000). Dir. William Friedkin. Warner Brothers.
[94] http://www.the numbers.com/movies (accessed 9/8/08).
[95] *Cleopatra.* (1963). Dir. Joseph L. Mankiewicz, Twentieth Century Fox.
[96] *The Andromeda Strain,* (1971). Dir. Robert Wise, Metro Goldwyn Mayer.
[97] *Gods and Monsters* (1998). Dir: Bill Condon, Lions Gate Films.
[98] *Khadak* (2006**).** Dirs: Peter Brosens and Jessica Hope Woodworth**.** BoFilms.br ba
[99] *The Terminal Man* (1974). Dir: Michael Hodges. Warner Bros.
[100] *La Bete Humaine* (1938). Dir: Jean Renoir Paris Film.
[101] *The Flying Camel* (1994). Dir: Rami Na'aman. Tranfax Film Productions.
[102] *To What Red Hell* (1929). Dir: Edwin Greenwood. Twickenham Studios (gb).
[103] *I Pugni in Tasca* (Fists in the Pockets) (1965). Dir: Marco Bellocchio. Doria.
[104] Schoonover, K. (2006). Fists in the Pocket. http://archive.sensesofcinema.com/contents/cteq/06/40/Fists-in-the-Pockets.html. (accessed 12/28/08).
[105] *Othello* (1995). Dir: Oliver Parker. Castle Rock.
[106] *El Aura* (2005). Dir: Fabian Bielinsky. Aura Films.
[107] *Disappearing Acts* (2000) (TV). Dir: Gina Prince-Bythewood. Amen Ra Films.
[108] *Les Pactes des Loups* (2001). Dir: Christofer Gans. David Films.
[109] Baxendale, S. and Fisher, J. (2008). Moonstruck? The effect of the lunar cycle on seizures. *Epilepsy and Behavior* 13:549-550.
[110] *Kaos.* (1984). Dirs: Paolo and Vittorio Taviani. Filmtre.
[111] Benbadis, S.R., Chang, S., Hunter, J. and Wang, W. (2004). The influence of the full moon on seizure frequency: Myth or reality. *Epilepsy and Behavior* Aug 5(4):596-97.

[112] *Drugstore Cowboy* (1989). Dir: Gus VanSant. Avenue Pictures Production.
[113] *Angela's Ashes* (1999). Dir: Alan Parker. Paramount.
[114] *Face/Off* (1997). Dir: John Woo. Paramount.
[115] *The Fugitive* (1993). Dir: Andrew Davis. Warner Bros.
[116] *Leap Year* (1921). Dir: James Cruze. Paramount Pictures.
[117] *Passion d'amore* (1981). Dir: Ettore Scola. Cocinor.fr
[118] *Priest* (1994). Dir: Antonia Bird. BBC.
[119] Whacked (5/16/05). *CSI-Miami* 3:23. Dir: Scott Lautanan. CBS.
[120] Janghwa, Hongryeon (2003). Dir: JiWoon Kim. Masulpiri ilms (kr).
[121] Deception (12/13/05). *House* 31. Dir: Deran Sarfian. FOX.
[122] *Deceiver*. (1997). Dirs: Josh Pate and Jonas Pate. Netro Goldwyn Mayer.
[123] .*The X Files: I Want to Believe*. (2008). Dir. Chris Carter. Crying Box Productions.
[124] *Kong Que* (2005). Dir: Changwei Gu, Asian Union Film and Entertainment
[125] *Lust for Life*. (1956). Dir: Vincent Minelli. Metro-Goldwyn-Mayer (MGM).
[126] Irving Stone. 1934. *Lust for Life*. Longmans.
[127] *Van Gogh*. (1991). Dir. Maurice Pialat. CNC.
[128] *Let Him Have It* (1991). Dir: Peter Medak. British Screen (gb)
[129] In *Bekenntuisse des Hochstaplers Felix Krull*. (aka *The Confessions of Felix Krull*). (1957). Dir: Kurt Hoffman. Filmaufbau (de), there is a scene in which Felix is declared unfit for service because he fakes a seizure in the office to which he has been called.
[130] See particularly, www.derekbentley.com (accessed 1/17/09).
[131] http://www.elviscostello.info/lyricsspike.html (accessed 1/17/09).
[132] Personal communication, Stefan Heiner, 2005.
[133] *Requiem* (2006). Dir: Hans Christian Schmid. 23/5 Filmprodektion GmbH.
[134] The Exorcism of Emily Rose (2005). Dir: Scott Derrickson. Lakeshore Productions.
[135] The Exorcism of Emily Rose::RogerEbert.com. (accessed 1/18/09).
[136] Anneliese Michel. YouTube.com/watch?v=92_XYLPrUMO. Real exorcism of Anneliese Michel. www.youtube.com/watch?v=x4n9vkO_mdk. (accessed 1/18/09)
[137] Ackerman, W. video.google.com/videoplay?dicod=1589685460865559 83. (accesses 1/18/09).
[138] Helft, Miguel. (2009). At first, funny videos. Now, a reference tool. *New York Times* (1/18): 4.
[139] Stealing from Saturn. (9/18/05). *Rome* 4:1. Dir: Julian Farino. HBO.
[140] Maps Don't Talk II (4/2/06). *Huff*.2:2. Dir: Scott Winant. Showtime. Whipped Doggie (4/9/06). *Huff* 2:3. Dir: Dan Lerner, Showtime Sweet Release (4/16/06).*Huff* 2:4. Dir: Sarah Pia Anderson. Showtime. Used, Abused, Unenthused (4/23/06). *Huff* 2:5. Dir: Steve Gomer. Showtime.
[141] Chaplin, C. (3/30/01). Accurate Treatment of Epilepsy. *Los Angeles Times* F2.
[142] Tyger, tyger (1/16/64, 1/23/64). Dr Kildare 3:16, 3:17. Dir:John Newland, NBC.
[143] Two Tonys (3/704). *The Sopranos* 5:1. Dir: Tim Van Patten, HBO.
[144] *JFK* (1991). Dir: Oliver Stone. Alcor Films.
[145] The Trial of Jack McCall (4/18/04) *Deadwood* 1:5. Dir: Ed Bianchi. Plague, (4/25/04) *Deadwood* 1:6. Dir: Davis Guggenheim. Sold under sin (6/13/04). *Deadwood* 1:12. Dir: Davis Guggenheim. The Whores can come (5/15/05). *Deadwood* 2:11. Dir: Gregg Feinberg.
[146] Lidz, F. (12/14/08). Villain of the afternoon, 28 years later. *New York Times* p. 26.

[147] Kerson, T. S. Lasting impressions of seizures in film and on television. *The Epilepsy Report*. 2: 7-13.
[148] *Carnage* (2001). Dir: Dephine Gleize. France 3 Cinema.fr.
[149] *Les Amants du Nil* (2002). Dir: Eric Heumann. Centre national de la Cinematographie.fr.
[150] *A Matter of Life or Death* ((1946). Dirs: Michael Powell and Eric Pressburger. J. Arthur Rank.
[151] *La Redingote Epileptique* (1913). Dir: Romeo Bosetti. Pathe Freres.
[152] Gamson, et al., op. cit., p 391.
[153] Implacable images: Why epileptiform events continue to be featured in film and television (with L.A. Kerson) *Epileptic Disorders*. 8(2):1-11. also published as La representation de l'epilepsie au cinema et a la television aux etats-unis, (2007) *La Lettre de Liaison de L'Epilepsie*-France Juin(5): 27-38 ; an abstract, Living in Harmony: Promoting Creative synergy in a stressful world (p. 32). 5th International Conference on Social Work in Health and Mental Health, Hong Kong, China.
[154] Kerson T. S, Kerson J. F., and Kerson L. A. (2000). *She'll have a seizure maybe: Then we can watch*. op. cit.
[155] Kobau R, Price P. (2003). Knowledge of epilepsy and familiarity with this disorder in the U.S. population: Results from the 2002 HealthStyles survey. *Epilepsia* 2003; 44:1149-1454.
[156] Van Brakel, W. H. (2006). Measuring health-related stigma – A literature review. *Psychology, Health and Medicine*: 11(3): 307-334.

INDEX

A

B

C

D

E

F

I

J

K

L

M

N

O

P

Q

R

S

T

W

Y

Z